Microbial Biofilms in Healthcare

Microbial Biofilms in Healthcare

Formation, Prevention and Treatment

Special Issue Editor
Karen Vickery

MDPI • Basel • Beijing • Wuhan • Barcelona • Belgrade • Manchester • Tokyo • Cluj • Tianjin

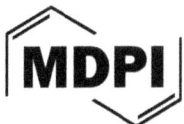

Special Issue Editor
Karen Vickery
Macquarie University
Australia

Editorial Office
MDPI
St. Alban-Anlage 66
4052 Basel, Switzerland

This is a reprint of articles from the Special Issue published online in the open access journal *Materials* (ISSN 1996-1944) (available at: https://www.mdpi.com/journal/materials/special_issues/microbial_biofilm_healthcare).

For citation purposes, cite each article independently as indicated on the article page online and as indicated below:

LastName, A.A.; LastName, B.B.; LastName, C.C. Article Title. *Journal Name* **Year**, *Article Number*, Page Range.

ISBN 978-3-03928-410-8 (Pbk)
ISBN 978-3-03928-411-5 (PDF)

© 2020 by the authors. Articles in this book are Open Access and distributed under the Creative Commons Attribution (CC BY) license, which allows users to download, copy and build upon published articles, as long as the author and publisher are properly credited, which ensures maximum dissemination and a wider impact of our publications.

The book as a whole is distributed by MDPI under the terms and conditions of the Creative Commons license CC BY-NC-ND.

Contents

About the Special Issue Editor vii

Preface to "Microbial Biofilms in Healthcare: Formation, Prevention and Treatment" ix

Karen Vickery
Special Issue: Microbial Biofilms in Healthcare: Formation, Prevention and Treatment
Reprinted from: *Materials* **2019**, *12*, 2001, doi:10.3390/ma12122001 1

Shamaila Tahir, Matthew Malone, Honghua Hu, Anand Deva and Karen Vickery
The Effect of Negative Pressure Wound Therapy with and without Instillation on Mature Biofilms In Vitro
Reprinted from: *Materials* **2018**, *11*, 811, doi:10.3390/ma11050811 5

Lasserre Jérôme Frédéric, Brecx Michel and Toma Selena
Oral Microbes, Biofilms and Their Role in Periodontal and Peri-Implant Diseases
Reprinted from: *Materials* **2018**, *11*, 1802, doi:10.3390/ma11101802 17

Maria Mempin, Honghua Hu, Durdana Chowdhury, Anand Deva and Karen Vickery
The A, B and C's of Silicone Breast Implants: Anaplastic Large Cell Lymphoma, Biofilm and Capsular Contracture
Reprinted from: *Materials* **2018**, *11*, 2393, doi:10.3390/ma11122393 35

Marie Beitelshees, Andrew Hill, Charles H. Jones and Blaine A. Pfeifer
Phenotypic Variation during Biofilm Formation: Implications for Anti-Biofilm Therapeutic Design
Reprinted from: *Materials* **2018**, *11*, 1086, doi:10.3390/ma11071086 47

Katarzyna Ledwoch and Jean-Yves Maillard
Candida auris Dry Surface Biofilm (DSB) for Disinfectant Efficacy Testing
Reprinted from: *Materials* **2019**, *12*, 18, doi:10.3390/ma12010018 65

Nor Fadhilah Kamaruzzaman, Tan Li Peng, Khairun Anisa Mat Yazid, Shamsaldeen Ibrahim Saeed, Ruhil Hayati Hamdan, Choong Siew Shean, Wong Weng Kin, Alexandru Chivu and Amanda Jane Gibson
Targeting the Bacterial Protective Armour; Challenges and Novel Strategies in the Treatment of Microbial Biofilm
Reprinted from: *Materials* **2018**, *11*, 1705, doi:10.3390/ma11091705 75

Phillip A. Laycock, John J. Cooper, Robert P. Howlin, Craig Delury, Sean Aiken and Paul Stoodley
In Vitro Efficacy of Antibiotics Released from Calcium Sulfate Bone Void Filler Beads
Reprinted from: *Materials* **2018**, *11*, 2265, doi:10.3390/ma11112265 103

Muhammad Yasir, Mark Duncan Perry Willcox and Debarun Dutta
Action of Antimicrobial Peptides against Bacterial Biofilms
Reprinted from: *Materials* **2018**, *11*, 2468, doi:10.3390/ma11122468 119

Bindu Subhadra, Dong Ho Kim, Kyungho Woo, Surya Surendran and Chul Hee Choi
Control of Biofilm Formation in Healthcare: Recent Advances Exploiting Quorum-Sensing Interference Strategies and Multidrug Efflux Pump Inhibitors
Reprinted from: *Materials* **2018**, *11*, 1676, doi:10.3390/ma11091676 135

About the Special Issue Editor

Karen Vickery graduated from Veterinary Science with honors in 1979 and worked in general veterinary practice in Australia and the United Kingdom. She obtained her Ph.D. in 1996 investigating hepatitis B virus (HBV) and developed the method for biocide efficacy testing against HBV for disinfectant registration referenced by the Australian Therapeutic Goods Administration. She is the Scientific Director of the Surgical Infection Research Group at Macquarie University, Australia and is primarily responsible for investigating medically important biofilms. Her research aims to prevent healthcare associated infections by focusing on both surgical strategies for preventing biofilm infection of medical implants, treating biofilm infections of chronic wounds, and strategies that improve instrument and environmental decontamination.

Preface to "Microbial Biofilms in Healthcare: Formation, Prevention and Treatment"

An estimated 99% of the world's bacteria live in close proximity with other bacteria in a biofilm. In a biofilm, the bacteria are enclosed in exopolymeric substances (EPS) and are generally attached to a surface. The biofilm phenotype and the surrounding EPS increase the tolerance of bacteria to desiccation and biocide action, resulting in bacterial persistence on surfaces long after free-swimming or planktonic bacteria are killed. In this book, we investigate the role of biofilms in breast and dental implant disease and cancer. We include in vitro models for investigating treatment of chronic wounds and disinfectant action against Candida sp. Also included are papers on the most recent strategies for treating biofilm infection ranging from antibiotics incorporated into bone void fillers to antimicrobial peptides and quorum sensing.

Karen Vickery
Special Issue Editor

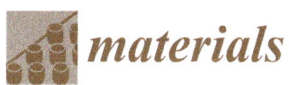

Editorial

Special Issue: Microbial Biofilms in Healthcare: Formation, Prevention and Treatment

Karen Vickery

Surgical Infection Research Group, Faculty of Medicine and Health Sciences, Macquarie University, Sydney 2109, Australia; karen.vickery@mq.edu.au

Received: 19 June 2019; Accepted: 21 June 2019; Published: 22 June 2019

Abstract: Biofilms are a structured community of microorganisms that are attached to a surface. Individual bacteria are embedded in a bacterial-secreted matrix. Biofilms have significantly increased tolerance to removal by cleaning agents and killing by disinfectants and antibiotics. This special issue is devoted to diagnosis and treatment of biofilm-related diseases in man. It highlights the differences between the biofilm and planktonic (single cell) lifestyles and the diseases biofilms cause from periodontitis to breast implant capsular contracture. Biofilm-specific treatment options are detailed in experimental and review manuscripts.

Keywords: biofilms; dry surface biofilms; periodontitis; breast implants; *Candida auris*; calcium sulphate; antibiotic; topical negative pressure wound therapy; antimicrobial peptides

Introduction

Biofilms are ubiquitous with an estimated 99% of the world's bacteria living enclosed in a biofilm. The problems that biofilm cause in industry have been well documented and methods to reduce their impact have been explored since before the middle of the last century. However, the extent to which biofilms play a significant detrimental role in chronic disease and implantable medical device failure has only been acknowledged over the past few decades whilst the role they play in surface and surgical instrument decontamination failure has only recently been highlighted.

Biofilms are a structured community of microorganisms that are attached to a surface. In healthcare, environmental biofilms take three forms: traditional hydrated biofilms which form in wet areas such as showers, water pipes and sinks; biofilms that form on dry surfaces such as benchtops and curtains, called dry surface biofilms (DSB); and build-up biofilms (BUB) that form on surgical instruments subjected to cycles of use, decontamination (cleaning and disinfection) and drying during storage. In addition, biofilm forms in human tissue such as the lung of cystic fibrosis sufferers and in chronic wounds, and biofilms on implantable medical devices lead to their failure. The importance of biofilms in healthcare arises due to biofilms' increased tolerance to biocides and increased tolerance to desiccation when compared with planktonic organisms of the same species.

Biofilms' increased tolerance to desiccation means that they can survive dry conditions which readily kills planktonic bacteria. DSB have been shown to survive over 12 months in a sterile container, on a bench without any nutrition, and they are particularly tolerant to disinfectants [1,2]. DSB have been detected on over 90% of dry hospital surfaces in four countries (Australia, Brazil, Saudi Arabia and the United Kingdom) [1,3–5]. In this special issue, Ledwoch and Maillard investigated the efficacy of 12 commercial disinfectants and 1000 ppm sodium hypochlorite (recommended as the disinfectant of choice by Public Health England) against DSB composed of *Candida auris* [6]. They initially developed a DSB model of this emerging pathogen and then used this model DSB in a modification of the ASTM2967-15 Wiperator test to measure decrease in *C. auris* viability, transfer of *C. auris* and biofilm re-growth following treatment. Similar to bacterial DSB, *C. auris* DSB showed increased tolerance to common disinfectant agents.

Bacteria can attach to host tissue and any implantable medical device. In this issue, Kamaruzzaman et al. review the bacterial species that are principally isolated from healthcare associated infection, the body sites where biofilms cause disease, diagnosis and treatment options [7]. They go on to describe the mechanisms of antimicrobial tolerance and evasion of host immune response which biofilm exhibits. Mempin et al. review the surface characteristics of different types of breast implants and how this affects bacterial attachment [8]. They also describe how biofilm formation on breast implants leads to capsular contracture and its possible role in the potentiation of breast implant associated Anaplastic Large Cell Lymphoma (ALCL). Frédéric et al. review the role that oral biofilm plays in periodontitis and peri-implantitis and the limitations of treatment options [9]. The poor response of chronic wounds to treatment promoted Tahir et al. to investigate whether physically altering biofilms' architecture increased its sensitivity to biocides [10]. They did this by utilizing their topical negative pressure wound therapy model. In this special issue, other treatment options that were experimentally explored included Laycock et al.'s work on the efficacy of antibiotic release from calcium sulphate bone void filler beads [11]. As calcium sulphate is completely biocompatible and absorbed by the body, combining it with antibiotics and using this combination locally would serve to increase antibiotic release at fracture sites and reduce the need for high dose systemic use of antibiotics.

In this special issue, three reviews address various antibiofilm treatment strategies. Biofilm formation and maturation can be stopped by preventing bacterial attachment or by interfering with bacterial quorum sensing. Once formed, biofilm removal can be induced by use of chemical and quorum sensing dispersal agents. Beitelshees et al. reviewed biofilm formation and how bacterial phenotype changes during biofilm development [12]. They relate bacterial phenotype to the anti-biofilm strategy. Yasir et al. reviewed the major antibiofilm mechanisms of the action of antimicrobial peptides and how these prevent biofilm formation and disrupt mature biofilms [13]. Subhadra et al. reviewed the recent advances in preventing biofilm formation and inducing its dispersal by interfering with quorum sensing [14].

Conflicts of Interest: The author declares no conflict of interest.

References

1. Hu, H.; Johani, K.; Gosbell, I.B.; Jacombs, A.; Almatroudi, A.; Whiteley, G.S.; Deva, A.K.; Jensen, S.; Vickery, K. Intensive care unit environmental surfaces are contaminated by multiresistant bacteria in biofilms: Combined results of conventional culture, pyrosequencing, scanning electron microscopy and confocal laser microscopy. *J. Hosp. Infect.* **2015**, *91*, 35–44. [CrossRef] [PubMed]
2. Almatroudi, A.; Gosbell, I.; Hu, H.; Jensen, S.; Espedido, B.; Tahir, S.; Glasbey, T.; Legge, P.; Whiteley, G.; Deva, A.; et al. Staphylococcus aureus dry-surface biofilms are not killed by sodium hypochlorite: Implications for infection control. *J. Hosp. Infect.* **2016**, *93*, 263–270. [CrossRef] [PubMed]
3. Costa, D.; Johani, K.; Melo, D.S.; Lopes, L.; Lima, L.L.; Tipple, A.; Hu, H.; Vickery, K.; Costa, D.D.M.; Lopes, L.K.D.O.; et al. Biofilm contamination of high-touched surfaces in intensive care units: Epidemiology and potential impacts. *Lett. Appl. Microbiol.* **2019**, *68*, 269–276. [CrossRef] [PubMed]
4. Johani, K.; Abualsaud, D.; Costa, D.M.; Hu, H.; Whiteley, G.; Deva, A.; Vickery, K. Characterization of microbial community composition, antimicrobial resistance and biofilm on intensive care surfaces. *J. Infect. Public Health* **2018**, *11*, 418–424. [CrossRef] [PubMed]
5. Ledwoch, K.; Dancer, S.; Otter, J.; Kerr, K.; Roposte, D.; Rushton, L.; Weiser, R.; Mahenthiralingam, E.; Muir, D.; Maillard, J.-Y. Beware biofilm! Dry biofilms containing bacterial pathogens on multiple healthcare surfaces; a multi-centre study. *J. Hosp. Infect.* **2018**, *100*, e47–e56. [CrossRef] [PubMed]
6. Ledwoch, K.; Maillard, J.-Y. Candida auris Dry Surface Biofilm (DSB) for Disinfectant Efficacy Testing. *Materials* **2018**, *12*, 18. [CrossRef] [PubMed]
7. Kamaruzzaman, N.F.; Tan, L.P.; Yazid, K.A.M.; Saeed, S.I.; Hamdan, R.H.; Choong, S.S.; Wong, W.K.; Chivu, A.; Gibson, A.J.; Yazid, K.M. Targeting the Bacterial Protective Armour; Challenges and Novel Strategies in the Treatment of Microbial Biofilm. *Materials* **2018**, *11*, 1705. [CrossRef] [PubMed]

8. Mempin, M.; Hu, H.; Chowdhury, D.; Deva, A.; Vickery, K. The A, B and C's of Silicone Breast Implants: Anaplastic Large Cell Lymphoma, Biofilm and Capsular Contracture. *Materials* **2018**, *11*, 2393. [CrossRef] [PubMed]
9. Lasserre, J.F.; Brecx, M.C.; Toma, S.; Frédéric, L.J.; Michel, B.; Selena, T. Oral Microbes, Biofilms and Their Role in Periodontal and Peri-Implant Diseases. *Materials* **2018**, *11*, 1802.
10. Tahir, S.; Malone, M.; Hu, H.; Deva, A.; Vickery, K. The Effect of Negative Pressure Wound Therapy with and without Instillation on Mature Biofilms In Vitro. *Materials* **2018**, *11*, 811. [CrossRef] [PubMed]
11. Laycock, P.A.; Cooper, J.J.; Howlin, R.P.; Delury, C.; Aiken, S.; Stoodley, P. In Vitro Efficacy of Antibiotics Released from Calcium Sulfate Bone Void Filler Beads. *Materials* **2018**, *11*, 2265. [CrossRef] [PubMed]
12. Beitelshees, M.; Hill, A.; Jones, C.H.; Pfeifer, B.A. Phenotypic Variation during Biofilm Formation: Implications for Anti-Biofilm Therapeutic Design. *Materials* **2018**, *11*, 1086. [CrossRef] [PubMed]
13. Yasir, M.; Willcox, M.D.P.; Dutta, D. Action of Antimicrobial Peptides against Bacterial Biofilms. *Materials* **2018**, *11*, 2468. [CrossRef]
14. Subhadra, B.; Kim, D.H.; Woo, K.; Surendran, S.; Choi, C.H. Control of Biofilm Formation in Healthcare: Recent Advances Exploiting Quorum-Sensing Interference Strategies and Multidrug Efflux Pump Inhibitors. *Materials* **2018**, *11*, 1676. [CrossRef]

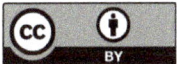

© 2019 by the author. Licensee MDPI, Basel, Switzerland. This article is an open access article distributed under the terms and conditions of the Creative Commons Attribution (CC BY) license (http://creativecommons.org/licenses/by/4.0/).

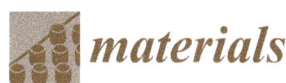

Article

The Effect of Negative Pressure Wound Therapy with and without Instillation on Mature Biofilms In Vitro

Shamaila Tahir [1,*], Matthew Malone [2,3,4], Honghua Hu [1], Anand Deva [1] and Karen Vickery [1]

1. Surgical Infection Research Group, Faculty of Medicine and Health Sciences, Macquarie University, Sydney 2109, Australia; helen.hu@mq.edu.au (H.H.); anand.deva@mq.edu.au (A.D.); karen.vickery@mq.edu.au (K.V.)
2. Infectious Diseases and Microbiology, School of Medicine, Western Sydney University, Sydney 2751, Australia; matthew.malone@westernsydney.edu.au
3. Liverpool Diabetes Collaborative Research Unit, Ingham Institute of Applied Medical Research, Sydney 2170, Australia
4. High Risk Foot Service, Liverpool Hospital, South West Sydney LHD, Sydney 2170, Australia
* Correspondence: shamaila.tahir@students.mq.edu.au

Received: 15 March 2018; Accepted: 14 May 2018; Published: 16 May 2018

Abstract: Background: To investigate the effect of negative pressure wound therapy (NPWT) with and without instillation (NPWTi) on in vitro mature biofilm. Methods: Mature biofilms of *Pseudomonas aeruginosa* and *Staphylococcus aureus* were grown under shear (130 rpm) on polycarbonate coupons in a CDC biofilm reactor for 3 days. Coupons containing biofilms were placed in a sterile petri dish and sealed using NPWT or NPWTi. Coupons were exposed to treatment for 24 h with NPWT alone or with instillation of: Povidone iodine solution (PVP-I) (10% w/v equivalent to 1% w/v available iodine, BETADINE®, Mundipharma, Singapore), surfactant based antimicrobial solution with polyhexamethylene biguanide (SBPHMB) (Prontosan®, B Braun Medical, Melsungen, Germany), Gentamicin 1 µg/mL (GM) (G1264 Sigma-Aldrich Pty Ltd., Castle Hill, Australia) Rifampicin 24 µg/mL (RF) (R3501 Sigma-Aldrich Pty Ltd., Castle Hill, Australia) and NaCl 0.9% (Baxter, Deerfield, IL, USA). Bacterial cell viability and biofilm architecture pre-and post-treatment were assessed using colony forming units (cfu), Live/Dead viability staining, confocal laser scanning microscopy (CLSM) and scanning electron microscopy (SEM). Results: Significant reductions were obtained in *S. aureus* biofilm thickness (65%) and mass (47%) when treated with NPWTi as compared to NPWT only. NPWTi with instillation of SBPHMB, PVP-I and RF achieved between 2 and 8 $\log_{10}$ reductions against *S. aureus* biofilm ($p < 0.05$–0.001). Conversely, PVP-I and SBMO achieved a 3.5 $\log_{10}$ reduction against *P. aeruginosa* ($p < 0.05$). Conclusions: NPWT alters biofilm architecture by reducing biofilm thickness and mass, but this does not affect bacterial cell viability. NPWT with instillation of certain antimicrobials solutions may provide a further synergistic effect in reducing the number of viable biofilm microorganisms. Our in vitro model may be used for screening the effectiveness of antimicrobials used under instillation prior to animal or human studies.

Keywords: biofilm; chronic wounds; instillation therapy; in vitro

1. Introduction

The causality of a wound that experiences a delay in healing can be multifactorial and attributed to factors such as local tissue hypoxia/poor perfusion, repetitive ischemia-reperfusion injury [1], microbial infection [2], inadequate offloading or compression therapy [3]. Perhaps the most significant of these factors are the cases where chronic wounds become complicated by pathogenic microorganisms. These may exist as planktonic rapidly dividing cells that invade host tissues and induce an acute infection [4]. Conversely, some microorganisms that complicate chronic wounds may alter their phenotype, differing markedly in both their physiology and activity. These microorganisms are sessile, attach to surfaces or other microorganisms, form aggregates, and regulate the production of an extracellular polymeric substance (biofilm) [5]. The hallmark features of these microorganisms are their tolerance to antimicrobials, the host immune responses and environmental stresses.

These wounds are a challenge for any clinician and ensuring their resolution can often involve a complex array of pathways that may involve surgical or sharp conservative debridement of any infected non-viable tissue. Even in this scenario the ability for a surgeon/clinician to remove all non-viable tissue and any microorganisms not visible to the naked eye is likely not possible [6]. Post-surgical debridement wound care is therefore a critical step to ensure a newly 'acute' wound continues through the orderly continuum of repair. To augment this process negative pressure wound therapy with instillation (NPWTi) and dwell time is an adjunctive treatment modality for selected complex wounds complicated by invasive infection or extensive biofilm [7,8].

Evidence for NPWT with or without instillation/dwell time on the microbial load of wounds is limited [9–11] with little data available for its action/s against microbial biofilms [12]. Previously our group demonstrated that NPWT resulted in a physical disruption to biofilm architecture [13]. This change resulted in a synergism between NPWT and a solid dressing (silver impregnated foam) eradicating an in vitro biofilm [14]. In this study we aim to test the effectiveness of NPWT with instillation and dwell time of topical antimicrobial solutions, against 3-day mature *S. aureus* and *P. aeruginosa* biofilms. We hypothesize that NPWT alters biofilm architecture and thus improves penetration of antimicrobials through the extracellular polymeric substance of biofilm forming microorganisms.

2. Materials and Methods

2.1. Bacterial Test Strains

Biofilm forming reference strains utilized in vitro were *S. aureus* (ATCC® 25923™), (methicillin-sensitive *S. aureus* (MSSA) and *P. aeruginosa* (ATCC® 25619™).

2.2. Solutions Used for Instillation Therapy

Details regarding the solutions used, any incorporated antimicrobials and tested concentration levels, and their respective manufacturers are noted in the Supplementary Materials (Table S1). Briefly, surfactant based antimicrobial solution with polyhexamethylene biguanide (SBPHMB; Prontosan®, B Braun Medical, Melsungen, Germany), povidone iodine (PVP-I) antimicrobial solution 10% w/v equivalent to 1% w/v available iodine (BETADINE®, Mundipharma, Singapore), Saline (NaCl) 0.9% (Baxter, Deerfield, IL, USA). The systemic antimicrobials tested were, gentamicin (GM) 1 µg/mL and Rifampicin (RF) 24 µg/mL, both diluted in NaCl 0.9% (Baxter International, Deerfield, IL, USA).

2.3. In Vitro CDC Biofilm Reactor

P. aeruginosa and *S. aureus* were grown separately under shear (130 rpm) at 35 °C on 24 removable polycarbonate coupons in a CDC biofilm reactor (BioSurface Technologies Corp., Bozeman, MT, USA). *S. aureus* biofilm was grown in 15 g/L (50%) tryptone soya broth (TSB) (Sigma Aldrich, St. Louis, MO, USA) in batch phase for 24 h and then replaced with fresh media 6 g/L (20% TSB) flowing through the chamber at 80 mL/h for a further 48 h. *P. aeruginosa* was grown in 600 mg/L (2%) TSB in batch phase for 24 h and then with fresh media (TSB 2%) flowing through the chamber at 80 mL/h for a further 48 h. Coupons were harvested by washing gently, three times, in phosphate buffered saline (PBS) to remove loosely attached and planktonic bacteria. The number of bacteria per coupon was 3.52×10^7 and 2.3×10^7 for *S. aureus* and *P. aeruginosa*, respectively. Bacterial biofilm was gently scraped off from the outer side of each coupon using a 12.5% sodium hypochlorite-soaked paper towel, and then again washed three times in TSB to remove residual chlorine.

2.4. In Vitro NPWTi Model

The NPWTi utilized in this study was the V.A.C. Ulta negative pressure wound therapy system (Acelity, San Antonio, TX, USA) incorporating the V.A.C. Veraflo therapy that allows the controlled instillation of topical solutions. Modifications to the system were necessary due to the tubular shape of the V.A.C. Veraflo dressing system, in keeping with previously published reports [13].

Five biofilm containing coupons were placed on top of 3% bacteriological agar (Thermo Scientific, Basingstoke, UK) in a sterile petri dish. The sterile NPWT dressing (V.A.C.® GRANUFOAM™) were added on top of the coupons until the petri dish was completely full, thus ensuring equal pressure application to all five biofilm covered coupons. An airtight seal was produced using a sterile semi-impervious dressing (V.A.C.® dressing system). In order to emulate wound exudate, coupons were bathed with TSB (30 g/L) at a flow rate of 40 mL/h via an inflow channel [15,16]. Excess fluid was drained via a gravity drainage tube, situated on the opposite side from the nutrition in-flow, for chambers not subjected to NPWT and via a centrally placed V.A.C.® Veralink Cassette for chambers subjected to NPWT (Figure 1).

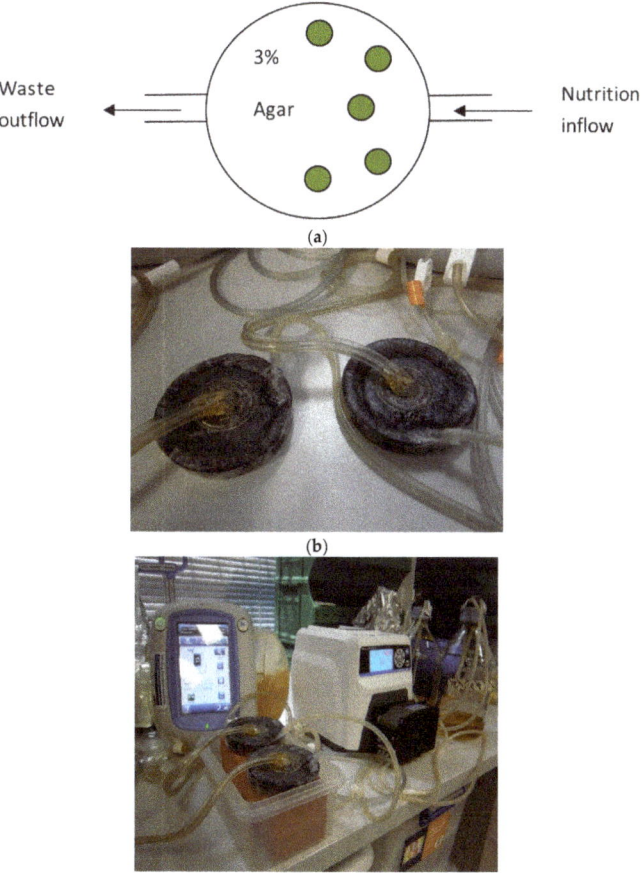

Figure 1. (a) Schematic presentation of modified wound model with polycarbonate coupons (green). (b) New wound model with Veraflo dressing system. (c) Experimental setup of instillation + V.A.C. therapy. Green circles represent biofilm coated polycarbonate coupons.

Five coupons for each test antimicrobial solution were exposed to the following treatment variables: (i) control with no treatment; (ii) NPWT alone with no instillation; (iii) instillation of antimicrobial plus continuous NPWT at 125 mmHg (except during the 20 min instillation treatment periods); and (iv) instillation of antimicrobial solution with no NPWT. The instillation cycles were as follows: instillation every 6 h with 35 mL of saline or test antimicrobial with a 20 min dwell time in a 24 h time period. Instillation with TSB was then continued for another 6 h before harvesting.

2.5. Bacterial Viability cfu/log$_{10}$

At the end of each treatment period, the numbers of residual bacterial colony forming units (cfu) per coupon were tested in triplicate by sonication in an ultrasonic bath (Soniclean, Stepney, Australia) for 10 min with a sweeping frequency of 42–47 kH at 20 °C.

Coupons were then vortexed for two min in 2 mL of PBS followed by sequential 10-fold dilution and plate count. Pre- and post-exposure average cfu/coupon was expressed as log$_{10}$.

2.6. Confocal Laser Scanning Microscopy

Bacterial cell viability pre- and post-exposure was also assessed using *Bac*Light™ (Live/Dead Bacterial Viability Kit, 7012, Molecular Probes, Invitrogen, Carlsbad, CA, USA) in conjunction with confocal laser scanning microscopy (CLSM) (Olympus FluoView™ FV1000, Tokyo, Japan). Following staining, coupons were fixed with 4% paraformaldehyde for 1 h and washed thrice with PBS for 10 min. 2D images were obtained within 24–48 h of staining. 3D images were obtained from three separate areas per coupon. Images were built with 0.2 μm optical sections and analyzed for average thickness, biofilm mass and percentage of viable cells, using the IMARIS 7.7.2 software (Bitplane, Zurich, Switzerland) and ImageJ program (scriptable Java application for scientific image processing). A 63× water immersion objective lens was used to capture images with reduced background noise at 10×, 20× and 40× magnifications. To minimize image artefacts these dual labelled (Syto-9 and propidium iodide) samples were sequentially scanned at 488 nm fluorescence excitation (green emission) and then at 543 nm (red emission) collected in the green and red regions, respectively. Line averaging (×2) was used to capture images with reduced noise.

Biofilm architecture was analyzed using IMARIS (Bitplane AG, Zurich, Switzerland) software to quantify 3-D CLSM images by: (1) Average thickness is the distance (μm) between the top of a biofilm and the substratum on which the biofilm resides. It provides a measure of the spatial size of biofilm; (2) Average biofilm biomass (μm^3), is defined as the volume of bacterial cells below μm^2 area. The value excludes the non-cellular components (e.g., EPS and water channels) of biofilm volume.

2.7. Scanning Electron Microscopy

For SEM, one coupon each from selected antimicrobial treatment were fixed in 3% glutaraldehyde, dehydrated through serial dilutions of ethanol and then immersed in hexamethyldisilazane (Polysciences Inc., Warrington, FL, USA) for 10 min before being aspirated dry and air dried for at least 48 h. Coupons were then mounted on specimen stubs, gold coated and examined at low and high magnifications (JOEL 6480LA SEM, Tokyo, Japan).

Statistical Analysis

Statistical analysis on cfu data was performed using the Sigma Plot 11 statistical program (Scientific Graphing Software: SigmaPlot® Version 11 by Systat Software, Inc., San Jose, CA, USA). Pre and post bacterial viability between treatment groups were analyzed by performing one-way analysis of variance (ANOVA). For non-normally distributed data a Kruskal-Wallis one-way analysis of variance on ranks was performed, and if significant, the Tukey test for all pair wise multiple comparisons were conducted to determine which treatment groups were significantly different from each other.

3. Results

All experiments were conducted over a 24 h test period. Control coupons of *S. aureus* and *P. aeruginosa* receiving no treatment increased in the number of biofilm bacteria from a starting cfu of 7.4 $\log_{10}$ cfu/coupon to 8.3 $\log_{10}$ cfu/coupon (0.9 $\log_{10}$ cfu/coupon increase, $p = 1.0$). The effects of NPWT, NPWTi and instillation alone on bacterial viability after 24 h are reported.

3.1. NPWT on Bacterial Viability cfu/$\log_{10}$

NPWT had little effect on *S. aureus* biofilms demonstrating a 1.2 $\log_{10}$ cfu/coupon reduction (control no treatment = 7.4 $\log_{10}$ cfu/coupon vs. NPWT = 6.2 $\log_{10}$ cfu/coupon $p > 1.0$) while numbers increased in the case of *P. aeruginosa* by 0.7 $\log_{10}$ cfu/coupon (control no treatment = 7.4 $\log_{10}$ cfu/coupon vs. NPWT = 8.1 $\log_{10}$ cfu/coupon $p > 1.0$).

3.2. Instillation Alone vs. NPWTi on Bacterial Viability cfu/$\log_{10}$

Bacterial viability of *S. aureus* and *P. aeruginosa* following Instillation or NPWTi are reported in Figures 2 and 3 and Table S2. Instillation with NaCl or PVP-I 1/10 demonstrated an equal reduction in *S. aureus* biofilms (0.8 $\log_{10}$ cfu/coupon, $p = 0.2$). When challenged against *P. aeruginosa* biofilms, NaCl reduced cfu by 0.6 $\log_{10}$ per coupon and PVP-I reduced cfu by 1.6 $\log_{10}$ per coupon ($p = 0.1$). SBPHMB was highly effective in reducing both *S. aureus* (5.6 $\log_{10}$ cfu/coupon $p < 0.001$) and *P. aeruginosa* biofilms (5.4 $\log_{10}$ cfu/coupon $p = 0.01$). RF achieved a 1.7 $\log_{10}$ cfu/coupon reduction against *S. aureus* ($p = 0.09$) and GM achieved a 1.22 log reduction cfu/coupon against *P. aeruginosa* ($p = 0.1$).

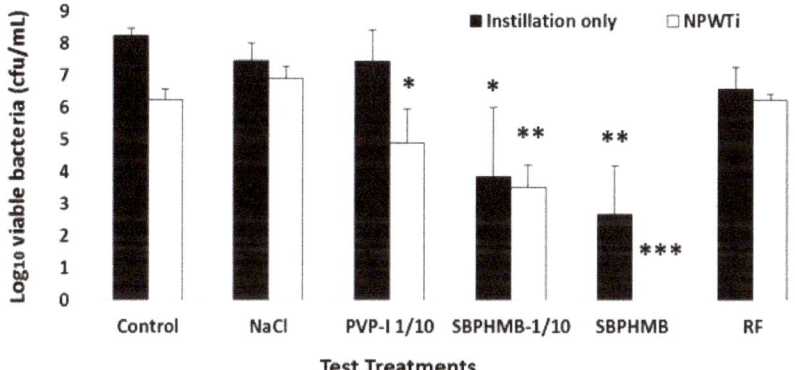

Figure 2. Mean $\log_{10}$ reduction of colony forming units (cfu) of *S. aureus* remaining on coupons following treatment with instillation alone or negative pressure wound therapy with instillation (NPWTi). Statistically significant from controls is shown by *, p value < 0.001 = (***), p value < 0.01 = (**), p value < 0.05 = (*).

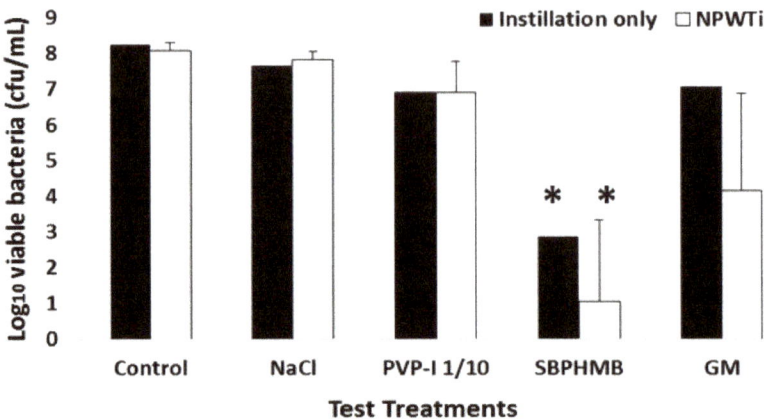

Figure 3. Mean $\log_{10}$ reduction of cfu of *P. aeruginosa* remaining on coupons following treatment with ($n = 5$) and without ($n = 5$) application of topical negative pressure. Statistically significant from controls is shown by p value $< 0.01 = (**)$.

NPWTi demonstrated significant increases in effectiveness against both *S. aureus* and *P. aeruginosa* when compared to instillation alone. When challenged against *S. aureus*, NPWTi using NaCl demonstrated a 1.4 $\log_{10}$ cfu/coupon reduction, ($p = 0.1$), PVP-I a 3.4 $\log_{10}$ cfu/coupon reduction ($p = 0.05$), SBPHMB an 8.3 $\log_{10}$ cfu/coupon reduction ($p = 0.001$) and RF a 2.1 $\log_{10}$ cfu/coupon reduction ($p = 0.05$). For *P. aeruginosa*, NPWTi using NaCl demonstrated a 0.4 $\log_{10}$ cfu/coupon ($p = 0.1$), PVP-I a 1.3 $\log_{10}$ cfu/coupon reduction ($p = 0.2$), SBPHMB a 7.3 $\log_{10}$ cfu/coupon reduction ($p < 0.0001$) and GM a 4.1 $\log_{10}$ cfu/coupon reduction ($p = 0.01$).

3.3. Microscopy

Given that SBPHMB demonstrated a greater efficacy than all other antimicrobials used in our biofilm models, we explored this agent in greater detail using both SEM and confocal microscopy with LIVE/DEAD stain. SEM images of *S. aureus* and *P. aeruginosa* biofilms from coupons undergoing instillation only with SBPHMB or NPWTi using SBPHMB are depicted in Figure 4. Minimal changes in biofilm structure of *S. aureus* and *P. aeruginosa* are noted in the SEM images (Figure 4a,c) following instillation of SBPHMB for 24 h. SEM identified dense coccoid and rod shaped microbial aggregates, respectively, embedded in a thick continuous EPS. Therefore, post-treatment with instillation only was ineffective. In contrast, SEM images of NPWTi using SBPHMB treated coupons showed significant reductions in biofilm EPS and in the number of microbial aggregates (Figure 4b,d). This was particularly evident for *S. aureus* biofilms, which demonstrated complete eradication of cocci aggregates and extracellular polymeric substance (EPS) (Figure 4b).

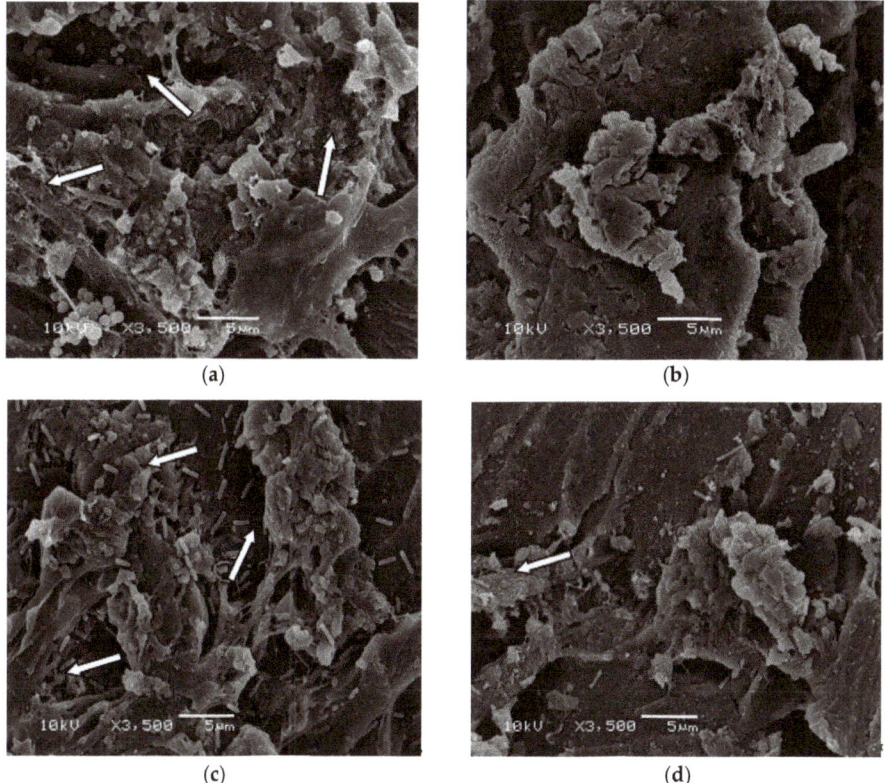

Figure 4. (**a**) SEM images of *S. aureus* biofilm coupon using SBPHMB/Instillation only for 24-h identifies dense coccoid bacteria embedded in EPS after treatment; (**b**) demonstrates an overall reduction in *S. aureus* biofilm after 24-h treatment with NPWTi using SBPHMB; (**c**) illustrates *P. aeruginosa* biofilm coupon using SPHMB/Instillation only for 24-h; (**d**) after 24-h treatment with NPWTi using SBPHMB. Arrows indicate biofilm aggregates.

Bacterial cell viability pre- and post-exposure of NPWTi with SBPHMB were analyzed using LIVE/DEAD stain with CLSM. This identified up to 97% reduction in live cells while live cells reduced by 3% in NPWT only treated *S. aureus* biofilm (Figure 5). The effects of NPWT with or without instillation on biofilm thickness and biomass are noted in Figures 6 and 7. Control coupons receiving no treatment had an average biofilm thickness of 57 µm and an average biomass of 1,264,111 µm^3. Coupons with *S. aureus* biofilms treated with NPWT alone had average thickness of 41 µm and biomass of 1,081,458 µm^3. In comparison, coupons with *S. aureus* biofilms treated with NPWTi SBPHMB experienced a 65% reduction in biofilm thickness (pre-treatment biofilm thickness = 57 µm versus post-treatment biofilm thickness = 19.8 µm, $p < 0.0003$), and a 48% reduction in total biofilm biomass (pre-treatment biofilm biomass = 1,264,111 µm^3 versus post-treatment biofilm biomass = 770,968 µm^3, $p = 0.05$).

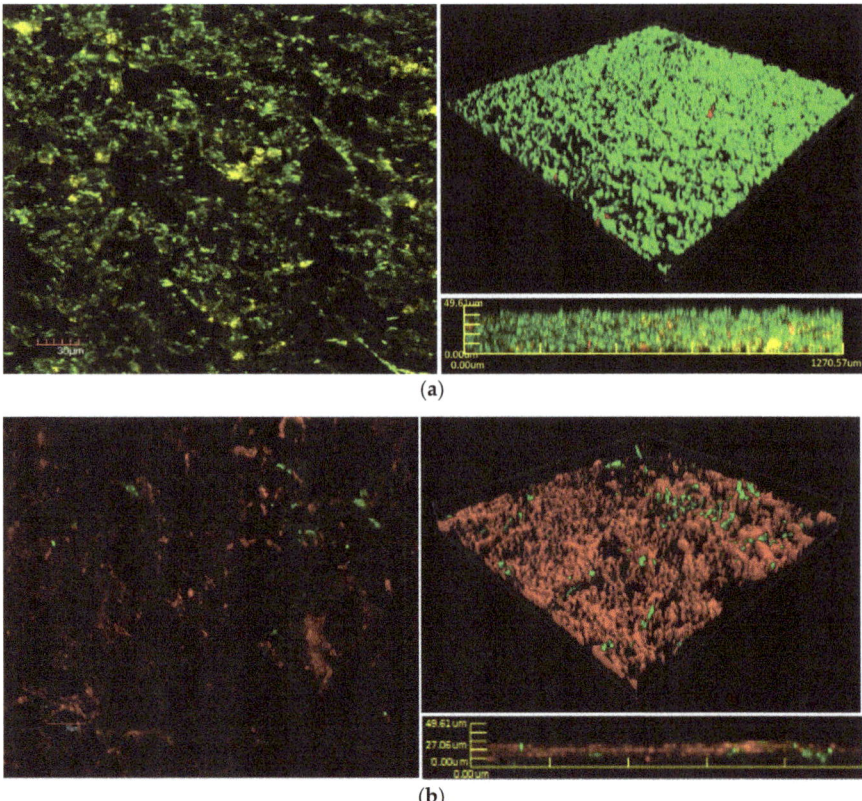

Figure 5. CLSM (30 μm) images of *S. aureus* biofilm with LIVE/DEAD® BacLight™ Bacterial Viability Kit, (**a**) pre-treatment with NPWTi using SBPHMB and (**b**) post-treatment with NPWTi using SBPHMB. Live bacteria are stained green and dead bacteria are stained red.

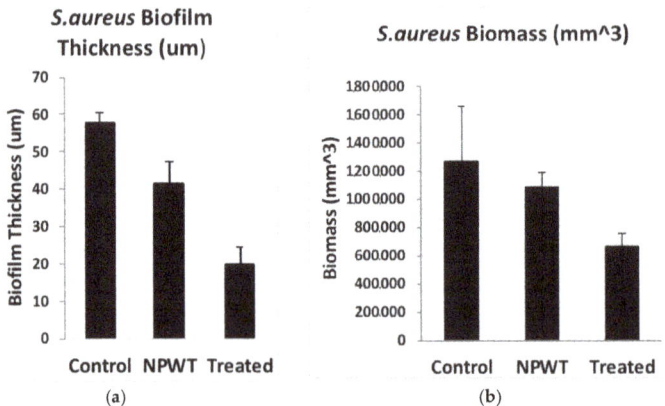

Figure 6. Demonstrates >60% reduction in *S. aureus* biofilm thickness (**a**) and >45% reduction in *S. aureus* biofilm biomass (**b**). *S. aureus* biofilm biomass pre-treatment NPWTi using SBPHMB.

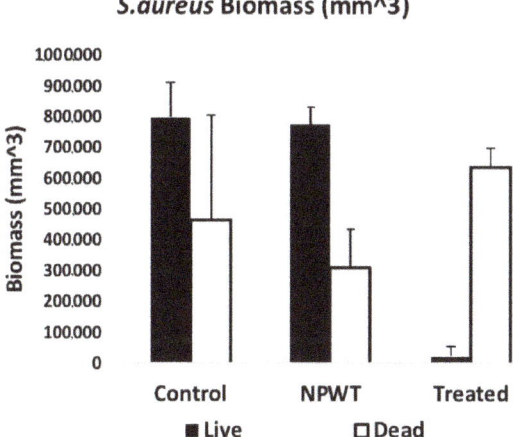

Figure 7. Demonstrates a 97% reduction in *S. aureus* biomass of live/dead cells after NPWTi using SBPHMB.

4. Discussion

NPWTi is reported to improve wound healing over NPWT alone, by enhancing autolytic and mechanical debridement and reducing the microbial load [17]. However there has been limited information detailing the increased efficacy of NPWTi over standard negative pressure with respect to microbial biofilms. The outcomes of this study confirm our previous work [13] and clearly demonstrate that NPWT alters in vitro biofilm architecture, reduces biofilm thickness and biomass, and decreases the diffusion distances for the penetration of antimicrobials through biofilms. We suggest that this action likely creates a synergy with antimicrobial solutions used under NPWTi (some antimicrobials have higher efficacy than others).

Given there has been a tremendous surge in research exploring anti-biofilm strategies for use in healthcare associated chronic infections, various agents have been explored that have included peptides, antiseptics, oral and topical antimicrobials. The methods of delivering these treatments have also varied and have included coatings, drug eluting, wound gels, nanoparticles, irrigations, and solutions. To complicate the picture, various methodologies to quantify outcomes measures have been used both in vitro and in animal models, and this lack of standardization makes comparing the results of different studies difficult [18]. The in vitro model utilized in this study is standardized, reproducible and easy-to-use. Furthermore this in vitro model offers a useful screening tool to identify potential antimicrobial solutions with greater efficacy against microbial biofilms when used under NPWTi, prior to undertaking animal or human studies.

These studies are often more complex requiring both a skilled laboratory/research group in addition to being costly. This has likely contributed to the limited studies to date (either in vitro or animal models), which have explored NPWTi using saline solutions or antimicrobial solutions against mature biofilms. Singh et al. [19] used an in vivo animal model to demonstrate the role of NPWT with antimicrobial instillation (Prontosan®, B Braun Medical, Melsungen, Germany) against clearance of infection and biofilm formation of infected spinal implants compared to traditional treatment modalities. A biofilm-forming methicillin-resistant *S. aureus* strain was grown for seven days in vivo, on implanted titanium rods that were then subjected to either wet to dry dressings (control arm) or NPWTi for a further seven days. The mean bacterial loads and presence of biofilm were lower in pigs receiving NPWTi (the experimental group was 6647 cfus/mL and 13,303 cfus/mL in the control group and SEM revealed the presence of uniform biofilm formation across the surface of control group instrumentation, the experimental group was positive for biofilm formation but with many skipped areas with no biofilm).

In another porcine skin explant model using NPWTi of various antimicrobial solutions, Phillips et al. [12] identified that SBPHMB and PVP-I reduced 3-day mature biofilms of *P. aeruginosa* by 4 $\log_{10}$ and 5 $\log_{10}$ respectively. In concluding, the authors hypothesize the potential synergy experienced was due to macrodistortion/microdistortion forces produced by negative pressure therapy, altering the biofilm EPS matrix structure sufficiently to enhance the penetration of the antimicrobial agents into the biofilm.

This can be clearly demonstrated by our confocal microscopy and in previous work by our group [13], which illustrates changes to biofilm architecture under negative pressure. We illustrate that NPWT significantly reduced biofilm thickness but has no effect on biomass which is concordance with viability results showing no reduction in bacterial numbers. In other words, the NPWT physically disrupts biofilm architecture by compressing it but does not kill the bacteria. In comparison, NPWTi significantly reduced both *S. aureus* biofilm thickness (reduced by 65%) and total biofilm mass (reduced by 48%), which was mirrored by a significant reduction in cell viability. This suggests a potential synergism between NPWT and the antimicrobial solution. The study results reflect that the synergism between antimicrobials and NPWT seems dependent upon bacterial species in addition to the type of antimicrobial used. For example, at the concentrations used for Rifampicin during instillation only, there was little to no effect on *S. aureus* biofilms even when RF was used under NPWTi.

5. Conclusions

With regards to wound care products in general, the majority of data on anti-biofilm strategies have been undertaken in vitro. This represents a challenge for clinicians where in vitro data may be based on laboratory methods that lack both standardized approaches and clinical relevance. The results obtained from in vitro testing which identify an effective wound care product, may therefore not translate into the same efficacy or outcomes when used clinically in vivo. Our in vitro model allows the simple and effective screening of antimicrobial solutions that may be used by clinicians as part of NPWTi therapy. However, the in vitro data generated from this model are a necessary precursor to further testing in more clinically relevant scenarios (that are often significantly more expensive) such as animal models or human studies, where results can be correlated.

Supplementary Materials: The following are available online at http://www.mdpi.com/1996-1944/11/5/811/s1, Table S1: Biocide clinical concentration and concentration used for in vitro wound model efficacy testing. Betadine and Prontosan concentration expressed as dilution of commercially available product. Table S2: Mean number of *S. aureus* and *P. aeruginosa* remaining on no treatment coupons and treatment coupons following four instillations of saline or biocide in 24 h with and without application of NPWT. Controls for *S. aureus* is 4.23×10^7 and for *P. aeruginosa* is 2.3×10^7. Number of samples, $n = 5$. Statistically significant from controls is shown by *, p value < 0.001 = (***), p value < 0.01 = (**), p value < 0.05 = (*).

Author Contributions: "S.T., K.V. and A.D. conceived and designed the experiments; S.T. and H.H. performed the experiments; S.T. and K.V. analyzed the data; M.M. wrote the paper." Authorship must be limited to those who have contributed substantially to the work reported.

Acknowledgments: We would like to thank KCI Medical Pty. Ltd. for providing the V.A.C.® machines and consumables. Shamaila Tahir was in receipt of Australian postgraduate award (APA). A/Professor Vickery was in receipt of a Macquarie University Vice Chancellor Innovation Fellowship.

Conflicts of Interest: None of the authors here have any conflict of interest or financial interest or otherwise in any component of the experimental work presented here.

References

1. Sen, C.K. Wound healing essentials: Let there be oxygen. *Wound Repair Regen.* **2009**, *17*, 1–18. [CrossRef] [PubMed]
2. Malone, M.; Johani, K.; Jensen, S.O.; Gosbell, I.B.; Dickson, H.G.; Hu, H.; Vickery, K. Next generation DNA sequencing of tissues from infected diabetic foot ulcers. *EBioMedicine* **2017**, *21*, 142–149. [CrossRef] [PubMed]

3. Armstrong, D.G.; Boulton, A.J.M.; Bus, S.A. Diabetic foot ulcers and their recurrence. *N. Engl. J. Med.* **2017**, *376*, 2367–2375. [CrossRef] [PubMed]
4. Lipsky, B.A.; Aragón-Sánchez, J.; Diggle, M.; Embil, J.; Kono, S.; Lavery, L.; Senneville, É.; Urbančič-Rovan, V.; Van Asten, S.; Peters, E.J.G.; et al. IWGDF guidance on the diagnosis and management of foot infections in persons with diabetes. *Diabetes Metab. Res. Rev.* **2016**, *32*, 45–74. [CrossRef] [PubMed]
5. Burmølle, M.; Thomsen, T.R.; Fazli, M.; Dige, I.; Christensen, L.; Homøe, P.; Tvede, M.; Nyvad, B.; Tolker-Nielsen, T.; Givskov, M.; et al. Biofilms in chronic infections—A matter of opportunity—Monospecies biofilms in multispecies infections. *FEMS Immunol. Med. Microbiol.* **2010**, *59*, 324–336. [CrossRef] [PubMed]
6. Schwartz, J.A.; Goss, S.G.; Facchin, F.; Avdagic, E.; Lantis, J.C. Surgical debridement alone does not adequately reduce planktonic bioburden in chronic lower extremity wounds. *J. Wound Care* **2014**, *23*, S4–S13. [CrossRef] [PubMed]
7. Gupta, S.; Gabriel, A.; Lantis, J.; Téot, L. Clinical recommendations and practical guide for negative pressure wound therapy with instillation. *Int. Wound J.* **2016**, *13*, 159–174. [CrossRef] [PubMed]
8. Andros, G.; Armstrong, D.G.; Attinger, C.E.; Boulton, A.J.; Frykberg, R.G.; Joseph, W.S.; Lavery, L.A.; Morbach, S.; Niezgoda, J.A.; Toursarkissian, B. Tuscon expert consensus conference. Consensus statement on negative pressure wound therapy (V.A.C therapy) for management of diabetic foot wounds. *Ostomy Wound Manag.* **2006**, *18*, 1–32.
9. Mouës, C.M.; Vos, M.C.; Van Den Bemd, G.-J.C.M.; Stijnen, T.; Hovius, S.E.R. Bacterial load in relation to vacuum-assisted closure wound therapy: A prospective randomized trial. *Wound Repair Regen.* **2004**, *12*, 11–17. [CrossRef] [PubMed]
10. Weed, T.; Ratliff, C.; Drake, D.B. Quantifying bacterial bioburden during negative pressure wound therapy: Does the wound VAC enhance bacterial clearance? *Ann. Plast. Surg.* **2004**, *52*, 276–279. [CrossRef] [PubMed]
11. Yusuf, E.; Jordan, X.; Clauss, M.; Borens, O.; Mäder, M.; Trampuz, A. High bacterial load in negative pressure wound therapy (NPWT) foams used in the treatment of chronic wounds. *Wound Repair Regen.* **2013**, *21*, 677–681. [CrossRef] [PubMed]
12. Phillips, P.L.; Yang, Q.; Schultz, G.S. The effect of negative pressure wound therapy with periodic instillation using antimicrobial solutions on pseudomonas aeruginosa biofilm on porcine skin explants. *Int. Wound J.* **2013**, *10*, 48–55. [CrossRef] [PubMed]
13. Ngo, Q.D.; Vickery, K.; Deva, A.K. The effect of topical negative pressure on wound biofilms using an in vitro wound model. *Wound Repair Regen.* **2012**, *20*, 83–90. [CrossRef] [PubMed]
14. Valente, P.M.D.S.; Deva, A.; Ngo, Q.; Vickery, K. The increased killing of biofilms in vitro by combining topical silver dressings with topical negative pressure in chronic wounds. *Int. Wound J.* **2016**, *13*, 130–136. [CrossRef] [PubMed]
15. Goeres, D.M.; Loetterle, L.R.; Hamilton, M.A.; Murga, R.; Kirby, D.W.; Donlan, R.M. Statistical assessment of a laboratory method for growing biofilms. *Microbiology* **2005**, *151*, 757–762. [CrossRef] [PubMed]
16. Hadi, R.; Vickery, K.; Deva, A.; Charlton, T. Biofilm removal by medical device cleaners: Comparison of two bioreactor detection assays. *J. Hosp. Infect.* **2010**, *74*, 160–167. [CrossRef] [PubMed]
17. Goss, S.G.; Schwartz, J.A.; Facchin, F.; Avdagic, E.; Gendics, C.; Lantis, J.C. Negative pressure wound therapy with instillation (NPWTI) better reduces post-debridement bioburden in chronically infected lower extremity wounds than NPWT alone. *J. Am. Coll. Clin. Wound Spec.* **2012**, *4*, 74–80. [CrossRef] [PubMed]
18. Malone, M.; Goeres, D.M.; Gosbell, I.; Vickery, K.; Jensen, S.; Stoodley, P. Approaches to biofilm-associated infections: The need for standardized and relevant biofilm methods for clinical applications. *Expert Rev. Anti-Infect. Ther.* **2017**, *15*, 147–156. [CrossRef] [PubMed]
19. Singh, D.P.; Gowda, A.U.; Chopra, K.; Tholen, M.; Chang, S.; Mavrophilipos, V.; Semsarzadeh, N.; Rasko, Y.; Holton, L., III. The Effect of Negative Pressure Wound Therapy with Antiseptic Instillation on Biofilm Formation in a Porcine Model of Infected Spinal Instrumentation. *Wounds* **2017**, *28*, 175–180. [PubMed]

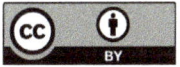

© 2018 by the authors. Licensee MDPI, Basel, Switzerland. This article is an open access article distributed under the terms and conditions of the Creative Commons Attribution (CC BY) license (http://creativecommons.org/licenses/by/4.0/).

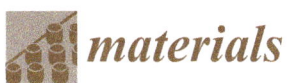

Review

Oral Microbes, Biofilms and Their Role in Periodontal and Peri-Implant Diseases

Jérôme Frédéric Lasserre *, Michel Christian Brecx and Selena Toma

Department of Periodontology, Université catholique de Louvain, 1348 Louvain-la-Neuve, Belgium; brecxparo@gmail.com (M.C.B.); selena.toma@uclouvain.be (S.T.)
* Correspondence: jerome.lasserre@uclouvain.be

Received: 20 August 2018; Accepted: 20 September 2018; Published: 22 September 2018

Abstract: Despite many discoveries over the past 20 years regarding the etio-pathogenesis of periodontal and peri-implant diseases, as well as significant advances in our understanding of microbial biofilms, the incidence of these pathologies still continues to rise. This review presents a general overview of the main protagonists and phenomena involved in oral health and disease. A special emphasis on the role of certain keystone pathogens in periodontitis and peri-implantitis is underlined. Their capacity to bring a dysregulation of the homeostasis with their host and the microbial biofilm lifestyle are also discussed. Finally, the current treatment principles of periodontitis and peri-implantitis are presented and their limits exposed. This leads to realize that new strategies must be developed and studied to overcome the shortcomings of existing approaches.

Keywords: periodontitis; peri-implantitis; biofilms; oral bacteria

1. Introduction

1.1. Microbes and Their Human Hosts

Humans are usually colonized from birth by many microbes that usually live in harmony with their host as commensal or symbiotic communities [1]. Among these, bacteria live in or on the human body, on mucosal surfaces or on the skin, and contribute in many ways to the host's life [2]. Indeed, in the healthy state, the commensal microbiota plays a protective role, like an invisible shield, against exogenous pathogens. Microbes also participate in food digestion, contribute to the synthesis of certain vitamins, and can educate our immune system [2,3]. It is estimated that the number of bacteria covering the human body is ten times greater than that of the eukaryotic cells of which we are composed [2,4]. Humans have, most likely, co-evolved with these microbes that have provided us with genetic and metabolic attributes [5]. Consequently, they are defined as "metaorganisms" [3]. Most of the microorganisms in humans are located in the gastrointestinal tract, where their concentration reaches its highest level in the colon with approximately 10^{11}–10^{12} cells/mL [6]. In fact, these indigenous microbes are usually essential in maintaining a healthy state, contrary to what was previously believed.

1.2. The Oral Microbiome

At the entrance of the upper digestive tract is the oral cavity (mouth), which is a very complex ecosystem that can harbor more than 150 different species of bacteria in one individual [7], as well as other types of microbes including archaea, fungi, protozoa and viruses [8]. More than 700 bacterial species have been isolated and identified from oral samples. They normally act as symbiotic communities with the host [9] but are also able to initiate a number of diseases in certain situations. The difference between a commensal and a symbiotic microbiota is subtle but important to clarify. The term commensal refers to partners that can live together but have no obvious mutual benefits [1]. A symbiosis is more than that; it is a relationship where both individuals (host and microbes) live in harmony and co-dependently. It is a real cooperation, a host–microbe mutualism [5]. For instance, periodontal pockets provide an ideal habitat for anaerobic proteolytic bacteria to grow, with anaerobic conditions and nutrients like peptides secreted in the gingival crevicular fluid [10]. Conversely, humans can also take advantage of the presence of oral microbes in various ways. First, commensals act as a natural barrier against exogenous or opportunistic pathogens. This barrier of resistance towards colonization is well illustrated when oral candidiasis develops after an antibiotic regimen [11]. Another example is the capability of the oral microbiota to metabolize inorganic nitrate from green vegetables, which is beneficial to the human body. Oral bacteria reduce inorganic nitrate into nitrite, which is then absorbed in the stomach before entering the blood stream [12]. There, it is transformed into nitric oxide, which is antihypertensive and vasoprotective [13]. Bacterial nitrite production by oral nitrate-reducing bacteria has also been shown to have antimicrobial effects against acidogenic bacteria such as *Streptococcus mutans* and to consequently reduce bacterial acid production and contribute to caries prevention [14]. These examples illustrate the mutual benefits between oral microbes and their human host.

Approximately 60% of the bacterial species that inhabit the oral cavity are not cultivable [15]. Culture-independent methods developed in the last two decades, such as checkerboard DNA–DNA hybridization or 16S rRNA gene sequencing, have provided considerable additional knowledge on the nature of the microbiotas associated with oral health and disease [16,17]. In the mouth, various types of tissues, growth conditions and nutrients are encountered in the development of different communities. Indeed, some bacteria are much more prevalent in some environments of the oral cavity than in others because they find ideal conditions to survive. For instance, the microbiota of the saliva resembles that of the tongue and differs significantly from that present on teeth and root surfaces [18,19]. Microbial community differences also occur between different people, even in health [15].

At present, the oral microbiota is one of the best-characterized microbiotas in humans because saliva and biofilms are easily harvested from oral surfaces. Its analysis is important for our understanding of its role in the development and pathogenesis of infectious oral diseases. It has been studied in various sites and conditions, such as around teeth or oral implants, and significant differences in its constitution have been demonstrated between health and disease states [15,17,20–24]. The principal findings of these studies showed that archaea, a group of single-celled microorganisms, were restricted to a small number of methanogen species, whereas more than 700 oral bacterial species belonging to different phyla (Actinobacteria, Bacteroidetes, Firmicutes, Proteobacteria, Spirochaetes, Synergistetes and Tenericutes and the uncultured divisions GN02, SR1 and TM7) were observed [8].

1.3. Oral Microbial-Shift Diseases

Oral health is linked to the equilibrium between the host and its commensal microbiota. Qualitative and/or quantitative shifts of the oral microbiome can lead to dysbiosis, an imbalance that is responsible for the development of microbe-related pathologies [25]. For instance, various oral diseases like periodontitis and peri-implantitis are strongly associated with dysbiotic microbial communities [26]. Some studies also reported a more relative but interesting association between some oral bacteria and *a priori* non-infectious disease like oral cancer. Hence, *Porphyromonas gingivalis* and *Fusobacterium nucleatum* have potential antigens like FimA and FadA adhesins that could lead to the development and progression of carcinomas (epithelial cell cancers) [27]. Additionally, a clinical study revealed an association between inadequate dental hygiene and an increased risk of oral cancer, especially in heavy alcohol consumers [28]. The authors of that report proposed that the risk could be related to the production of acetaldehyde; indeed, oral bacteria in saliva can metabolize ethanol into acetaldehyde, a known carcinogen. Furthermore, non-oral infections such as endocarditis, brain or lung abscesses, hip arthroplasty infections, and septicemias have also been correlated to oral bacteria that can access the blood stream through untreated caries lesions or via the periodontal/peri-implant pockets [29]. Finally, several systemic conditions like diabetes, preterm birth and cardiovascular diseases have been associated with periodontal disease and their microbiota in epidemiological studies [30–32]. Many human diseases are thus caused or influenced, directly or indirectly, by the oral microbiome. The present article will focus on two important infectious oral diseases: periodontal and peri-implant diseases.

2. Periodontal and Peri-Implant Diseases

2.1. Definition

Periodontitis and peri-implantitis are two major oral diseases that we have to deal with in periodontal practice. They are polymicrobial inflammatory diseases that lead to the destruction of the tissue supporting the tooth/implant. Without treatment, they result in tooth/implant loss.

2.2. Epidemiology

Periodontitis is one of the most frequent infections in humans and is often recognized as the leading cause of tooth loss in adults [25]. It can lead to oral and potentially systemic disabilities. Recent epidemiological data from the Global Burden of Disease (GBD) 2010 study suggest that periodontitis is the sixth-most prevalent condition in the world [33]. Its frequency has increased slightly since 1990 and ranges between 10.5% and 12% of the population, depending on the region [34]. Additional information from the National Health and Nutrition Survey (NHANES) 2009–2010 presents the periodontal health status of adults in the U.S.; nearly 4000 patients (aged >30 years) were examined, and periodontitis was observed in more than 47% of the sample [35]. More precisely, 8.7%, 30.0% and 8.5% had mild, moderate and severe periodontitis, respectively. The prevalence was significantly higher in older participants (periodontitis was present in around 25% of young adults versus 70% of patients older than 65 years).

The epidemiology of peri-implantitis, a biological complication of oral implants, is less well studied compared to that of periodontal diseases because of the relatively recent development of this disease. Two important Swedish cross-sectional studies of 662 and 216 subjects evaluated the prevalence of peri-implantitis on Brånemark System® implants with a documented function time of at least 5 years. The recorded values of peri-implantitis were 28% and 16% for the studied patients, and 12% and 7% at the implant level, respectively [36,37]. However, it was stated at the sixth European Workshop on Periodontology, organized by the European Federation of Periodontology in 2008, that very few epidemiological data of peri-implant diseases were available and that research should be conducted in a way that establishes accurate estimations of the disease and associated risk factors [38]. Since then, several studies have evaluated the prevalence and incidence of peri-implantitis in various populations, implant systems and clinical situations [39–45]. The values varied widely between the studies, from 9% to 47% at the patient level. These differences were partly due to the definition of peri-implantitis, which differed between the studies, and to the mean function time of the implants. The incidence of peri-implantitis tended to increase in patients without supportive therapy [46] and with time of function [42]. A recent systematic review, which evaluated the current epidemiology of peri-implant diseases, retained only 15 articles reporting on the topic and meeting the inclusion criteria [47]. In that review, no limits on function time were applied but at least 100 patients had to be included and subject-level data had to be reported for the study to be eligible. Weighted mean prevalence of mucositis and peri-implantitis at the patient level was 43% and 22%, respectively. Although the first consequence of these biological complications is implant loss, the systemic effects of such infections are still unknown.

2.3. Etiology

An emerging concept is the strong association between oral dysbiosis and oral disease [48]. In the healthy mouth, teeth are surrounded by the periodontium. This entity represents the tooth-supporting tissues and is composed of five elements: the gingiva, the alveolar mucosa, the alveolar bone, the periodontal ligament and the cementum (Figure 1). Each of these components is essential for maintaining the proper attachment and function of the teeth. All the structures found in the mouth (including teeth and implants) are permanently soaked in saliva containing billions of microorganisms (bacteria, viruses, archaea, protozoa, fungi; 10^8 cells/mL) [49]. In the healthy mouth, conditions are appropriate for these microbes, which live in harmony with the host and participate in many physiological reactions. Using various saliva proteins, they can adhere to biotic and abiotic surfaces, and form oral biofilms. On mucosal surfaces, the shedding mechanism occurring during oral epithelial turnover is a natural effective means of reducing microbial adhesion. But this protective phenomenon does not occur on tooth or implant surfaces, where the dental biofilm can accumulate in the periodontal/peri-implant crevice and stay in contact with the gingival epithelium (Figure 1).

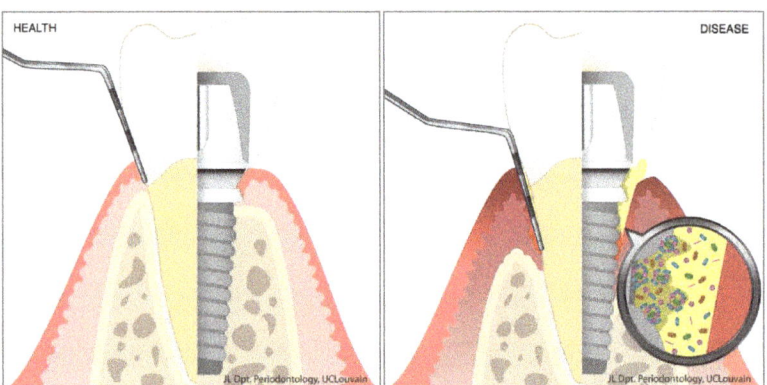

Figure 1. Periodontal/peri-implant tissues in health and disease. In the diseased state, the dysbiotic oral biofilm (yellow) that accumulates on the tooth/implant surface is responsible for the destruction of the supporting tissues through unresolved inflammation. This leads to the formation of periodontal/peri-implant pockets.

In susceptible patients, if dysbiotic, these sticky microbial communities elicit an inflammatory host response that can damage the surrounding tissues including the alveolar bone. The precise pathogenic pathways that lead to tissue destruction are still poorly understood but research conducted during the past decade has provided significant insight into this old enigma [25,50]. For example, the dysbiotic oral microbiota involved in these pathologies can induce direct tissue destruction through proteolytic enzymes. Additionally, the periodontal/peri-implant tissues will be damaged because of a non-resolving innate and acquired immunity response [25].

The microbial etiology of periodontal disease was first proposed in the late 1800s, when the germ theory changed the world's understanding of disease. However, specific pathogens remained elusive at this time, which led in the mid-1920s–1930s to the suggestion of other causes like trauma or disuse atrophy. Then, in the late 1950s, when it was observed that gingival inflammation resolved after routine cleaning and dental plaque removal, the belief returned that microbes were non-specifically involved in the etiology of periodontal disease: the so-called "non-specific plaque hypothesis" [51]. This theory placed importance on the entire community as a causative entity, rather than potential specific periodontal pathogens. Later, in the 1970s and 1980s, detailed cultural studies characterized dental plaque bacterial composition and revealed significant differences between healthy mouths and those with periodontitis [52]. This led to the "specific plaque hypothesis", in which the disease was strongly believed to be associated with the presence of certain pathogenic microorganisms [53] because these species were not (or were hardly) detectable by culture in healthy subjects. Considerable research efforts were then engaged to identify pathogens responsible for periodontal disease, and molecular technologies allowed the manufacturing of DNA probes. In 1998, a landmark study was performed in 185 volunteers (25 healthy; 160 with periodontitis) using whole genomic probes and the DNA–DNA checkerboard hybridization technique [16]. The researchers collected 13,261 subgingival plaque samples and identified three major pathogenic bacteria that were very often encountered together and strongly associated with severe periodontitis. These bacteria, namely *Porphyromonas gingivalis*, *Tannerella forsythia* and *Treponema denticola*, were called the "red complex" bacteria and accepted as strong etiological agents of periodontal disease. However, although these periopathogens were identified as potential causative agents of periodontitis at this time using microarray techniques, data collected since the early 2000s, during a period that saw enormous advances in microbiome characterization—first with Sanger sequencing and then with next generation sequencing—demonstrated that the situation is much more complex than that. Indeed, many works during the past 15 years have focused on the precise characterization of microbial profiles associated with oral health, and periodontal and peri-implant diseases using these novel technologies that sequence the bacterial 16s rRNA gene for microbial identification [15,17,21,23,24,54]. New information came out of these studies: first, the well-known microorganisms of the red complex could be found in sites and subjects in the absence of disease; second, new potential periopathogens emerged, some of which were not necessarily Gram-negative (*Filifactor alocis*, *Peptostreptococcus spp.*). These new candidates also outnumber the classical red complex species in the diseased sites but their pathogenic properties remain to be discovered [55].

The current model of periodontal/peri-implant disease, the "polymicrobial synergy and dysbiosis" model, tries to integrate the numerous theories from the past. It is based on the hypothesis that disease is provoked by a dysbiotic community shaped progressively by the introduction (even at low abundance) of keystone pathogens like *Porphyromonas gingivalis* [56]. In some clinical situations (physical disruption of the epithelium, antibiotic regimen, pathogen infection, host genetic defects, bacterial gene modification, tobacco smoking), these kinds of pathogens could colonize and develop into the commensal community by immune subversion, and then influence the whole symbiotic microbiota to become more pathogenic and initiate disease [20,48]. The microbiota is then progressively shaped by environmental changes into a more inflammophilic community composed of large proportions of pathobionts capable of maintaining dysbiosis and subsequent disease [57–59]. This model combines the previous "polymicrobial disruption of homeostasis" [25] and the "keystone pathogen hypothesis" [60]. According to this model, the key pathogens do not directly cause disease (as specific pathogens), but manipulate, through bacterial communication, the commensal microbiota that globally changes its metabolic activities to increase its pathogenicity.

2.4. Microbial Ecology of Dental Plaque

Saliva contains thousands of free-floating bacteria per milliliter that progressively deposit and adhere to dental/implant surfaces, first by non-specific physicochemical means and then by specific interactions with surface-adsorbed saliva proteins. The initial colonizers of early dental plaque in the first few days are essentially composed of Gram-positive bacteria, mostly cocci. The population then becomes increasingly complex, shifting progressively to a largely Gram-negative community with the appearance of rods, filamentous organisms, vibrios and spirochetes [61]. This maturation of undisturbed dental plaque is very important because it is associated with the clinical development of gingival and peri-implant mucosal inflammation [62,63]. This microbial succession is mediated by coaggregation between different bacterial species that corresponds to intergeneric specific cell-to-cell recognition via surface adhesins and receptors (Figure 2) [64].

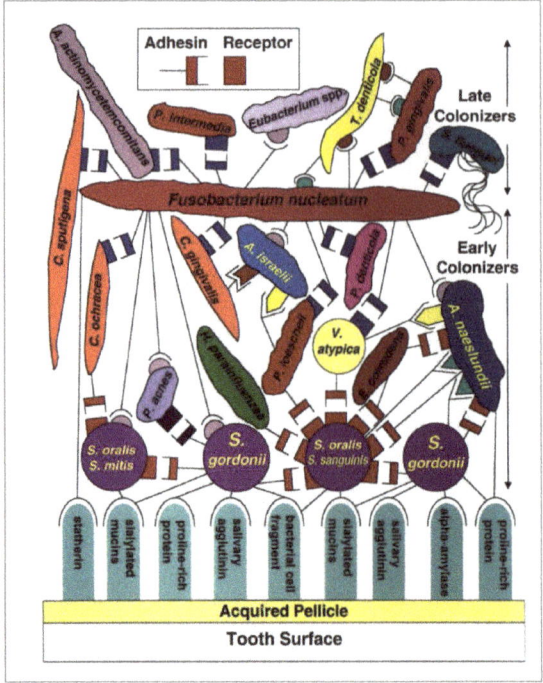

Figure 2. Intergeneric coaggregation among oral bacteria [64].

Later, in more advanced disease states such as periodontitis, the diversity of the periodontal microbiota increases further. It is composed supragingivally of a dense filament-containing plaque and subgingivally of flagellated bacteria, spirochetes and small Gram-negative bacteria [65]. More recent studies analyzing the initial composition of early dental plaque have confirmed, with molecular techniques, that most of the early colonizers were Gram-positive and belonged to the genera *Streptococcus spp.* and *Actinomyces*. Some Gram-negative genera, like *Neisseria* (aerobes) or *Veillonella* (anaerobes), were also observed [66,67]. Nevertheless, these culture-independent methods have demonstrated that even in healthy situations and in early dental plaque, some peripathogens like those of the red complex or *Aggregatibacter actinomycetemcomitans* could be found. This was also the case in the pockets of newly abutment-connected dental implants [68]. Surprisingly, these studies highlighted real differences in the microbial profiles of the participants, demonstrating a significant subject-specificity of the initial dental plaque biofilm.

After a few days, the accumulation of dental plaque biofilms in the periodontal or peri-implant sulcus induces clinical signs of inflammation, including increases in probing pocket depths, gingival index and gingival crevicular fluid (GCF) flow [62,63]. Thus, the early colonizers, mainly Gram-positive aerobes composed of *Streptococcus spp.* and *Actinomyces spp.*, influence the local environment, which, in turn, becomes suitable for secondary colonizers such as *Fusobacterium nucleatum*. This bacterium acts as a "bridging species". Indeed, through coaggregation, it allows the adhesion of late colonizers and peripathogens like *Porphyromonas gingivalis* [10,64]. This succession during the colonization of the periodontal/peri-implant crevice shows how the accumulation of commensal bacteria can induce (if important and undisturbed) a change in the local habitat (↑pH, ↑GCF, ↓Eh (Redox potential), ↓O_2) that allows peripathogens to colonize the periodontal/peri-implant crevice. This shift from a symbiotic microbial community to a more complex and aggressive microbiota is a risk predisposing the site to disease. This sequence is in accordance with what has been called the "ecological plaque hypothesis" of periodontal disease (Figure 3) [69].

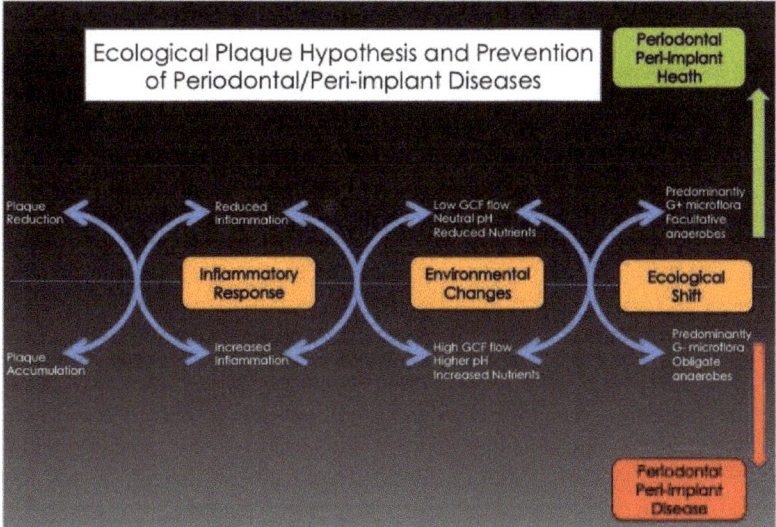

Figure 3. The ecological plaque hypothesis (Adapted from [69]).

It is now well accepted that dental biofilms play a key role in the initiation and progression of periodontal and peri-implant diseases. However, the precise mechanisms leading to homeostasis disruption and the detailed pathways of pathogenesis are still unclear.

2.5. Pathogenesis of Periodontal and Peri-Implant Diseases

Although the etiology of periodontal and peri-implant diseases is bacterial, and some well-characterized pathogens display destructive virulence factors, the pathogenesis of periodontitis and peri-implantitis is essentially mediated by the host response [70]. Certain advances in the past 15 years instilled a new appreciation of pathogenesis. Indeed, it has been demonstrated that even in health, the periodontal or peri-implant tissues that are in close contact with the dental biofilm show an active immune response, which is physiological. This low-grade inflammation is complex and involves both innate and acquired immunity as well as the complement system, the major link between the two arms of the immune system [71,72]. Dysregulation in the production of inflammatory mediators in response to the dysbiotic microbial challenge leads to the production of toxic products by the host cells. When produced in excess, these toxic products are responsible for tissue destruction around teeth and oral implants [70]. Additionally, the identification of Toll-like receptors (TLRs) highlighted how both commensal and pathogenic bacteria can initiate innate immune responses [73,74]. Finally, the discovery that most bacteria live in biofilms as tenacious multicellular communities has been important for our understanding of how microorganisms could resist the host immune response and even some conventional anti-infective approaches [25]. Figure 4 illustrates the pathogenesis of periodontal and peri-implant diseases.

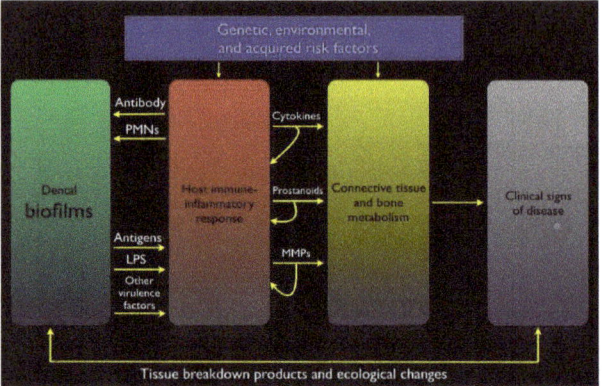

Figure 4. Schematic of the pathogenesis of periodontal and peri-implant diseases (PMNs: polymorphonuclear neutrophils; MMPs: matrix metalloproteinases; LPS: lipopolysaccharides). (Adapted from [75]).

To cope with constant contact with microorganisms and their virulence factors in the periodontal and peri-implant pockets, the host orchestrates the expression of defense mediators. First, direct recognition of bacteria (or virulence factors) by resident cells occurs through interaction between the TLR and bacteria, and this mediates the production of chemokines. Thereafter, intercellular adhesion molecules and E-selectin are produced at the surface of local endothelial cells. These molecules initiate the transit of polymorphonuclear neutrophils (PMNs) from the gingival vessels to the junctional epithelium, where they act as the first line of defense in the periodontium and peri-implant mucosae. This migration is guided by a gradient of interleukin (IL)-8, a cytokine produced in abundance by gingival epithelial cells [76]. PMNs are essential in maintaining periodontal health, as individuals with congenital diseases characterized by a deficiency of PMNs, such as leukocyte adhesion deficiencies or neutropenia, systematically develop periodontal diseases [77]. To eliminate aggressive pathobionts, PMNs employ various antimicrobial strategies, including phagocytosis, reactive oxygen species production and intra- or extracellular degranulation of specific enzymes [78]. In addition to IL-8, the host also expresses other mediators that contribute to innate immunity and that are encountered in the gingival or junctional epithelia. Of these innate molecules, β-defensins, CD14 and lipopolysaccharide-binding protein play a role in the neutralization of oral pathogens as well as TLRs [74] and neutrophil extracellular traps (NETs) [79]. TLRs are host-cell receptors that recognize commensal and pathogenic microbes and launch immune reaction pathways to defend the host against microbial invasion. NETs form a web-like structure of decondensed nuclear chromatin or mitochondrial DNA that is released in the extracellular spaces by PMNs and is associated with an array of antimicrobial molecules, including peptides. Their aim is to eliminate invading periodontal or peri-implant pathogens. In parallel to this innate immunity, periodontal and peri-implant tissues produce numerous cytokine and chemokine molecules that, in a refined equilibrium, help maintain a healthy situation. However, some of them—like IL-1β, tumor necrosis factor (TNF)-α, IL-6 and IL-17—are known as strong pro-inflammatory molecules that, without appropriate control, can lead to tissue destruction. Indeed, these signaling molecules stimulate the activation of enzymes and transcription factors that in turn recruit more immune cells and degrade the surrounding tissues by maintaining a continual loop of local inflammation [71,75]. Three protein pathways—nuclear factor kappa B (NF-κB), cyclo-oxygenase (COX) and lipo-oxygenase (LOX)—are activated in periodontal and peri-implant diseases and play key roles in maintaining inflammation and bone resorption. COX and LOX produce lipid mediators such as prostaglandins and leukotrienes (eicosanoids) by the oxidation of arachidonic acid. These lipid signaling molecules are pro-inflammatory, and the consequence of the prolonged elevation of their concentration is alveolar bone resorption [70]. The NF-κB pathway is another system probably related to bone resorption in periodontitis and peri-implantitis. Normally, the mechanisms that regulate bone deposition and resorption during remodeling are mediated through the refined equilibrium between the expression of two molecules: receptor activator of NF-κB ligand (RANKL) and osteoprotegerin (OPG) [25]. Indeed, RANKL, produced by several cell types, interacts with its receptor, RANK, located on the membrane of osteoclast precursors. This interaction allows them to finish their differentiation into active osteoclasts that will resorb the alveolar bone. OPG is a soluble RANKL receptor that is secreted by osteoblasts and, at high concentrations, prevents RANK–RANKL interaction and limits bone resorption. OPG formation is regulated by transforming growth factor β, and RANKL is induced by pro-inflammatory cytokines like IL-1β and TNF-α. Together, this demonstrates how the production of pro-inflammatory mediators can influence the RANKL/OPG ratio and contribute to periodontitis and peri-implantitis (Figure 5).

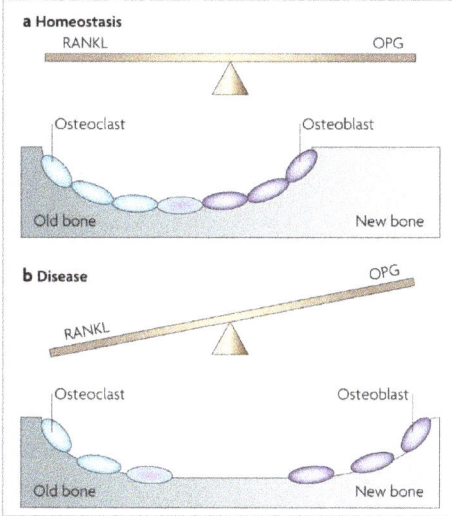

Figure 5. The NF-κB model of bone resorption during periodontal and peri-implant diseases [25].

Periodontitis and peri-implantitis also involve the destruction of the connective tissues including collagens, proteoglycans and other components of the extracellular matrix. The degradation of this extracellular matrix is performed by matrix metalloproteinases, a group of enzymes including collagenases. They are released locally by immune cells (macrophages or PMNs) or resident tissue cells (mostly gingival fibroblasts, because of their high number) [75]. All these immune and inflammatory reactions that lead to periodontal and peri-implant diseases are induced by the microorganisms that develop on enamel and titanium surfaces as microbial biofilms in close contact with the junctional and sulcular epithelia of their host. The biofilm mode of growth of dental plaque is likely to influence the pathogenicity of oral microbes.

3. Current Treatment Principles of Periodontitis and Peri-Implantitis

Despite all the discoveries of the past 20 years regarding the etio-pathogenesis of periodontal and peri-implant diseases, as well as the significant advances in our understanding of microbial biofilms, the incidence of these pathologies continues to rise [34,80]. Even though peri-implant diseases present some physio-pathological specificities [81,82] histo-pathological particularities [83] and are associated with microbiomes that seems to differ from those of periodontitis [23,84], they are recognized as biofilm-induced inflammatory diseases. They are often, and in many ways, compared to periodontitis. Both diseases are thus related to a switch from a symbiotic to a dysbiotic microbiota [56].

The main objective of peri-implantitis treatment is hence anti-infective as it is for periodontitis [85]. Control of the subgingival dysbiotic dental biofilm to restore homeostasis between the microbial community and its host remains the main purpose of currently available clinical treatments for these pathologies. This primarily involves giving instructions for proper oral hygiene, as well as nonsurgical mechanical debridement of the periodontal and peri-implant pockets. If performed carefully, these noninvasive mechanical therapeutic approaches most often allow the control of inflammation and disease in periodontitis [86]. Unfortunately, for advanced lesions with probing pocket depths of ≥7 mm, these treatments are less efficient, with about 15% showing no improvement [87]. Results of such treatment on furcation-involved teeth are also less beneficial, requiring more aggressive (surgical flaps) or alternative anti-infective approaches [88].

Few studies have investigated the efficacy of treatments of peri-implantitis lesions, but recent clinical trials and systematic reviews have shown that a nonsurgical mechanical approach is not sufficient for controlling the disease [89–93]. The relative failure of mechanical treatments in these clinical situations can be related to the fact that the disinfection is insufficient, leading to recolonization of the affected pocket and continued disease progression. Some local factors, such as a deep pocket, unfavorable root anatomy, or a rough surface threads, can explain the difficulty of achieving complete and efficient mechanical debridement. The recolonization of the periodontal or peri-implant pocket by a dysbiotic community can also come from pathogens that had previously infiltrated the dentin tubuli [94] or the periodontal/peri-implant tissues [95]. To improve clinical results, some authors proposed the use of conventional antibiotics or local antiseptics as adjunctive methods to the mechanical debridement of diseased pockets. Indeed, the clinical benefits of antibiotics used in this way have been demonstrated, and their use is now recommended for the treatment of aggressive periodontitis [96]. The use of antibiotics has also been suggested for severe periodontitis, though only when necessary, as the body of evidence for this is weaker [97]. However, considering the increase in incidence of microbial resistance (and the mild risk of the patient developing an allergy), the use of antibiotics should be kept to a minimum.

Subgingival irrigation as a nonsurgical treatment of periodontal and peri-implant diseases remains controversial [98], with a lack of randomized controlled clinical trials, and data that do not allow the discrimination between the relative efficacy of various available methods [99]. Therefore, the development of new strategies to better treat severe periodontitis and peri-implantitis is still needed. To this end, two distinct approaches can be considered. The first would try to improve the host's immune/inflammatory response to the microbial challenge. The second would investigate new pre-clinical and clinical strategies to control more efficiently the periodontal and peri-implant biofilms and pathogens associated with periodontitis and peri-implantitis.

4. New or Recent Antibiofilm Strategies

It is estimated that 99% of bacteria on earth live in biofilm aggregates [100] and most infectious diseases (65%) are related to the development of such sessile communities [101]. To counteract the natural resistance/tolerance of microbial biofilms against antimicrobial agents and to mitigate their pathologic consequences, new strategies are being considered and studied. They can be classified into four main categories according to Bjarnsholt et al. [102]: (a) prevention, (b) weakening, (c) disruption, and (d) killing (Figure 6).

The first approach, (a), aims to prevent biofilm formation through antibiotic prophylaxis or by modifying surface characteristics using antimicrobial or anti-adhesive coatings. For instance, silver nanoparticles on titanium surfaces are currently being evaluated for use in dentistry [103].

Weakening, (b), refers to interfering with signaling molecules, virulence factors and/or biofilm-forming properties to make the biofilm more susceptible to conventional antimicrobial agents and to the natural host defense system. To achieve this, quorum sensing inhibitors, inhibitors of small RNAs (messengers involved in biofilm formation), specific antibodies against virulence factors, or metabolically inactive metal ions that can interfere with iron metabolism are being tested in vitro [102].

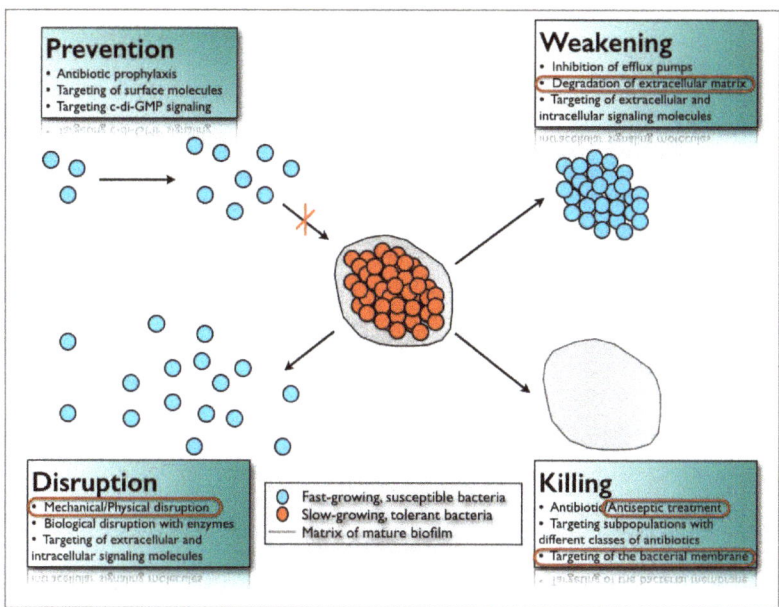

Figure 6. The four anti-biofilm strategies. (Adapted from [102]).

The third antibiofilm approach, (c), aims to disorganize the biofilm structure in order to disrupt the communication network between its cells and to make them more susceptible to antimicrobials. For example, Alhede et al. [104] showed that vortexing *Pseudomonas aeruginosa* biofilms was a valuable in vitro method of increasing their sensitivity towards tobramycin. Another method for the same purpose is to use biological molecules such as enzymes (DNAses or dispersin B) that target the extracellular matrix components of the biofilm that are responsible, in part, for its cohesive property [105,106]. Nevertheless, the most efficient method for treating a biofilm infection is by mechanically or surgically removing the biofilm. Two basic examples of biofilm removal are tooth brushing and scaling, and root planning. These mechanical methods are the first choice when the contaminated surface can be accessed. Unfortunately, this is not always possible and innovative antibiofilm approaches need to be developed.

The fourth strategy for controlling microbial aggregates, (d), is by killing biofilm cells by specific and/or nonspecific anti-infective means. New synergistic approaches involving small molecules (2-aminoimidazoles) capable of dispersing biofilm bacteria, and conventional antibiotics, have been proposed to better combat biofilm aggregates [107]. Furthermore, the use of bacteriophages (viruses that contaminate bacterial cells) [108], antimicrobial peptides [109] or photodynamic therapy [110] have also been investigated in the past decade as innovative antibiofilm strategies. Finally, among the numerous antibiofilm approaches that have been suggested, an interesting electrical enhancement of the effects of several antibiotics and industrial biocides have been described against different types of bacterial biofilms [111–113]. Electric currents have also been reported to have a bactericidal effect [114] in addition to detaching adherent bacteria [115] and preventing their adhesion [116]. The mechanisms by which these phenomena occur have not been elucidated in detail, but may be related to a better diffusion of antimicrobials through the biofilm [117], the electrolytic generation of oxygen [118] or the electrochemical formation of antimicrobial oxidants [119]. Electric currents might also lead to the degradation of the bacterial membrane, resulting in the leakage of the cytoplasmic constituents [114]. They could potentially have another physical effect on the charged extracellular matrix, which would induce a weakening of its structure. These antibiofilm phenomena, which have been described as bioelectric and electricidal effects, could be of great interest to the field of oral care, particularly in the treatment of advanced or refractory periodontal and peri-implant infections.

5. Concluding Remarks

Periodontitis and peri-implantitis are two major biofilm-induced inflammatory diseases that lead to the loss of teeth and oral implants if left untreated. These diseases are also associated with systemic conditions such as diabetes or cardiovascular diseases. Unfortunately, currently available treatments are not always successful, so innovative antibiofilm approaches need to be developed. Many strategies have been developed in that way and tested in vitro, as outlined above, but their clinical applicability is sometimes difficult. Considerable research efforts are needed, and additional anti-inflammatory approaches should be investigated to improve treatment efficacy.

Funding: This research received no external funding.

Acknowledgments: The authors are very grateful to Professor Gaëtane Leloup (Université catholique de Louvain, Belgium), to Professor Anton Sculean (Bern Universität, Switzerland) and to Professor Henri Tenenbaum (Université de Strasbourg, France) for their precious advice and discussions.

Conflicts of Interest: The authors declare no conflicts of interest.

References

1. Hooper, L.V.; Gordon, J.I. Commensal host-bacterial relationships in the gut. *Science* **2001**, *292*, 1115–1118. [CrossRef] [PubMed]
2. Maynard, C.L.; Elson, C.O.; Hatton, R.D.; Weaver, C.T. Reciprocal interactions of the intestinal microbiota and immune system. *Nature* **2012**, *489*, 231–241. [CrossRef] [PubMed]
3. Candela, M.; Maccaferri, S.; Turroni, S.; Carnevali, P.; Brigidi, P. Functional intestinal microbiome, new frontiers in prebiotic design. *Int. J. Food Microbiol.* **2010**, *140*, 93–101. [CrossRef] [PubMed]
4. Ley, R.E.; Peterson, D.A.; Gordon, J.I. Ecological and evolutionary forces shaping microbial diversity in the human intestine. *Cell* **2006**, *124*, 837–848. [CrossRef] [PubMed]
5. Backhed, F.; Ley, R.E.; Sonnenburg, J.L.; Peterson, D.A.; Gordon, J.I. Host-bacterial mutualism in the human intestine. *Science* **2005**, *307*, 1915–1920. [CrossRef] [PubMed]
6. Whitman, W.B.; Coleman, D.C.; Wiebe, W.J. Prokaryotes: The unseen majority. *Proc. Natl. Acad. Sci. USA* **1998**, *95*, 6578–6583. [CrossRef] [PubMed]
7. Moore, W.E.; Moore, L.V. The bacteria of periodontal diseases. *Periodontology 2000* **1994**, *5*, 66–77. [CrossRef] [PubMed]
8. Wade, W.G. The oral microbiome in health and disease. *Pharmacol. Res.* **2013**, *69*, 137–143. [CrossRef] [PubMed]
9. Dewhirst, F.E.; Chen, T.; Izard, J.; Paster, B.J.; Tanner, A.C.; Yu, W.H.; Lakshmanan, A.; Wade, W.G. The human oral microbiome. *J. Bacteriol.* **2010**, *192*, 5002–5017. [CrossRef] [PubMed]
10. Socransky, S.S.; Haffajee, A.D. Periodontal microbial ecology. *Periodontology 2000* **2005**, *38*, 135–187. [CrossRef] [PubMed]
11. Sullivan, Å.; Edlund, C.; Nord, C.E. Effect of antimicrobial agents on the ecological balance of human microflora. *Lancet Infect. Dis.* **2001**, *1*, 101–114. [CrossRef]
12. Lundberg, J.M. An audience with... Jan M. Lundberg. *Nat. Rev. Drug Discov.* **2005**, *4*, 452. [CrossRef] [PubMed]
13. Kapil, V.; Milsom, A.B.; Okorie, M.; Maleki-Toyserkani, S.; Akram, F.; Rehman, F.; Arghandawi, S.; Pearl, V.; Benjamin, N.; Loukogeorgakis, S.; et al. Inorganic nitrate supplementation lowers blood pressure in humans: Role for nitrite-derived NO. *Hypertension* **2010**, *56*, 274–281. [CrossRef] [PubMed]
14. Doel, J.J.; Hector, M.P.; Amirtham, C.V.; Al-Anzan, L.A.; Benjamin, N.; Allaker, R.P. Protective effect of salivary nitrate and microbial nitrate reductase activity against caries. *Eur. J. Oral Sci.* **2004**, *112*, 424–428. [CrossRef] [PubMed]
15. Aas, J.A.; Paster, B.J.; Stokes, L.N.; Olsen, I.; Dewhirst, F.E. Defining the normal bacterial flora of the oral cavity. *J. Clin. Microbiol.* **2005**, *43*, 5721–5732. [CrossRef] [PubMed]

16. Socransky, S.S.; Haffajee, A.D.; Cugini, M.A.; Smith, C.; Kent, R.L., Jr. Microbial complexes in subgingival plaque. *J. Clin. Periodontol.* **1998**, *25*, 134–144. [CrossRef] [PubMed]
17. Abusleme, L.; Dupuy, A.K.; Dutzan, N.; Silva, N.; Burleson, J.A.; Strausbaugh, L.D.; Gamonal, J.; Diaz, P.I. The subgingival microbiome in health and periodontitis and its relationship with community biomass and inflammation. *ISME J.* **2013**, *7*, 1016–1025. [CrossRef] [PubMed]
18. Mager, D.L.; Ximenez-Fyvie, L.A.; Haffajee, A.D.; Socransky, S.S. Distribution of selected bacterial species on intraoral surfaces. *J. Clin. Periodontol.* **2003**, *30*, 644–654. [CrossRef] [PubMed]
19. Paster, B.J.; Olsen, I.; Aas, J.A.; Dewhirst, F.E. The breadth of bacterial diversity in the human periodontal pocket and other oral sites. *Periodontology 2000* **2006**, *42*, 80–87. [CrossRef] [PubMed]
20. Mason, M.R.; Preshaw, P.M.; Nagaraja, H.N.; Dabdoub, S.M.; Rahman, A.; Kumar, P.S. The subgingival microbiome of clinically healthy current and never smokers. *ISME J* **2015**, *9*, 268–272. [CrossRef] [PubMed]
21. Griffen, A.L.; Beall, C.J.; Campbell, J.H.; Firestone, N.D.; Kumar, P.S.; Yang, Z.K.; Podar, M.; Leys, E.J. Distinct and complex bacterial profiles in human periodontitis and health revealed by 16S pyrosequencing. *ISME J.* **2012**, *6*, 1176–1185. [CrossRef] [PubMed]
22. Zaura, E.; Mira, A. Editorial: The oral microbiome in an ecological perspective. *Front. Cell. Infect. Microbiol.* **2015**, *5*, 39. [CrossRef] [PubMed]
23. Kumar, P.S.; Mason, M.R.; Brooker, M.R.; O'Brien, K. Pyrosequencing reveals unique microbial signatures associated with healthy and failing dental implants. *J. Clin. Periodontol.* **2012**, *39*, 425–433. [CrossRef] [PubMed]
24. Paster, B.J.; Boches, S.K.; Galvin, J.L.; Ericson, R.E.; Lau, C.N.; Levanos, V.A.; Sahasrabudhe, A.; Dewhirst, F.E. Bacterial diversity in human subgingival plaque. *J. Bacteriol.* **2001**, *183*, 3770–3783. [CrossRef] [PubMed]
25. Darveau, R.P. Periodontitis: A polymicrobial disruption of host homeostasis. *Nat. Rev. Microbiol.* **2010**, *8*, 481–490. [CrossRef] [PubMed]
26. Duran-Pinedo, A.E.; Frias-Lopez, J. Beyond microbial community composition: Functional activities of the oral microbiome in health and disease. *Microbes Infect.* **2015**, *17*, 505–516. [CrossRef] [PubMed]
27. Whitmore, S.E.; Lamont, R.J. Oral bacteria and cancer. *PLoS Pathog.* **2014**, *10*, e1003933. [CrossRef] [PubMed]
28. Homann, N.; Tillonen, J.; Rintamaki, H.; Salaspuro, M.; Lindqvist, C.; Meurman, J.H. Poor dental status increases acetaldehyde production from ethanol in saliva: A possible link to increased oral cancer risk among heavy drinkers. *Oral Oncol.* **2001**, *37*, 153–158. [CrossRef]
29. Parahitiyawa, N.B.; Jin, L.J.; Leung, W.K.; Yam, W.C.; Samaranayake, L.P. Microbiology of odontogenic bacteremia: Beyond endocarditis. *Clin. Microbiol. Rev.* **2009**, *22*, 46–64. [CrossRef] [PubMed]
30. Seymour, G.J.; Ford, P.J.; Cullinan, M.P.; Leishman, S.; Yamazaki, K. Relationship between periodontal infections and systemic disease. *Clin. Microbiol. Infect.* **2007**, *13*, 3–10. [CrossRef] [PubMed]
31. Rautemaa, R.; Lauhio, A.; Cullinan, M.P.; Seymour, G.J. Oral infections and systemic disease—An emerging problem in medicine. *Clin. Microbiol. Infect.* **2007**, *13*, 1041–1047. [CrossRef] [PubMed]
32. Rakoto-Alson, S.; Tenenbaum, H.; Davideau, J.L. Periodontal diseases, preterm births, and low birth weight: Findings from a homogeneous cohort of women in Madagascar. *J. Periodontol.* **2010**, *81*, 205–213. [CrossRef] [PubMed]
33. Marcenes, W.; Kassebaum, N.J.; Bernabe, E.; Flaxman, A.; Naghavi, M.; Lopez, A.; Murray, C.J. Global burden of oral conditions in 1990-2010: A systematic analysis. *J. Dent. Res.* **2013**, *92*, 592–597. [CrossRef] [PubMed]
34. Kassebaum, N.J.; Bernabe, E.; Dahiya, M.; Bhandari, B.; Murray, C.J.; Marcenes, W. Global burden of severe periodontitis in 1990–2010: A systematic review and meta-regression. *J. Dent. Res.* **2014**, *93*, 1045–1053. [CrossRef] [PubMed]
35. Eke, P.I.; Dye, B.A.; Wei, L.; Thornton-Evans, G.O.; Genco, R.J.; Cdc Periodontal Disease Surveillance Workgroup. Prevalence of periodontitis in adults in the United States: 2009 and 2010. *J. Dent. Res.* **2012**, *91*, 914–920. [CrossRef] [PubMed]
36. Fransson, C.; Lekholm, U.; Jemt, T.; Berglundh, T. Prevalence of subjects with progressive bone loss at implants. *Clin. Oral Implants Res.* **2005**, *16*, 440–446. [CrossRef] [PubMed]
37. Roos-Jansaker, A.M.; Lindahl, C.; Renvert, H.; Renvert, S. Nine- to fourteen-year follow-up of implant treatment. Part II: Presence of peri-implant lesions. *J. Clin. Periodontol.* **2006**, *33*, 290–295. [CrossRef] [PubMed]
38. Lindhe, J.; Meyle, J.; Group D of European Workshop on Periodontology. Peri-implant diseases: Consensus Report of the Sixth European Workshop on Periodontology. *J. Clin. Periodontol.* **2008**, *35*, 282–285. [CrossRef] [PubMed]

39. Koldsland, O.C.; Scheie, A.A.; Aass, A.M. Prevalence of peri-implantitis related to severity of the disease with different degrees of bone loss. *J. Periodontol.* **2010**, *81*, 231–238. [CrossRef] [PubMed]
40. Marrone, A.; Lasserre, J.; Bercy, P.; Brecx, M.C. Prevalence and risk factors for peri-implant disease in Belgian adults. *Clin. Oral Implants Res.* **2013**, *24*, 934–940. [CrossRef] [PubMed]
41. Mir-Mari, J.; Mir-Orfila, P.; Figueiredo, R.; Valmaseda-Castellon, E.; Gay-Escoda, C. Prevalence of peri-implant diseases. A cross-sectional study based on a private practice environment. *J. Clin. Periodontol.* **2012**, *39*, 490–494. [CrossRef] [PubMed]
42. Meijer, H.J.; Raghoebar, G.M.; de Waal, Y.C.; Vissink, A. Incidence of peri-implant mucositis and peri-implantitis in edentulous patients with an implant-retained mandibular overdenture during a 10-year follow-up period. *J. Clin. Periodontol.* **2014**, *41*, 1178–1183. [CrossRef] [PubMed]
43. Schwarz, F.; Becker, K.; Sahm, N.; Horstkemper, T.; Rousi, K.; Becker, J. The prevalence of peri-implant diseases for two-piece implants with an internal tube-in-tube connection: A cross-sectional analysis of 512 implants. *Clin. Oral Implants Res.* **2015**. [CrossRef] [PubMed]
44. Derks, J.; Schaller, D.; Hakansson, J.; Wennstrom, J.L.; Tomasi, C.; Berglundh, T. Effectiveness of Implant Therapy Analyzed in a Swedish Population: Prevalence of Peri-implantitis. *J. Dent. Res.* **2016**, *95*, 43–49. [CrossRef] [PubMed]
45. Tenenbaum, H.; Bogen, O.; Severac, F.; Elkaim, R.; Davideau, J.L.; Huck, O. Long-term prospective cohort study on dental implants: Clinical and microbiological parameters. *Clin. Oral Implants Res.* **2016**, *28*, 86–94. [CrossRef] [PubMed]
46. Costa, F.O.; Takenaka-Martinez, S.; Cota, L.O.; Ferreira, S.D.; Silva, G.L.; Costa, J.E. Peri-implant disease in subjects with and without preventive maintenance: A 5-year follow-up. *J. Clin. Periodontol.* **2012**, *39*, 173–181. [CrossRef] [PubMed]
47. Derks, J.; Tomasi, C. Peri-implant health and disease. A systematic review of current epidemiology. *J. Clin. Periodontol.* **2015**, *42*, S158–S171. [CrossRef] [PubMed]
48. Jiao, Y.; Hasegawa, M.; Inohara, N. The Role of Oral Pathobionts in Dysbiosis during Periodontitis Development. *J. Dent. Res.* **2014**, *93*, 539–546. [CrossRef] [PubMed]
49. Marsh, P.D.; Do, T.; Beighton, D.; Devine, D.A. Influence of saliva on the oral microbiota. *Periodontology 2000* **2016**, *70*, 80–92. [CrossRef] [PubMed]
50. Curtis, M. The oral commensal microbiota bites back through Nod1. *Cell Host Microbe* **2013**, *13*, 503–505. [CrossRef] [PubMed]
51. Schultz-Haudt, S.; Bruce, M.A.; Bibby, B.G. Bacterial factors in nonspecific gingivitis. *J. Dent. Res.* **1954**, *33*, 454–458. [CrossRef] [PubMed]
52. Socransky, S.S. Microbiology of periodontal disease—Present status and future considerations. *J. Periodontol.* **1977**, *48*, 497–504. [CrossRef] [PubMed]
53. Loesche, W.J. Clinical and microbiological aspects of chemotherapeutic agents used according to the specific plaque hypothesis. *J. Dent. Res.* **1979**, *58*, 2404–2412. [CrossRef] [PubMed]
54. Faveri, M.; Figueiredo, L.C.; Shibli, J.A.; Perez-Chaparro, P.J.; Feres, M. Microbiological diversity of peri-implantitis biofilms. *Adv. Exp. Med. Biol.* **2015**, *830*, 85–96. [CrossRef] [PubMed]
55. Kumar, P.S.; Griffen, A.L.; Moeschberger, M.L.; Leys, E.J. Identification of candidate periodontal pathogens and beneficial species by quantitative 16S clonal analysis. *J. Clin. Microbiol.* **2005**, *43*, 3944–3955. [CrossRef] [PubMed]
56. Hajishengallis, G.; Lamont, R.J. Beyond the red complex and into more complexity: The polymicrobial synergy and dysbiosis (PSD) model of periodontal disease etiology. *Mol. Oral Microbiol.* **2012**, *27*, 409–419. [CrossRef] [PubMed]
57. Hajishengallis, G. The inflammophilic character of the periodontitis-associated microbiota. *Mol. Oral Microbiol.* **2014**, *29*, 248–257. [CrossRef] [PubMed]
58. Maekawa, T.; Krauss, J.L.; Abe, T.; Jotwani, R.; Triantafilou, M.; Triantafilou, K.; Hashim, A.; Hoch, S.; Curtis, M.A.; Nussbaum, G.; et al. Porphyromonas gingivalis manipulates complement and TLR signaling to uncouple bacterial clearance from inflammation and promote dysbiosis. *Cell Host Microbe* **2014**, *15*, 768–778. [CrossRef] [PubMed]
59. Hajishengallis, G.; Lamont, R.J. Breaking bad: Manipulation of the host response by Porphyromonas gingivalis. *Eur. J. Immunol.* **2014**, *44*, 328–338. [CrossRef] [PubMed]

60. Hajishengallis, G.; Darveau, R.P.; Curtis, M.A. The keystone-pathogen hypothesis. *Nat. Rev. Microbiol.* **2012**, *10*, 717–725. [CrossRef] [PubMed]
61. Theilade, E.; Wright, W.H.; Jensen, S.B.; Loe, H. Experimental gingivitis in man. II. A longitudinal clinical and bacteriological investigation. *J. Periodontal. Res.* **1966**, *1*, 1–13. [CrossRef] [PubMed]
62. Loe, H.; Theilade, E.; Jensen, S.B. Experimental Gingivitis in Man. *J. Periodontol.* **1965**, *36*, 177–187. [CrossRef] [PubMed]
63. Zitzmann, N.U.; Berglundh, T.; Marinello, C.P.; Lindhe, J. Experimental peri-implant mucositis in man. *J. Clin. Periodontol.* **2001**, *28*, 517–523. [CrossRef] [PubMed]
64. Kolenbrander, P.E.; Palmer, R.J., Jr.; Rickard, A.H.; Jakubovics, N.S.; Chalmers, N.I.; Diaz, P.I. Bacterial interactions and successions during plaque development. *Periodontology 2000* **2006**, *42*, 47–79. [CrossRef] [PubMed]
65. Listgarten, M.A.; Hellden, L. Relative distribution of bacteria at clinically healthy and periodontally diseased sites in humans. *J. Clin. Periodontol.* **1978**, *5*, 115–132. [CrossRef] [PubMed]
66. Diaz, P.I.; Chalmers, N.I.; Rickard, A.H.; Kong, C.; Milburn, C.L.; Palmer, R.J., Jr.; Kolenbrander, P.E. Molecular characterization of subject-specific oral microflora during initial colonization of enamel. *Appl. Environ. Microbiol.* **2006**, *72*, 2837–2848. [CrossRef] [PubMed]
67. Li, J.; Helmerhorst, E.J.; Leone, C.W.; Troxler, R.F.; Yaskell, T.; Haffajee, A.D.; Socransky, S.S.; Oppenheim, F.G. Identification of early microbial colonizers in human dental biofilm. *J. Appl. Microbiol.* **2004**, *97*, 1311–1318. [CrossRef] [PubMed]
68. Quirynen, M.; Vogels, R.; Pauwels, M.; Haffajee, A.D.; Socransky, S.S.; Uzel, N.G.; van Steenberghe, D. Initial Subgingival Colonization of 'Pristine' Pockets. *J. Dent. Res.* **2005**, *84*, 340–344. [CrossRef] [PubMed]
69. Marsh, P.D. Microbial ecology of dental plaque and its significance in health and disease. *Adv. Dent. Res.* **1994**, *8*, 263–271. [CrossRef] [PubMed]
70. Van Dyke, T.E.; Serhan, C.N. Resolution of inflammation: A new paradigm for the pathogenesis of periodontal diseases. *J. Dent. Res.* **2003**, *82*, 82–90. [CrossRef] [PubMed]
71. Cekici, A.; Kantarci, A.; Hasturk, H.; Van Dyke, T.E. Inflammatory and immune pathways in the pathogenesis of periodontal disease. *Periodontology 2000* **2014**, *64*, 57–80. [CrossRef] [PubMed]
72. Ricklin, D.; Hajishengallis, G.; Yang, K.; Lambris, J.D. Complement: A key system for immune surveillance and homeostasis. *Nat. Immunol.* **2010**, *11*, 785–797. [CrossRef] [PubMed]
73. Benakanakere, M.; Abdolhosseini, M.; Hosur, K.; Finoti, L.S.; Kinane, D.F. TLR2 promoter hypermethylation creates innate immune dysbiosis. *J. Dent. Res.* **2015**, *94*, 183–191. [CrossRef] [PubMed]
74. Gay, N.J.; Symmons, M.F.; Gangloff, M.; Bryant, C.E. Assembly and localization of Toll-like receptor signalling complexes. *Nat. Rev. Immunol.* **2014**, *14*, 546–558. [CrossRef] [PubMed]
75. Page, R.C.; Offenbacher, S.; Schroeder, H.E.; Seymour, G.J.; Kornman, K.S. Advances in the pathogenesis of periodontitis: Summary of developments, clinical implications and future directions. *Periodontology 2000* **1997**, *14*, 216–248. [CrossRef] [PubMed]
76. Tonetti, M.S.; Imboden, M.A.; Lang, N.P. Neutrophil migration into the gingival sulcus is associated with transepithelial gradients of interleukin-8 and ICAM-1. *J. Periodontol.* **1998**, *69*, 1139–1147. [CrossRef] [PubMed]
77. Hajishengallis, G.; Moutsopoulos, N.M. Etiology of leukocyte adhesion deficiency-associated periodontitis revisited: Not a raging infection but a raging inflammatory response. *Expert Rev. Clin. Immunol.* **2014**, *10*, 973–975. [CrossRef] [PubMed]
78. Jaillon, S.; Galdiero, M.R.; Del Prete, D.; Cassatella, M.A.; Garlanda, C.; Mantovani, A. Neutrophils in innate and adaptive immunity. *Semin. Immunopathol.* **2013**, *35*, 377–394. [CrossRef] [PubMed]
79. White, P.C.; Chicca, I.J.; Cooper, P.R.; Milward, M.R.; Chapple, I.L. Neutrophil Extracellular Traps in Periodontitis: A Web of Intrigue. *J. Dent. Res.* **2016**, *95*, 26–34. [CrossRef] [PubMed]
80. Tarnow, D.P. Increasing Prevalence of Peri-implantitis: How Will We Manage? *J. Dent. Res.* **2016**, *95*, 7–8. [CrossRef] [PubMed]
81. Lang, N.P.B.T. Working Group 4 of Seventh European Workshop on P. 2011. Periimplant diseases: Where are we now?—Consensus of the Seventh European Workshop on Periodontology. *J. Clin. Periodontol.* **2011**, *38*, 178–181. [CrossRef] [PubMed]

82. Becker, S.T.; Beck-Broichsitter, B.E.; Graetz, C.; Dorfer, C.E.; Wiltfang, J.; Hasler, R. Peri-implantitis versus periodontitis: Functional differences indicated by transcriptome profiling. *Clin. Implant Dent. Relat. Res.* **2014**, *16*, 401–411. [CrossRef] [PubMed]
83. Carcuac, O.; Berglundh, T. Composition of human peri-implantitis and periodontitis lesions. *J. Dent. Res.* **2014**, *93*, 1083–1088. [CrossRef] [PubMed]
84. Lafaurie, G.I.; Sabogal, M.A.; Castillo, D.M.; Rincón, M.V.; Gómez, L.A.; Lesmes, Y.A.; Chambrone, L. Microbiome and microbial biofilm profiles of peri-implantitis: A systematic review. *J. Periodontol.* **2017**, *88*, 1066–1089. [CrossRef] [PubMed]
85. Lasserre, J.F.; Toma, S.; Bourgeois, T.; El Khatmaoui, H.; Marichal, E.; Brecx, M.C. Influence of low direct electric currents and chlorhexidine upon human dental biofilms. *Clin. Exp. Dent. Res.* **2016**, *2*, 146–154. [CrossRef] [PubMed]
86. Badersten, A.; Nilveus, R.; Egelberg, J. Effect of nonsurgical periodontal therapy. I. Moderately advanced periodontitis. *J. Clin. Periodontol.* **1981**, *8*, 57–72. [CrossRef] [PubMed]
87. Badersten, A.; Nilveus, R.; Egelberg, J. Effect of nonsurgical periodontal therapy. II. Severely advanced periodontitis. *J. Clin. Periodontol.* **1984**, *11*, 63–76. [CrossRef] [PubMed]
88. Adriaens, P.A.; Adriaens, L.M. Effects of nonsurgical periodontal therapy on hard and soft tissues. *Periodontology 2000* **2004**, *36*, 121–145. [CrossRef] [PubMed]
89. Karring, E.S.; Stavropoulos, A.; Ellegaard, B.; Karring, T. Treatment of peri-implantitis by the Vector system. *Clin. Oral Implants Res.* **2005**, *16*, 288–293. [CrossRef] [PubMed]
90. Renvert, S.; Roos-Jansaker, A.M.; Claffey, N. Non-surgical treatment of peri-implant mucositis and peri-implantitis: A literature review. *J. Clin. Periodontol.* **2008**, *35*, 305–315. [CrossRef] [PubMed]
91. Renvert, S.; Samuelsson, E.; Lindahl, C.; Persson, G.R. Mechanical non-surgical treatment of peri-implantitis: A double-blind randomized longitudinal clinical study. I: Clinical results. *J. Clin. Periodontol.* **2009**, *36*, 604–609. [CrossRef] [PubMed]
92. Renvert, S.; Lindahl, C.; Roos Jansaker, A.M.; Persson, G.R. Treatment of peri-implantitis using an Er:YAG laser or an air-abrasive device: A randomized clinical trial. *J. Clin. Periodontol.* **2011**, *38*, 65–73. [CrossRef] [PubMed]
93. Schwarz, F.; Becker, K.; Renvert, S. Efficacy of air polishing for the non-surgical treatment of peri-implant diseases: A systematic review. *J. Clin. Periodontol.* **2015**. [CrossRef] [PubMed]
94. Adriaens, P.A.; Edwards, C.A.; De Boever, J.A.; Loesche, W.J. Ultrastructural observations on bacterial invasion in cementum and radicular dentin of periodontally diseased human teeth. *J. Periodontol.* **1988**, *59*, 493–503. [CrossRef] [PubMed]
95. Lamont, R.J.; Chan, A.; Belton, C.M.; Izutsu, K.T.; Vasel, D.; Weinberg, A. Porphyromonas gingivalis invasion of gingival epithelial cells. *Infect. Immun.* **1995**, *63*, 3878–3885. [PubMed]
96. Keestra, J.A.; Grosjean, I.; Coucke, W.; Quirynen, M.; Teughels, W. Non-surgical periodontal therapy with systemic antibiotics in patients with untreated aggressive periodontitis: A systematic review and meta-analysis. *J. Periodontal Res.* **2015**, *50*, 689–706. [CrossRef] [PubMed]
97. Keestra, J.A.; Grosjean, I.; Coucke, W.; Quirynen, M.; Teughels, W. Non-surgical periodontal therapy with systemic antibiotics in patients with untreated chronic periodontitis: A systematic review and meta-analysis. *J. Periodontal Res.* **2015**, *50*, 294–314. [CrossRef] [PubMed]
98. Greenstein, G.; Research, S.; Therapy Committee of the American Academy of, P. Position paper: The role of supra- and subgingival irrigation in the treatment of periodontal diseases. *J. Periodontol.* **2005**, *76*, 2015–2027. [CrossRef] [PubMed]
99. Esposito, M.; Grusovin, M.G.; Worthington, H.V. Interventions for replacing missing teeth: Treatment of peri-implantitis. *Cochrane Database Syst. Rev.* **2012**, *1*, Cd004970. [CrossRef] [PubMed]
100. Potera, C. Studying slime. *Environ. Health Perspect.* **1998**, *106*, A604–A606. [CrossRef] [PubMed]
101. Potera, C. Forging a link between biofilms and disease. *Science* **1999**, *283*, 1837–1839. [CrossRef] [PubMed]
102. Bjarnsholt, T.; Ciofu, O.; Molin, S.; Givskov, M.; Hoiby, N. Applying insights from biofilm biology to drug development—Can a new approach be developed? *Nat. Rev. Drug Discov.* **2013**, *12*, 791–808. [CrossRef] [PubMed]

103. Zhong, X.; Song, Y.; Yang, P.; Wang, Y.; Jiang, S.; Zhang, X.; Li, C. Titanium Surface Priming with Phase-Transited Lysozyme to Establish a Silver Nanoparticle-Loaded Chitosan/Hyaluronic Acid Antibacterial Multilayer via Layer-by-Layer Self-Assembly. *PLoS ONE* **2016**, *11*, e0146957. [CrossRef] [PubMed]
104. Alhede, M.; Kragh, K.N.; Qvortrup, K.; Allesen-Holm, M.; van Gennip, M.; Christensen, L.D.; Jensen, P.O.; Nielsen, A.K.; Parsek, M.; Wozniak, D.; et al. Phenotypes of non-attached Pseudomonas aeruginosa aggregates resemble surface attached biofilm. *PLoS ONE* **2011**, *6*, e27943. [CrossRef] [PubMed]
105. Shields, R.C.; Mokhtar, N.; Ford, M.; Hall, M.J.; Burgess, J.G.; ElBadawey, M.R.; Jakubovics, N.S. Efficacy of a marine bacterial nuclease against biofilm forming microorganisms isolated from chronic rhinosinusitis. *PLoS ONE* **2013**, *8*, e55339. [CrossRef] [PubMed]
106. Izano, E.A.; Wang, H.; Ragunath, C.; Ramasubbu, N.; Kaplan, J.B. Detachment and killing of *Aggregatibacter actinomycetemcomitans* biofilms by dispersin B and SDS. *J. Dent. Res.* **2007**, *86*, 618–622. [CrossRef] [PubMed]
107. Rogers, S.A.; Huigens, R.W., 3rd; Cavanagh, J.; Melander, C. Synergistic effects between conventional antibiotics and 2-aminoimidazole-derived antibiofilm agents. *Antimicrob. Agents Chemother.* **2010**, *54*, 2112–2118. [CrossRef] [PubMed]
108. Pires, D.P.; Oliveira, H.; Melo, L.D.; Sillankorva, S.; Azeredo, J. Bacteriophage-encoded depolymerases: Their diversity and biotechnological applications. *Appl. Microbiol. Biotechnol.* **2016**, *100*, 2141–2151. [CrossRef] [PubMed]
109. Gorr, S.U.; Abdolhosseini, M. Antimicrobial peptides and periodontal disease. *J. Clin. Periodontol.* **2011**, *38*, 126–141. [CrossRef] [PubMed]
110. Bassetti, M.; Schar, D.; Wicki, B.; Eick, S.; Ramseier, C.A.; Arweiler, N.B.; Sculean, A.; Salvi, G.E. Anti-infective therapy of peri-implantitis with adjunctive local drug delivery or photodynamic therapy: 12-month outcomes of a randomized controlled clinical trial. *Clin. Oral Implants Res.* **2014**, *25*, 279–287. [CrossRef] [PubMed]
111. Blenkinsopp, S.A.; Khoury, A.E.; Costerton, J.W. Electrical enhancement of biocide efficacy against Pseudomonas aeruginosa biofilms. *Appl. Environ. Microbiol.* **1992**, *58*, 3770–3773. [PubMed]
112. Jass, J.; Lappin-Scott, H.M. The efficacy of antibiotics enhanced by electrical currents against Pseudomonas aeruginosa biofilms. *J. Antimicrob. Chemother.* **1996**, *38*, 987–1000. [CrossRef] [PubMed]
113. Haddad, P.A.; Mah, T.F.; Mussivand, T. In Vitro Assessment of Electric Currents Increasing the Effectiveness of Vancomycin Against Staphylococcus epidermidis Biofilms. *Artif. Organs* **2015**. [CrossRef]
114. del Pozo, J.L.; Rouse, M.S.; Mandrekar, J.N.; Steckelberg, J.M.; Patel, R. The electricidal effect: Reduction of Staphylococcus and pseudomonas biofilms by prolonged exposure to low-intensity electrical current. *Antimicrob. Agents Chemother.* **2009**, *53*, 41–45. [CrossRef] [PubMed]
115. Poortinga, A.T.; Smit, J.; van der Mei, H.C.; Busscher, H.J. Electric field induced desorption of bacteria from a conditioning film covered substratum. *Biotechnol. Bioeng.* **2001**, *76*, 395–399. [CrossRef] [PubMed]
116. Hong, S.H.; Jeong, J.; Shim, S.; Kang, H.; Kwon, S.; Ahn, K.H.; Yoon, J. Effect of electric currents on bacterial detachment and inactivation. *Biotechnol. Bioeng.* **2008**, *100*, 379–386. [CrossRef] [PubMed]
117. Costerton, J.W.; Ellis, B.; Lam, K.; Johnson, F.; Khoury, A.E. Mechanism of electrical enhancement of efficacy of antibiotics in killing biofilm bacteria. *Antimicrob. Agents Chemother.* **1994**, *38*, 2803–2809. [CrossRef] [PubMed]
118. Stewart, P.S.; Wattanakaroon, W.; Goodrum, L.; Fortun, S.M.; McLeod, B.R. Electrolytic generation of oxygen partially explains electrical enhancement of tobramycin efficacy against Pseudomonas aeruginosa biofilm. *Antimicrob. Agents Chemother.* **1999**, *43*, 292–296. [PubMed]
119. Mohn, D.; Zehnder, M.; Stark, W.J.; Imfeld, T. Electrochemical disinfection of dental implants—A proof of concept. *PLoS ONE* **2011**, *6*, e16157. [CrossRef] [PubMed]

© 2018 by the authors. Licensee MDPI, Basel, Switzerland. This article is an open access article distributed under the terms and conditions of the Creative Commons Attribution (CC BY) license (http://creativecommons.org/licenses/by/4.0/).

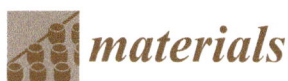

Review

The A, B and C's of Silicone Breast Implants: Anaplastic Large Cell Lymphoma, Biofilm and Capsular Contracture

Maria Mempin, Honghua Hu, Durdana Chowdhury, Anand Deva and Karen Vickery *

Faculty of Medicine and Health Sciences, Macquarie University, Macquarie Park, NSW, 2109, Australia; maria.mempin@mq.edu.au (M.M.); helen.hu@mq.edu.au (H.H.); Durdana.chowdhury@hdr.mq.edu.au (D.C.); anand.deva@mq.edu.au (A.D.)
* Correspondence: karen.vickery@mq.edu.au; Tel.: +61-298-502-773

Received: 5 November 2018; Accepted: 26 November 2018; Published: 28 November 2018

Abstract: Breast implantation either for cosmetic or reconstructive e purposes is one of the most common procedures performed in plastic surgery. Biofilm infection is hypothesised to be involved in the development of both capsular contracture and anaplastic large cell lymphoma (ALCL). Capsular contracture is one of the principal reasons for breast revision surgery and is characterised by the tightening and hardening of the capsule surrounding the implant, and ALCL is an indolent lymphoma found only in women with textured implants. We describe the types of breast implants available with regard to their surface characteristics of surface area and roughness and how this might contribute to capsular contracture and/or biofilm formation. The pathogenesis of capsular contracture is thought to be due to biofilm formation on the implant, which results in on-going inflammation. We describe the current research into breast implant associated ALCL and how implant properties may affect its pathogenesis, with ALCL only occurring in women with textured implants.

Keywords: biofilm; breast implant; textured: capsular contracture; anaplastic large cell lymphoma; BIA-ALCL

1. Introduction

Breast implantation, either for cosmetic or reconstructive purposes, is one of the most common procedures performed in plastic surgery. In 2015, in the United States of America alone, more than 280,000 women had breast enlargement surgery and an estimated 106,000 breast cancer patients underwent post-mastectomy breast reconstruction, which often involved insertion of implantable medical devices [1].

2. Breast Implants

Basic designed silicone breast implants were first introduced in the early 1960s [2]. As each new "generation" of implant has been introduced, their design has undergone major improvements. Modern breast implants can be divided into categories based on implant filling (silicone or saline), surface texture (textured or smooth), and shape (round or anatomic), each of which have slightly different properties [3,4].

Silicone or saline implant filling:

Saline implants are sold as empty silicone elastomer shells and are filled to the appropriate volume with sterile saline in the operating room. The silicone filling comes as either a "fluid form" that is not cohesive enough to maintain an anatomic shape or a "form-stable" more viscous and greater cross-linked silicone gel that has cohesive properties [5]. The cohesive gel increases form stability and correlates with better shape retention when compared with saline or fluid form silicone filled implants [6].

Textured or smooth outer surface:

Smooth breast implants move within the breast implant pocket to give a more natural movement [5], while aggressive texturisation of the implant surface improves integration between the living host and the implant by enhancing tissue adhesion, growth and proliferation of the host blood supply, enhancement of cellular migration, and fibroblast adhesion [7,8]. Texturisation is thought to increase device stability as it helps prevent rotation in the breast pocket or migration of implants [5].

Currently available breast implants can be categorised into 4 different surface types based on the 3D to 2D surface area ratio (high >5, intermediate 3–5, low 2–3 and minimal <2) and surface roughness expressed as a multiple of the value of smooth implants (high > 150, intermediate 75–150, low 25–75 and minimal <25) [9]. Figure 1 describes the implant surface classification system and representative scanning electron microscope pictures of breast implants.

Surface Type	4	3	2	1	1
3D :2D ratio	High	Intermediate	Low	Minimal	Minimal
Surface roughness	High	Intermediate	Low	Minimal	Minimal
Example	Silimed Polyurethane	Allergan Biocell	Mentor Siltex	Motiva Velvet	Smooth

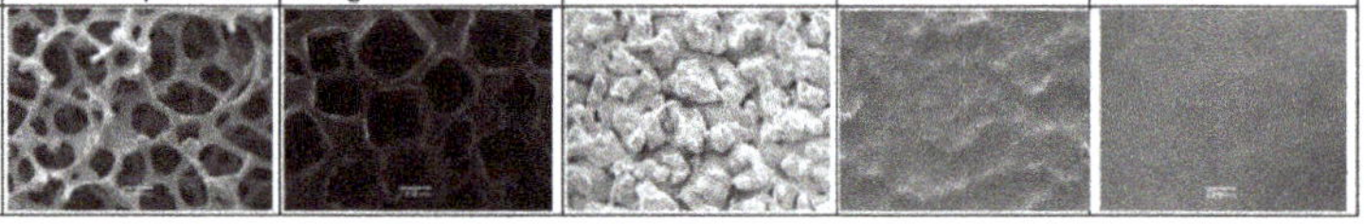

Figure 1. Implant surface classification and representative examples of implants.

The first textured implant, released in 1968, incorporated a 1.2–2 mm polyurethane foam (PU) coating on its outer surface, which adhered to the surrounding tissues, and subsequently delaminated from the silicon implant producing a relatively non-contractible capsule and thus reduced the risk of capsular contracture [10,11]. However, polyurethane (PU) coated silicone implants were voluntarily removed from the USA market in 1991, due to reporting of an association between polyurethane and the carcinogen 2,4-toluenediamine (TDA) [12]. This withdrawal lead to the development of alternative technologies to modify the outer silicone shell, including bonding the PU foam coating to the silicon surface, e.g., the Silimed PU implant, which retains the aggressive texture but prevents delamination [4]. This implant has been classified as surface type 4 (Figure 1) [9].

The salt-loss technique of producing a textured surface is produced by adding salt crystals to the silicone before curing, which are then washed from the surface leaving behind a pitted surface with randomly sized and arranged interconnected pores [13]. The pores promote adherence to the surrounding tissue [14–16] and make these devices relatively immobile [16]. Allergan Biocell is produced by the salt-loss technique and has pores with an average diameter of 600–800 μm and depth of 150–200 μm [15] and is an example of a surface type 3 implant (Figure 1) [9]. A micro textured implant (with an average pore size of 100 to 150 μm diameter) manufactured by Polytech Mesmo through a vulcanisation process that coats the surface of the uncured implant with ammonium carbonate [6,17] has also been classified as a surface type 3.

Negative contact imprinting, such as with Mentor Siltex, creates a less aggressive textured silicone surface by pressing the uncured silicone mandrel into PU foam. This results in an implant surface of type 2 with average pore diameters of 70–150 μm and depth of 60–275 μm and is meant to mimic the PU foam (Figure 1) [15]. In contrast to Silimed PU and Biocell, Siltex does not adhere to the surrounding tissue and is not immobile [10]. Motiva, using a propriety method of negative imprinting, manufacture the nanotextured SilkSurface and the micro-textured VelvetSurface (Figure 1). The pore depth on the VelvetSurface is 40–100 μm [18] which is shallower than Mentor Siltex. Along with smooth implants, nanotextured implants are classified as surface type 1 (Figure 1) [9].

3. Capsular Contracture

Complications of breast augmentation include hematoma, seroma, infection, altered nipple sensation, asymmetry, scarring, swelling, rupture, leakage and capsular contracture (CC) but CC is thought to be the most common complication and frequently requires surgical revision [19]. In 2015, 43,000 implant removal procedures were reported in the United States of America [1], and the Food and Drug Administration (FDA) reports that between 20 to 40% of augmentation patients and 40 to 70% of reconstruction patients had reoperations during the first eight to ten years after receiving their breast implants [20]. CC is a common reason for reoperation in Australia, being responsible for 38.9% of the 5290 breast implant revisions occurring between 2012 and 2016 [21]. Surgical revisions following CC result in poorer aesthetic outcome and a high rate of recurrence of CC [22,23].

Upon insertion of a breast implant, a foreign body reaction is induced, which is essentially an excessive fibrotic response that encloses the implant. CC is contracture of the peri-prosthetic capsule, which is characterised by the tightening and hardening of the tissue capsule around the breast implant. CC eventually leads to distortion of the implant [24,25]. Individual studies have reported incidence rates of CC ranging from 1.3 to 45% [23,26–30]. The wide range of CC rates is attributed to differences in follow-up times, as CC rate increases with time following implantation, as well as different type of implants and differing surgical techniques being used throughout the various studies [4].

The degree of CC is classified using the Baker clinical grading system which divides CC into four grades [31]. A grade I breast looks and feels natural, while grade II breasts have minimal contracture where the surgeon can tell surgery has been performed but there are no clinical symptoms. Grade III and IV are clinically significant and symptomatic, where grade III describes moderate contracture with some firmness felt by the patient, and grade IV describes severe contracture that is obvious from observation and symptomatic in the patient [31].

With each new implant generation, the incidence of CC has decreased, although whether this is due to implant design or better surgical technique, or a combination of both, is unclear. Historically, the type of fill was thought to influence the development of CC. Older generation silicone gel devices were characterised by higher gel bleeds and rupture rates compared to current generation implants [5,32,33]. The rates of CC were six-fold higher with these older devices than with devices containing low-bleed silicone gel fillings [34] or cohesive silicone gel fill implants [22,35–39].

The benefits of textured implants in reducing CC remains controversial. Systematic reviews of comparative clinical studies concluded texturisation may reduce the incidence of early capsular contracture if the implant was placed under the breast glandular tissue, but had no significant effect if placed under the pectoral muscle [29,40]. Smaller comparative or split breast studies, inserting one smooth and one textured implant in the same patient, are evenly divided as to the benefit of texturisation [41–48]. Many of these published reports lack adequate description of implant type, surgical technique, outcome assessment, and have short follow-up or the time period of follow-up is not stated. Several early randomised controlled trials reported textured implants had lower rates of clinically significant CC compared to smooth surface implants [42,45]. Similarly, some later prospective trials and metanalysis of 16 randomised controlled trials combined with two case-control studies, involving 4412 patients, have shown that smooth implants are more likely to develop CC [40,48,49]. However, the follow-up of most of these studies has been less than five years. When 715 of these patients were followed for 10 years there was no difference in the rate of CC [23]. It is likely that the effect of surface technology is of some benefit but is one of many factors that impact on clinical outcome, and the aetiopathogenesis of CC is likely to be multifactorial.

4. Aetiopathogenesis of Capsular Contracture (CC)

In 1981, Burkhardt and co-workers [50] were the first to propose that subclinical infection led to CC. However, the lack of culture positivity in many clinical studies of CC delayed the acceptance of this hypothesis. The detection of a *Staphylococcus epidermidis* biofilm in a patient with recurrent CC led to the hypothesis that the proposed subclinical infection is due to biofilm formation on the breast implant [51]. The presence of biofilm on implants obtained from CC patients was confirmed using scanning electron microscopy [25]. The likelihood of bacterial isolation was increased by mincing, sonication, and broth culture of a piece of implant or tissue, rather than using a swab to collect samples. Using this improved method of culture, the authors found a significant relationship between culture positivity ($p < 0.0006$) and the presence of *S. epidermidis* ($p < 0.01$) with CC. Subsequently, the degree of Baker grade CC has been shown to directly correlate with the number of bacteria in humans [52] and in the porcine model [53]. The biofilm hypothesis helps explain the lack of culture positivity in older studies where sonication was not employed, as biofilm bacteria are notoriously difficult to culture [54].

An alternative, to the biofilm hypothesis is that CC is purely an immunological response (reviewed in Headon [4]). The principal cell type within the capsule include activated macrophages, lymphocytes, and fibrocytes, and the number of lymphocytes and fibrocytes correlate with Baker grade [4]. However, the trigger for activating these cells is unknown. The presence of silicon particles has been postulated as a trigger. The amount of silicon in capsular macrophages is greater in higher grade CC and is associated with increased inflammation [55]. In contrast, the biofilm hypothesis proposes that the immunological response is activated by biofilm infection. The patient's endogenous flora or bacteria present at the time of surgery gain access to the breast implant during or following placement. Once in contact with the implant, they attach to the prosthetic surface and form a biofilm. If implants are contaminated with only low numbers of bacteria, the host can contain the biofilm to a level that produces minimal inflammation [53]. However, once bacterial numbers reach a critical point, the host response is overwhelmed, and the bacteria continue to proliferate and trigger a chronic inflammatory response, leading to subsequent fibrosis and accelerated CC [53].

Frequently, organisms that are part of the microflora of the skin or the breast, such as *Cutibacterium acnes* (formally *Proprionibacterium acnes*) and coagulase-negative staphylococci, particularly *S. epidermidis*, are commonly isolated from CC samples [25,50,52,56–59]; however, any bacterial species can be involved and multiple species can be grown from one breast [25,59].

Further evidence for bacterial involvement in CC aetiopathogenesis is provided by artificial inoculation of implants, resulting in increased CC development in animal models [56,60,61]. In the porcine model, breast pocket inoculation of *S. epidermidis* led to biofilm development, and biofilm formation was associated with a four-fold increased risk of developing contracture (odds ratio = 4.1667) [61].

Additional evidence to support the subclinical biofilm hypothesis is that strategies to prevent breast implant infection appear to be effective. Animal studies have shown that antimicrobial coated implants can significantly reduce the genesis of biofilm and subsequent CC [62,63], whilst clinical studies utilising antibiotic or antiseptic breast implant pocket irrigation at time of surgery have shown a significant reduction in CC [24,64]. The reduction in CC following biocide irrigation has been confirmed in two comparative clinical trials that showed a 10-fold reduction in CC utilising either betadine and/or topical antibiotics in pocket irrigation [65,66].

Other strategies to prevent bacterial contamination of the implant by modifying surgical technique have resulted in decreased CC rates (reviewed by Deva et al. [19]). These include modification of implantation site (subpectoral position reduces access of breast flora to the implant through the natural musculofascial barrier); avoiding periareolar and transaxillary incisions, which have higher rates of CC compared to submammary incisions; use of a nipple shield; and use of an introductory shield to prevent the implant touching the skin surface [19].

The occurrence of unilateral contracture following bilateral insertion of identical breast implants means that systemic or implant material-related causes are also less likely [52]. Thus, although contracture remains poorly understood, it is likely to be multifactorial in origin, and of all the theories on the potential aetiology of CC, the subclinical infection hypothesis remains the leading theory.

5. Breast Implant Associated Anaplastic Large Cell Lymphoma

In 2011, the FDA identified a possible association between textured breast implants and anaplastic large cell lymphoma (BIA-ALCL) [67], a rare T- or null-cell non-Hodgkin lymphoma first described by Stein and co-workers [68]. It was recognised as a distinct cancer by the World Health Organisation in 2016 [20]. As of 2017, over 500 cases were reported worldwide, and recent epidemiological studies suggest that the number will continue to rise [69–71]. Australia has a high incidence rate with 70 confirmed cases of BIA-ALCL, including four deaths by August 2016 [70,72]. The Australian Therapeutic Goods Administration estimates the risk of developing BIA-ALCL to be between 1:1000 and 1:10,000 for women with breast implants [70,72]. However, the true incidence of BIA-ALCL is likely to be higher due to under reporting and the lack of accurate breast implant sales figures.

BIA-ALCL generally presents as a localised late peri-implant seroma containing malignant cells in one breast and less commonly as a tumour mass attached to the capsule, and regional lymph node involvement is seen in around 5–10% of patients. In the Australian cohort, all patients were exposed to textured implants with 85% of cases associated with implants with a high surface area (surface type 3 or 4, Figure 1) [70]. BIA-ALCL occurs an average of seven to ten years after implant placement but can range from 0.4 to 20 years [70,73–75]. Treatment for the majority of patients consists of complete surgical excision of diseased tissue, implants, and the surrounding fibrosis capsule, while adjuvant chemotherapy is only recommended for patients with advanced disease (reviewed by Clemens and co-workers [76]).

BIA-ALCL seroma fluid is composed of large, pleomorphic cells with horseshoe-shaped nuclei and are anaplastic lymphoma kinase (ALK) negative. Immunophenotypically they are diffusely positive for CD30 and T-cell markers such as CD3, CD4 [76–80]. Additionally, in cell lines developed from clinical cases of BIA-ALCL antigen presentation markers (HLA-DR, CD80, CD86), IL-2 receptors (CD25, CD122) and IL-6 receptors are present [80–82]. BIA-ALCL cells show clonal TCR gene arrangement and/or the demonstration of phenotypic aberrancy, including CD4 and CD8 co-expression [76,79,80].

The aetiopathogenesis of BIA-ALCL is unknown, but it is thought that chronic inflammatory stimulus leads to T-cell dysplasia in patients that are genetically susceptible. It is postulated that a milieu rich in immune stimulatory cytokines, which promotes rapid division of host lymphocytes, may cause the initial tumorigenic changes that lead to BIA-ALCL in some patients. Autocrine production of IL-6 has been identified as a driver of tumorigenesis in some diffuse large B-cell lymphomas, as well as solid tumours, including breast, lung, and ovarian carcinomas [83–85]. The cytokine profile of BIA-ALCL cell lines, specifically IL-6, TGF-β and IL-10, has also been shown to induce immune suppressor cell populations (Tregs and myeloid-derived suppressor cells), which may inhibit host anti-tumour immunity and facilitate cancer development [86,87].

One theory is that biofilm infection, combined with host factors such as the patient's genetic background and their immune response, activate T-lymphocytes and trigger polyclonal proliferation and, with time, in some cases monoclonal proliferation and the eventual development of ALCL [88] Figure 2.

In support of the biofilm infection theory, chronic biofilm infection with *Helicobacter pylori*, and hence ongoing inflammation, is recognized as being the causal agent in the development of gastric lymphoma [89], and antibiotic treatment alone in patients with low grade malignancy results in remission in 80% [90]. Similarly, a phase II clinical trial showed regression of adnexal marginal zone lymphoma in 65% of patients given doxycycline monotherapy for the treatment of *Chlamydophila psittaci* (n = 34) [91]. Therefore, it is plausible that chronically infected breast implants may mediate similar inflammatory and neoplastic processes resulting in the development of a T cell lymphoma. In support of biofilm being the chronic inflammatory stimulus, significantly more bacteria attach to textured implants compared to smooth implants [9]. In the porcine model this correlated with a 63-fold increase in the number of lymphocytes attached to textured implants compared to smooth implants, whilst in clinical samples of CC the number of lymphocytes surrounding breast implants is positively and significantly correlated (r = 0.83) with the number of bacteria [53].

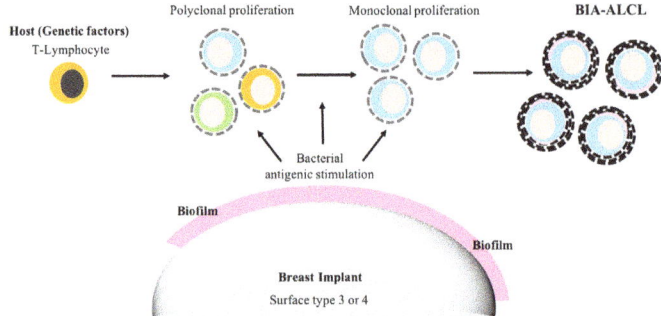

Figure 2. Suggested biofilm aetiopathogenesis of breast implant associated-anaplastic large cell lymphoma (BIA-ALCL).

The strongest support for the role of bacterial biofilm in the aetiopathogenesis of BIA-ALCL was the detection of biofilm in clinical samples using qPCR, with visual confirmation of biofilm presence using fluorescent in situ hybridisation and scanning electron microscopy [88]. Analysis of the microbiome (bacterial community genetic profile), using next generation sequencing, showed a significantly greater proportion of Gram-negative bacteria in BIA-ALCL specimens compared with non-tumour CC specimens (Figure 3), suggesting that different bacterial species may preferentially trigger lymphocyte activation [88].

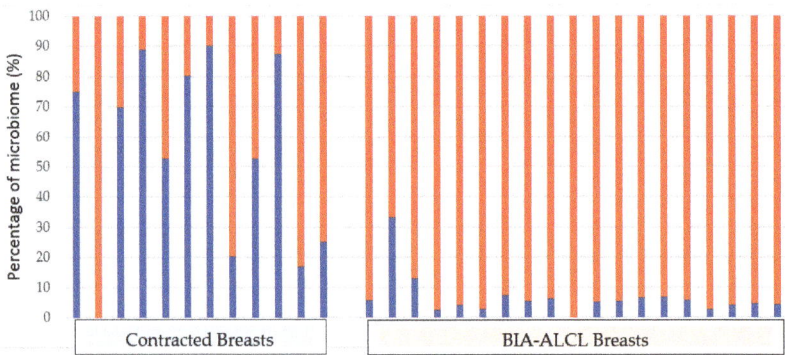

Figure 3. Percentage of Gram-positive (coloured blue) and Gram-negative (coloured red) organisms in capsules obtained from contracted breasts and in BIA-ALCL samples [88].

The development of BIA-ALCL is likely to be a complex process resulting from an interplay of host, implant and microbial factors, including the patient's genetic background, immune response, the textured implant surface, and bacterial phenotype. However, the rarity of BIA-ALCL presents a challenge for conducting meaningful epidemiologic studies, and although the pathogenesis of BIA-ALCL is undergoing active research, the drivers of this malignancy remains poorly understood.

Author Contributions: Writing—Original Draft Preparation, M.M. and K.V.; Writing—Review and Editing, K.V., H.H., and A.D.; Scanning Electron Microscopy, D.C.

Funding: This research received no external funding.

Conflicts of Interest: A.D. is a consultant, research coordinator, and educator to Allergan, Mentor (Johnson & Johnson), Sientra, Motiva and Acelity (KCI.) He has previously coordinated industry-sponsored research for these companies relating to both biofilms and breast prostheses. MM, DC, HH, and KV have no conflicts of interest.

References

1. ASPS. ASPS Plastic Surgery Statistics Report. Available online: www.plasticsurgery.org (accessed on 30 June 2018).
2. Cronin, T.D.; Gerow, F.J. Augmentation mammaplasty: A new "natural feel" prosthesis. In Proceedings of the Transactions of the Third International Congress of Plastic and Reconstructive Surgery, Washington, DC, USA, 13–18 October 1963; Excerpta Medica: Amsterdam, The Netherlands, 1964; pp. 41–49.
3. Namnoum, J.D.; Largent, J.; Kaplan, H.M.; Oefelein, M.G.; Brown, M.H. Primary breast augmentation clinical trial outcomes stratified by surgical incision, anatomical placement and implant device type. *J. Plast. Reconstr. Aesthet. Surg.* **2013**, *66*, 1165–1172. [CrossRef] [PubMed]
4. Headon, H.; Kasem, A.; Mokbel, K. Capsular contracture after breast augmentation: An update for clinical practice. *Archiv. Plast. Surg.* **2015**, *42*, 532–543. [CrossRef] [PubMed]
5. O'Shaughnessy, K. Evolution and update on current devices for prosthetic breast reconstruction. *Gland Surg.* **2015**, *4*, 97–110. [PubMed]
6. Henderson, P.W.; Nash, D.; Laskowski, M.; Grant, R.T. Objective Comparison of Commercially Available Breast Implant Devices. *Aesthet. Plast. Surg.* **2015**, *39*, 724–732. [CrossRef] [PubMed]
7. Clubb, F.J.; Ciapper, D.L.; Deferrari, D.A.; Hu, S.; Stare, W.J., Jr.; Capik, P.P.; Armstrong, J.; McGEE, M.G.; Bilings, L.A.; Fuqua, J.M. Surface texturing and coating of biomaterial implants: Effects on tissue integration and fibrosis. *ASAIO J.* **1999**, *45*, 281–287. [CrossRef] [PubMed]
8. Dalby, M.J.; Yarwood, S.J.; Riehle, M.O.; Johnstone, H.J.; Affrossman, S.; Curtis, A.S. Increasing fibroblast response to materials using nanotopography: Morphological and genetic measurements of cell response to 13-nm-high polymer demixed islands. *Exp. Cell Res.* **2002**, *276*, 1–9. [CrossRef] [PubMed]
9. Jones, P.; Mempin, M.; Hu, H.; Chowdhury, D.; Foley, M.; Cooter, R.; Adams, W.P., Jr.; Vickery, K.; Deva, A.K. The Functional Influence of Breast Implant Outer Shell Morphology on Bacterial Attachment and Growth. *Plast. Reconstr. Surg.* **2018**, *142*, 837–849. [CrossRef] [PubMed]
10. Ashley, F.L. Further studies on the natural-y breast prosthesis. *Plast. Reconstr. Surg.* **1972**, *49*, 414–419. [CrossRef] [PubMed]
11. Sinclair, T.M.; Kerrigan, C.L.; Buntic, R. Biodegradation of the polyurethane foam covering of breast implants. *Plast. Reconstr. Surg* **1993**, *92*, 1003–1013; discussion 1014. [CrossRef] [PubMed]
12. Chan, S.C.; Birdsell, D.C.; Gradeen, C.Y. Detection of toluenediamines in the urine of a patient with polyurethane-covered breast implants. *Clin. Chem.* **1991**, *37*, 756–758. [PubMed]
13. Barr, S.; Bayat, A. Breast surgery review article: Breast implant surface development: Perspectives on development and manufacture. *Aesthet. Surg. J.* **2011**, *31*, 56–67. [CrossRef] [PubMed]
14. Barone, F.E.; Perry, L.; Keller, T.; Maxwell, G.P. The biomechanical and histopathologic effects of surface texturing with silicone and polyurethane in tissue implantation and expansion. *Plast. Reconstr. Surg.* **1992**, *90*, 77–86. [CrossRef] [PubMed]
15. Danino, A.M.; Basmacioglu, P.; Saito, S.; Rocher, F.; Blanchet-Bardon, C.; Revol, M.; Servant, J.-M. Comparison of the capsular response to the Biocell RTV and Mentor 1600 Siltex breast implant surface texturing: A scanning electron microscopic study. *Plast. Reconstr. Surg.* **2001**, *108*, 2047–2052. [CrossRef] [PubMed]
16. Maxwell, G.P.; Hammond, D.C. Breast implants: Smooth versus textured. *Adv. Plast. Reconstr. Surg.* **1993**, *9*, 209–220.
17. Barr, S.; Hill, E.W.; Bayat, A. Functional biocompatibility testing of silicone breast implants and a novel classification system based on surface roughness. *J. Mech. Behav. Biomed. Mater.* **2017**, *75*, 75–81. [CrossRef] [PubMed]
18. Sforza, M.; Zaccheddu, R.; Alleruzzo, A.; Seno, A.; Mileto, D.; Paganelli, A.; Sulaiman, H.; Payne, M.; Maurovich-Horvat, L. Preliminary 3-Year Evaluation of Experience with SilkSurface and VelvetSurface Motiva Silicone Breast Implants: A Single-Center Experience with 5813 Consecutive Breast Augmentation Cases. *Aesthet. Surg. J.* **2018**, *38*, S62–S73. [CrossRef] [PubMed]
19. Deva, A.K.; Adams, W.P.; Vickery, K. The role of bacterial biofilms in device-associated infection. *Plast. Reconstr. Surg.* **2013**, *132*, 1319–1328. [CrossRef] [PubMed]
20. FDA. *Breast Implant- Associated Anaplastic Large Cell Lymphoma (BIA-ALCL)*; FDA: Silver Spring, MD, USA, 2018.

21. Hopper, I.; Parker, E.; Pelligrini, B.; Mulvany, C.; Pase, M.; Ahem, S.; Earnest, A.; McNeil, J. *The Australian Breast Device Registry 2016 Report*; Monash University: Melbourne, Australia, 2018.
22. Bengtson, B.P.; Van Natta, B.W.; Murphy, D.K.; Slicton, A.; Maxwell, G.P.; Style 410 U.S. Core Clinical Study Group. Style 410 highly cohesive silicone breast implant core study results at 3 years. *Plast. Reconstr. Surg.* **2007**, *120*, 40S–48S. [CrossRef] [PubMed]
23. Spear, S.L.; Murphy, D.K. Natrelle round silicone breast implants: Core study results at 10 years. *Plast. Reconstr. Surg.* **2014**, *133*, 1354–1361. [CrossRef] [PubMed]
24. Adams, W.P., Jr.; Rios, J.L.; Smith, S.J. Enhancing patient outcomes in aesthetic and reconstructive breast surgery using triple antibiotic breast irrigation: Six-year prospective clinical study. *Plast. Reconstr. Surg.* **2006**, *117*, 30–36. [CrossRef] [PubMed]
25. Pajkos, A.; Deva, A.K.; Vickery, K.; Cope, C.; Chang, L.; Cossart, Y.E. Detection of subclinical infection in significant breast implant capsules. *Plast. Reconstr. Surg.* **2003**, *111*, 1605–1611. [CrossRef] [PubMed]
26. Ersek, R.A. Rate and incidence of capsular contracture: A comparison of smooth and textured silicone double-lumen breast prostheses. *Plast. Reconstr. Surg.* **1991**, *87*, 879–884. [CrossRef] [PubMed]
27. Ersek, R.A.; Salisbury, A.V. Textured surface, nonsili- cone gel breast implants: Four years' clinical outcome. *Plast. Reconstr. Surg.* **1997**, *100*, 1729–1739. [CrossRef] [PubMed]
28. Handel, N.; Jensen, J.A.; Black, Q.; Waisman, J.R.; Silverstein, M.J. The fate of breast implants: A critical analysis of complications and outcomes. *Plast. Reconstr. Surg.* **1995**, *96*, 1521–1533. [CrossRef] [PubMed]
29. Barnsley, G.P.; Sigurdson, L.J.; Barnsley, S.E. Textured surface breast implants in the prevention of capsular contracture among breast augmentation patients: A meta-analysis of randomized controlled trials. *Plast. Reconstr. Surg.* **2006**, *117*, 2182–2190. [CrossRef] [PubMed]
30. Araco, A.; Caruso, R.; Araco, F.; Overton, J.; Gravante, G. Capsular contractures: A systematic review. *Plast. Reconstr. Surg.* **2009**, *124*, 1808–1819. [CrossRef] [PubMed]
31. Spear, S.L.; Baker, J.L., Jr. Classification of capsular contracture after prosthetic breast reconstruction. *Plast. Reconstr. Surg.* **1995**, *96*, 1119–1123; discussion 1124. [CrossRef] [PubMed]
32. Malata, C.M.; Varma, S.; Scott, M.; Liston, J.C.; Sharpe, D.T. Silicone breast implant rupture: Common/serious complication? *Med. Prog. Technol.* **1994**, *20*, 251–260. [PubMed]
33. Maxwell, G.P.; Gabriel, A. The evolution of breast implants. *Clin. Plast. Surg.* **2009**, *36*, 1–13. [CrossRef] [PubMed]
34. Chang, L.; Caldwell, E.; Reading, G.; Wray, R.C., Jr. A comparison of conventional and low-bleed implants in augmentation mammaplasty. *Plast. Reconstr. Surg.* **1992**, *89*, 79–82. [CrossRef] [PubMed]
35. Bogetti, P.; Boltri, M.; Balocco, P.; Spagnoli, G. Augmentation mammaplasty with a new cohesive gel prosthesis. *Aesthet. Plast. Surg.* **2000**, *24*, 440–444. [CrossRef] [PubMed]
36. Heden, P.; Jernbeck, J.; Hober, M. Breast augmentation with anatomical cohesive gel implants: The world's largest current experience. *Clin. Plast. Surg.* **2001**, *28*, 531–552. [PubMed]
37. Drever, J. Cohesive gel implants for breast augmentation. *Aesthet. Surg. J.* **2003**, *23*, 405–409. [CrossRef]
38. Brown, M.H.; Shenker, R.; Silver, S.A. Cohesive silicone gel breast implants in aesthetic and reconstructive breast surgery. *Plast. Reconstr. Surg.* **2005**, *116*, 768–779. [CrossRef] [PubMed]
39. Henriksen, T.F.; Fryzek, J.P.; Holmich, L.R.; McLaughlin, J.K.; Krag, C.; Karlsen, R.; Kjøller, K.; Olsen, J.H.; Friis, S. Reconstructive breast implantation after mastectomy for breast cancer: Clinical outcomes in a nationwide prospective cohort study. *Arch. Surg.* **2005**, *140*, 1152–1159. [CrossRef] [PubMed]
40. Wong, C.-H.; Samuel, M.; Tan, B.-K.; Song, C. Capsular contracture in subglandular breast augmentation with textured versus smooth breast implants: A systematic review. *Plast. Reconstr. Surg.* **2006**, *118*, 1224–1236. [CrossRef] [PubMed]
41. Coleman, D.J.; Foo, I.T.; Sharpe, D.T. Textured or smooth implants for breast augmentation? A prospective controlled trial. *Br. J. Plast. Surg.* **1991**, *44*, 444–448. [CrossRef]
42. Hakelius, L.; Ohlsen, L. Tendency to capsular contracture around smooth and textured gel-filled silicone mammary implants: A five-year follow-up. *Plast. Reconstr. Surg.* **1997**, *100*, 1566–1569. [CrossRef] [PubMed]
43. Burkhardt, B.R.; Demas, C.P. The effect of Siltex texturing and povidone-iodine irrigation on capsular contracture around saline inflatable breast implants. *Plast. Reconstr. Surg.* **1994**, *93*, 123–128; discussion 129–130. [CrossRef] [PubMed]

44. Burkhardt, B.R.; Eades, E. The effect of Biocell texturing and povidone-iodine irrigation on capsular contracture around saline-inflatable breast implants. *Plast. Reconstr. Surg.* **1995**, *96*, 1317–1325. [CrossRef] [PubMed]
45. Asplund, O.; Gylbert, L.; Jurell, G.; Ward, C. Textured or smooth implants for submuscular breast augmentation: A controlled study. *Plast. Reconstr. Surg.* **1996**, *97*, 1200–1206. [CrossRef] [PubMed]
46. Malata, C.M.; Feldberg, L.; Coleman, D.J.; Foo, I.T.; Sharpe, D.T. Textured or smooth implants for breast augmentation? Three year follow-up of a prospective randomised controlled trial. *Br. J. Plast. Surg.* **1997**, *50*, 99–105. [CrossRef]
47. Poeppl, N.; Schreml, S.; Lichtenegger, F.; Lenich, A.; Eisenmann-Klein, M.; Prantl, L. Does the surface structure of implants have an impact on the formation of a capsular contracture? *Aesthet. Plast. Surg.* **2007**, *31*, 133–139. [CrossRef] [PubMed]
48. Stevens, W.G.; Nahabedian, M.Y.; Calobrace, M.B.; Harrington, J.L.; Capizzi, P.J.; Cohen, R.; d'Incelli, R.C.; Beckstrand, M. Risk factor analysis for capsular contracture: A 5-year Sientra study analysis using round, smooth, and textured implants for breast augmentation. *Plast. Reconstr. Surg.* **2013**, *132*, 1115–1123. [CrossRef] [PubMed]
49. Liu, X.; Zhou, L.; Pan, F.; Gao, Y.; Yuan, X.; Fan, D. Comparison of the postoperative incidence rate of capsular contracture among different breast implants: A cumulative meta-analysis. *PLoS ONE* **2015**, *10*, e0116071. [CrossRef] [PubMed]
50. Burkhardt, B.R.; Fried, M.; Schnur, P.L.; Tofield, J.J. Capsules, infection, and intraluminal antibiotics. *Plast. Reconstr. Surg.* **1981**, *68*, 43–47. [CrossRef] [PubMed]
51. Deva, A.K.; Chang, L.C. Bacterial biofilms: A cause for accelerated capsular contracture? *Aesthet. Surg. J.* **1999**, *19*, 130–133. [CrossRef]
52. Rieger, U.; Mesina, J.; Kalbermatten, D.; Haug, M.; Frey, H.; Pico, R.; Frei, R.; Pierer, G.; Lüscher, N.; Trampuz, A. Bacterial biofilms and capsular contracture in patients with breast implants. *Br. J. Surg.* **2013**, *100*, 768–774. [CrossRef] [PubMed]
53. Hu, H.; Jacombs, A.; Vickery, K.; Merten, S.L.; Pennington, D.G.; Deva, A.K. Chronic biofilm infection in breast implants is associated with an increased T-cell lymphocytic infiltrate: Implications for breast implant-associated lymphoma. *Plast. Reconstr. Surg.* **2015**, *135*, 319–329. [CrossRef] [PubMed]
54. Fux, C.A.; Stoodley, P.; Hall-Stoodley, L.; Costerton, J.W. Bacterial biofilms: A diagnostic and therapeutic challenge. *Expert Rev. Antiinfect. Ther.* **2003**, *1*, 667–683. [CrossRef]
55. Prantl, L.; Pöppl, N.; Horvat, N.; Heine, N.; Eisenmann-Klein, M. Serologic and histologic findings in patients with capsular contracture after breast augmentation with smooth silicone gel implants: Is serum hyaluronan a potential predictor? *Aesthet. Plast. Surg.* **2005**, *29*, 510–518. [CrossRef] [PubMed]
56. Shah, Z.; Lehman, J.A., Jr.; Tan, J. Does Infection Play a Role in Breast Capsular Contracture? *Plast. Reconstr. Surg.* **1981**, *68*, 34–38. [CrossRef] [PubMed]
57. Virden, C.P.; Dobke, M.K.; Stein, P.; Parsons, C.L.; Frank, D.H. Subclinical infection of the silicone breast implant surface as a possible cause of capsular contracture. *Aesthet. Plast. Surg.* **1992**, *16*, 173–179. [CrossRef]
58. Netscher, D.T. Subclinical infection in breast capsules. *Plast. Reconstr. Surg.* **2004**, *114*, 818–820. [CrossRef] [PubMed]
59. Del Pozo, J.L.; Tran, N.V.; Petty, P.M.; Johnson, C.H.; Walsh, M.F.; Bite, U.; Clay, R.P.; Mandrekar, J.N.; Piper, K.E.; Steckelberg, J.M. Pilot study of association of bacteria on breast implants with capsular contracture. *J. Clin. Microbiol.* **2009**, *47*, 1333–1337. [CrossRef] [PubMed]
60. Marques, M.; Brown, S.A.; Cordeiro, N.D.; Rodrigues-Pereira, P.; Cobrado, M.L.; Morales-Helguera, A.; Queirós, L.; Luís, A.; Freitas, R.; Gonçalves-Rodrigues, A. Effects of coagulase-negative staphylococci and fibrin on breast capsule formation in a rabbit model. *Aesthet. Surg. J.* **2011**, *31*, 420–428. [CrossRef] [PubMed]
61. Tamboto, H.; Vickery, K.; Deva, A.K. Subclinical (biofilm) infection causes capsular contracture in a porcine model following augmentation mammaplasty. *Plast. Reconstr. Surg.* **2010**, *126*, 835–842. [CrossRef] [PubMed]
62. Darouiche, R.O.; Meade, R.; Mansouri, M.D.; Netscher, D.T. In vivo efficacy of antimicrobe-impregnated saline-filled silicone implants. *Plast. Reconstr. Surg.* **2002**, *109*, 1352–1357. [CrossRef] [PubMed]
63. Jacombs, A.; Allan, J.; Hu, H.; Valente, P.M.; Wessels, W.L.F.; Deva, A.K.; Vickery, K. Prevention of Biofilm-Induced Capsular Contracture with Antibiotic-Impregnated Mesh in a Porcine Model. *Aesthet. Surg. J.* **2012**, *32*, 886–891. [CrossRef] [PubMed]

64. Adams, W.P., Jr.; Conner, W.C.H.; Barton, F.E., Jr.; Rohrich, R.J. Optimizing breast-pocket irrigation: The post-Betadine era. *Plast. Reconstr. Surg.* **2001**, *107*, 1596–1601. [CrossRef] [PubMed]
65. Blount, A.L.; Martin, M.D.; Lineberry, K.D.; Kettaneh, N.; Alfonso, D.R. Capsular contracture rate in a low-risk population after primary augmentation mammaplasty. *Aesthet. Surg. J.* **2013**, *33*, 516–521. [CrossRef] [PubMed]
66. Giordano, S.; Peltoniemi, H.; Lilius, P.; Salmi, A. Povidone-iodine combined with antibiotic topical irrigation to reduce capsular contracture in cosmetic breast augmentation: A comparative study. *Aesthet. Surg. J.* **2013**, *33*, 675–680. [CrossRef] [PubMed]
67. FDA. *Anaplastic Large Cell Lymphoma (ALCL) in Women with Breast Implants: Preliminary FDA Findings and Analyses*; Center for Devices and Radiological Health: Silver Spring, MD, USA, 2011.
68. Stein, H.; Foss, H.-D.; Dürkop, H.; Marafioti, T.; Delsol, G.; Pulford, K.; Pileri, S.; Falini, B. CD30+ anaplastic large cell lymphoma: A review of its histopathologic, genetic, and clinical features. *Blood* **2000**, *96*, 3681–3695. [PubMed]
69. Knight, R.; Loch-Wilkinson, A.-M.; Wessels, W.; Papadopoulos, T.; Magnusson, M.; Lofts, J.; Connell, T.; Hopper, I.; Beath, K.; Lade, S. Epidemiology and risk factors for Breast implant-associated anaplastic large cell lymphoma (BIA-ALCL) in Australia & New Zealand. *Plast. Reconstr. Surg.* **2016**, *4*, 94–95.
70. Loch-Wilkinson, A.; Beath, K.J.; Knight, R.J.W.; Wessels, W.L.F.; Magnusson, M.; Papadopoulos, T.; Connell, T.; Lofts, J.; Locke, M.; Hopper, I.; et al. Breast Implant-Associated Anaplastic Large Cell Lymphoma in Australia and New Zealand: High-Surface-Area Textured Implants Are Associated with Increased Risk. *Plast. Reconstr. Surg.* **2017**, *140*, 645–654. [CrossRef] [PubMed]
71. Doren, E.L.; Miranda, R.N.; Selber, J.C.; Garvey, P.B.; Liu, J.; Medeiros, L.J.; Butler, C.E.; Clemens, M.W. US Epidemiology of Breast Implant–Associated Anaplastic Large Cell Lymphoma. *Plast. Reconstr. Surg.* **2017**, *139*, 1042–1050. [CrossRef] [PubMed]
72. TGA. *Breast Implants and Anaplastic Large Cell Lymphoma. Update—Additional Confirmed Cases of Anaplastic Large Cell Lymphoma*; TGA: Symonston, Australia, 2018.
73. Bishara, M.R.; Ross, C.; Sur, M. Primary anaplastic large cell lymphoma of the breast arising in reconstruction mammoplasty capsule of saline filled breast implant after radical mastectomy for breast cancer: An unusual case presentation. *Diagn. Pathol.* **2009**, *4*, 11. [CrossRef] [PubMed]
74. Thompson, P.A.; Lade, S.; Webster, H.; Ryan, G.; Prince, H.M. Effusion-associated anaplastic large cell lymphoma of the breast: Time for it to be defined as a distinct clinico-pathological entity. *Haematologica* **2010**, *95*, 1977–1979. [CrossRef] [PubMed]
75. Rupani, A.; Frame, J.D.; Kamel, D. Lymphomas Associated with Breast Implants: A Review of the Literature. *Aesthet. Surg. J.* **2015**, *35*, 533–544. [CrossRef] [PubMed]
76. Clemens, M.W.; Brody, G.S.; Mahabir, R.C.; Miranda, R.N. How to Diagnose and Treat Breast Implant-Associated Anaplastic Large Cell Lymphoma. *Plast. Reconstr. Surg.* **2018**, *141*, 586e–599e. [CrossRef] [PubMed]
77. Roden, A.C.; Macon, W.R.; Keeney, G.L.; Myers, J.L.; Feldman, A.L.; Dogan, A. Seroma-associated primary anaplastic large-cell lymphoma adjacent to breast implants: An indolent T-cell lymphoproliferative disorder. *Mod. Pathol.* **2008**, *21*, 455–463. [CrossRef] [PubMed]
78. Swerdlow, S.H. *WHO Classification of Tumours of Haematopoietic and Lymphoid Tissues*; WHO Classification of Tumours; WHO: Geneva, Switzerland, 2008; Volume 22008, p. 439.
79. Jewell, M.; Spear, S.L.; Largent, J.; Oefelein, M.G.; Adams, W.P., Jr. Anaplastic large T-cell lymphoma and breast implants: A review of the literature. *Plast. Reconstr. Surg.* **2011**, *128*, 651–661. [CrossRef] [PubMed]
80. Lechner, M.G.; Lade, S.; Liebertz, D.J.; Prince, H.M.; Brody, G.S.; Webster, H.R.; Epstein, A.L. Breast implant-associated, ALK-negative, T-cell, anaplastic, large-cell lymphoma: Establishment and characterization of a model cell line (TLBR-1) for this newly emerging clinical entity. *Cancer* **2011**, *117*, 1478–1489. [CrossRef] [PubMed]
81. Kadin, M.E.; Deva, A.; Xu, H.; Morgan, J.; Khare, P.; MacLeod, R.A.; Van Natta, B.W.; Adams, W.P., Jr.; Brody, G.S.; Epstein, A.L. Biomarkers Provide Clues to Early Events in the Pathogenesis of Breast Implant-Associated Anaplastic Large Cell Lymphoma. *Aesthet. Surg. J.* **2016**, *36*, 773–781. [CrossRef] [PubMed]

82. Lechner, M.G.; Megiel, C.; Church, C.H.; Angell, T.E.; Russell, S.M.; Sevell, R.B.; Jang, J.K.; Brody, G.S.; Epstein, A.L. Survival signals and targets for therapy in breast implant-associated ALK-anaplastic large cell lymphoma. *Clin. Cancer Res.* **2012**, *18*, 4549–4559. [CrossRef] [PubMed]
83. Grivennikov, S.; Karin, M. Autocrine IL-6 signaling: A key event in tumorigenesis? *Cancer Cell* **2008**, *13*, 7–9. [CrossRef] [PubMed]
84. Lam, L.T.; Wright, G.; Davis, R.E.; Lenz, G.; Farinha, P.; Dang, L.; Chan, J.W.; Rosenwald, A.; Gascoyne, R.D.; Staudt, L.M. Cooperative signaling through the signal transducer and activator of transcription 3 and nuclear factor-κB pathways in subtypes of diffuse large B-cell lymphoma. *Blood* **2008**, *111*, 3701–3713. [CrossRef] [PubMed]
85. Scuto, A.; Kujawski, M.; Kowolik, C.; Krymskaya, L.; Wang, L.; Weiss, L.M.; DiGiusto, D.; Yu, H.; Forman, S.; Jove, R. STAT3 inhibition is a therapeutic strategy for ABC-like diffuse large B-cell lymphoma. *Cancer Res.* **2011**, *71*, 3182–3188. [CrossRef] [PubMed]
86. Lechner, M.G.; Liebertz, D.J.; Epstein, A.L. Characterization of cytokine-induced myeloid-derived suppressor cells from normal human peripheral blood mononuclear cells. *J. Immunol.* **2010**, *185*, 2273–2284. [CrossRef] [PubMed]
87. Stewart, T.J.; Smyth, M.J. Improving cancer immunotherapy by targeting tumor-induced immune suppression. *Cancer Metastasis Rev.* **2011**, *30*, 125–140. [CrossRef] [PubMed]
88. Hu, H.; Johani, K.; Almatroudi, A.; Vickery, K.; Van Natta, B.; Kadin, M.E.; Brody, G.; Clemens, M.; Cheah, C.Y.; Lade, S.; et al. Bacterial Biofilm Infection Detected in Breast Implant-Associated Anaplastic Large-Cell Lymphoma. *Plast. Reconstr. Surg.* **2016**, *137*, 1659–1669. [CrossRef] [PubMed]
89. Wang, M.-Y.; Chen, C.; Gao, X.-Z.; Li, J.; Yue, J.; Ling, F.; Wang, X.-C.; Shao, S.-H. Distribution of Helicobacter pylori virulence markers in patients with gastroduodenal diseases in a region at high risk of gastric cancer. *Microb. Pathog.* **2013**, *59–60*, 13–18. [CrossRef] [PubMed]
90. Matysiak-Budnik, T.; Fabiani, B.; Hennequin, C.; Thieblemont, C.; Malamut, G.; Cadiot, G.; Bouché, O.; Ruskoné-Fourmestraux, A. Gastrointestinal lymphomas: French Intergroup clinical practice recommendations for diagnosis, treatment and follow-up (SNFGE, FFCD, GERCOR, UNICANCER, SFCD, SFED, SFRO, SFH). *Dig. Liver Dis.* **2018**, *50*, 124–131. [CrossRef] [PubMed]
91. Ferreri, A.J.M.; Govi, S.; Pasini, E.; Mappa, S.; Bertoni, F.; Zaja, F.; Montalbán, C.; Stelitano, C.; Cabrera, M.E.; Resti, A.G.; et al. Chlamydophila Psittaci eradication with doxycycline as first-line targeted therapy for ocular adnexae lymphoma: Final results of an international phase II trial. *J. Clin. Oncol.* **2012**, *30*, 2988–2994. [CrossRef] [PubMed]

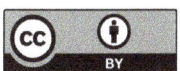

© 2018 by the authors. Licensee MDPI, Basel, Switzerland. This article is an open access article distributed under the terms and conditions of the Creative Commons Attribution (CC BY) license (http://creativecommons.org/licenses/by/4.0/).

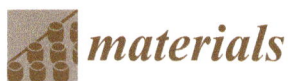

Review

Phenotypic Variation during Biofilm Formation: Implications for Anti-Biofilm Therapeutic Design

Marie Beitelshees [1], Andrew Hill [1,2], Charles H. Jones [2,*] and Blaine A. Pfeifer [1,3,*]

1. Department of Chemical and Biological Engineering, University at Buffalo, The State University of New York, Buffalo, NY 14260, USA; marie.beitelshees@abcombibio.com (M.B.); andrew.hill@abcombibio.com (A.H.)
2. Abcombi Biosciences Inc., 1576 Sweet Home Road, Amherst, NY 14228, USA
3. Department of Biomedical Engineering, University at Buffalo, The State University of New York, Buffalo, New York, NY 14260, USA
* Correspondence: charles.jones@abcombibio.com (C.H.J.); blainepf@buffalo.edu (B.A.P.); Tel: +1-(716)-213-8414 (C.H.J.); +1-(716)-645-1198 (B.A.P.)

Received: 20 April 2018; Accepted: 22 June 2018; Published: 26 June 2018

Abstract: Various bacterial species cycle between growth phases and biofilm formation, of which the latter facilitates persistence in inhospitable environments. These phases can be generally characterized by one or more cellular phenotype(s), each with distinct virulence factor functionality. In addition, a variety of phenotypes can often be observed within the phases themselves, which can be dependent on host conditions or the presence of nutrient and oxygen gradients within the biofilm itself (i.e., microenvironments). Currently, most anti-biofilm strategies have targeted a single phenotype; this approach has driven effective, yet incomplete, protection due to the lack of consideration of gene expression dynamics throughout the bacteria's pathogenesis. As such, this article provides an overview of the distinct phenotypes found within each biofilm development phase and demonstrates the unique anti-biofilm solutions each phase offers. However, we conclude that a combinatorial approach must be taken to provide complete protection against biofilm forming bacterial and their resulting diseases.

Keywords: bacterial biofilms; commensal bacteria; bacterial phenotypes; anti-biofilm strategies; anti-adhesion; dispersion

1. Introduction

Until recently, there was little appreciation for the relationship between a bacterial phenotype and the organism's pathogenesis. However, recent work has provided evidence that biofilms act as a primary stage of pathogenesis for up to 80% of bacterial diseases [1]. A list of common opportunistic pathogens can be found in Table 1. Interestingly, bacterial communities themselves are often asymptomatic and potentially beneficial (i.e., the microbiome). They can form on respiratory, digestive, skin, and urogenital epithelial cells, altogether colonizing a combined surface area of 300–400 m² of tissue in humans [2]. While these colonies do not normally cause disease directly, disturbances in the local environment, such as viral infections or mechanical disruption, can trigger a phenotypic shift, which causes the dispersion of virulent bacteria from the biofilm. This phenotypic shift has been associated with the upregulation of virulence factors that enable the bacteria to disseminate into normally sterile regions such as the middle ear, lungs, brain, and blood, thus causing clinical conditions including otitis media, pneumonia, bacterial meningitis, and bacteremia, respectively [3,4].

Diseases caused by these dispersed bacteria are currently regulated through the use of antibiotics. However, the increasing prevalence of antibiotic resistance highlights that these measures may be short lived. Furthermore, most antibiotics are unsuccessful at clearing recalcitrant bacterial biofilms, which have the ability to partially protect normally susceptible bacteria even from high levels of antibiotics [5]. Incomplete clearance can also leave behind metabolically dormant bacteria, such as persister cells, a distinct cell type which is unaffected by antibiotics [6]. This is of particular concern as biofilms have been implicated in chronic infections, inflammation, and various genetic conditions, thus further driving the need for alternative approaches [7]. For example, *Pseudomonas aeruginosa* colonies exacerbate complications such as chronic inflammation in patients suffering from cystic fibrosis, a genetic condition of the lungs [8,9].

Table 1. List of colonizing bacterial pathogens.

Pathogen	Disease	Colonization Site	Incidence Rate [A]	Fatality Rate [A]
Streptococcus pneumoniae	Pneumonia	Nasopharynx	9.5 [A]	1.14 [A]
Staphylococcus aureus (MRSA)	Skin infection	Nasopharynx, Skin	22.72 [A]	2.88 [A]
Group A Streptococcus	Strep throat	Pharynx	5.8 [A]	0.58 [A]
Haemophilus influenzae	Bacteremia	Nasopharynx	1.99 [A]	0.29 [A]
Neisseria meningitidis	Meningitis	Nasopharynx	0.12 [A]	0.01 [A]
Legionellosis	Atypical pneumonia	Lungs	1.42 [A]	0.1 [A]
Moraxella catarrhalis	Otitis media	Nasopharynx	N/A	0 [A]
Group B Streptococcus	Septicemia	Gastrointestinal tract	9.6 [A]	0.53 [A]
Porphyromonas gingivalis	Periodontal disease	Oral Cavity	9.24 [B]	-
Escherichia coli *Pseudomonas aeruginosa* *Klebsiella pneumoniae*	Catheter- Associated Urinary Tract Infection (CAUTI)	Bladder Catheter	3.3 [C]	17.3 [C]
	Ventilator-Associated Pneumonia (VAP)	Ventilator	3.3 [C]	15.2 [C]
Escherichia coli *Staphylococcus aureus* *Pseudomonas aeruginosa*	Prosthetic Joint Infections (PJI)	Prosthetic Joints (e.g., hip, knee)	1.5–2.5 [D]	2.5 [D]

[A] Incidence or Fatality rate of disease per 100,000 obtained from CDC's Active Bacterial Core Surveillance program. [B] [10]. [C] Incidence rate per 1000 Catheter/Ventilator-days; Fatality rate per 100 CATUI/VAP cases [11]. [D] Incidence rate per 100 arthroplasties; Fatality rate per 100 PJI cases [12].

One shortcoming of current antimicrobial strategies is the inability to compensate for the transcriptional and phenotypic differences present in unique phases of bacterial pathogenesis. For example, commercially available pneumococcal conjugate vaccines (PCVs) target capsular polysaccharides (CPs) that are expressed during the colonizing phase of *Streptococcus pneumoniae* infection. However, PCVs protect against only 13 of the >95 serotypes (serotypes correspond to different versions of CPs) of *S. pneumoniae* that cause disease in humans. Therefore, these vaccines are not capable of preventing colonization of non-vaccine type (NVT) *S. pneumoniae*, which has led to a marked global increase in infectious pneumococcal disease (IPD) caused by NVT serotypes [13]. Furthermore, these vaccines are ineffective at providing protection against virulent bacteria released from the biofilm which have shed their CPs [14]. Therefore, using PCVs as the example, further protection may be offered by taking into account characteristics of other phenotypes (e.g., biofilm-detached) observed during *S. pneumoniae* pathogenesis. However, the development of such therapeutics is further complicated by phenotype variation that results from the presence of microenvironments [15,16]. It should also be noted that the presence of multiple species can affect bacterial phenotype, which has been previously covered in detail [17] and will not be discussed in this review. Finally, even if a strategy succeeds in dispersing existing biofilms, the method of dispersion may result in virulent bacteria that are phenotypically distinct from both their planktonic and biofilm counterparts [18,19]. As these bacteria could result in the subsequent biofilm formation or infectious disease, this long neglected phenotype should be accounted for in anti-biofilm strategies.

In this review, we provide an overview of the various phenotypes that exist throughout the pathogenesis of single species bacterial biofilms and highlight those studies that have made use of this knowledge to develop specific antimicrobial therapies (Table 2). However, no solution presented below is likely to become a comprehensive anti-microbial. Instead, we contend that, by understanding the phenotypes observed in each phase of biofilm development, a comprehensive picture of a target pathogen can be leveraged to inform the development of next-generation therapeutics and vaccines.

Table 2. Summary of anti-biofilm strategies by biofilm phase.

Target	Bacteria	Anti-Microbial Strategy	Reference
Anti-Adhesion Phenotype Strategies			
Type I Pili	*Escherichia coli*	Pilicide ec240	[20]
		SAMan	[21]
P-fimbrate	*Escherichia coli*	Synthetic galabinose	[22]
Spy0128 and Spy0130	Group A Streptococcus	Vaccination	[23]
StrA	*Streptococcus mutans*	Morin	[24]
StrA	*Staphylococcus aureus*	pyrazolethione and pyridazinone	[25]
Anti-Biofilm Phenotype Strategies			
AHL Molecules	*Pseudomonas aeruginosa*	SsoPox-W263I	[26]
c-di-GMP	*Stenotrophomonas maltophilia*	BsmR	[27]
LuxS	*Streptococcus pneumoniae*	CRISPR	[28,29]
PIA	*Staphylococcus*	dispersin B	[30]
eDNA	*Pseudomonas aeruginosa*	DNAse I (Pulmozyme®)	[31]
PNAG	*S. aureus*	Monoclonal Antibody	[32]
Persister Cells	*Escherichia coli*	Mitomycin C	[33]
Persister Cells	*Pseudomonas aeruginosa*	Cisplatin	[34]
Persister Cells	*Pseudomonas aeruginosa* *Escherichia coli*	cis-2-Decenoic Acid	[35]
Anti-Dispersed Bacteria Phenotype Strategies			
GlpO	*Streptococcus pneumoniae*	Vaccine with GlpO Antigen	[36,37]
PncO	*Streptococcus pneumoniae*	Vaccine with PncO Antigen	[36,37]

2. Biofilm Development Overview

Upon entering a host, bacteria are confronted with several environmental challenges such as shear forces generated by bodily fluids, host immune responses, and shifts in nutrient availability. To survive, bacteria adapt by regulating gene transcription to exhibit more favorable phenotypes for the host environment, which often culminates in biofilm development [15,38–40]. However, throughout this process, a diversity of factors result in many phenotypes that differ between biofilm phases and within the biofilm itself [16]. As this results in inconsistently expressed therapeutic targets and changes in metabolic state, the heterogeneity of phenotypes present a distinct challenge for developing antimicrobial treatments.

The first step in biofilm formation involves the adherence of planktonic bacteria to anatomical surfaces, such as host epithelial cells, followed by their propagation into complex cellular communities. This process can be generalized into four stages: (1) reversible bacterial adhesion; (2) semi-irreversible attachment; (3) biofilm maturation; and (4) induced bacterial dispersion, all of which are represented by unique phenotypes [41]. Each phase offers many targets for anti-biofilm strategies (Figure 1). The first stage, initial reversible adhesion, is driven by locomotive appendages (i.e., flagella) and initiated as a response to environmental factors such as interactions with host immune cells, van der Waals and electrostatic interactions between bacterial and host surfaces, and shear forces within the body [42–44]. The second stage, semi-irreversible attachment, is driven by a variety of complex mechanisms that involve bacterial surface anchor proteins and macromolecule assemblies such as pili [45–47]. After a semi-irreversible attachment has been achieved, biofilm maturation is initiated with the production of an external matrix composed of extracellular polymeric substances (EPS) such as polysaccharides, extracellular DNA (eDNA), lipids, and proteins [48]. During or after biofilm maturation, environmental stimuli (i.e., changes in microenvironment, temperature, pH, nutrient concentration, microbial variability, and cell density) can induce the release of bacteria from the biofilm matrix (the last stage), which can then disseminate to new anatomical locations and cause disease [49].

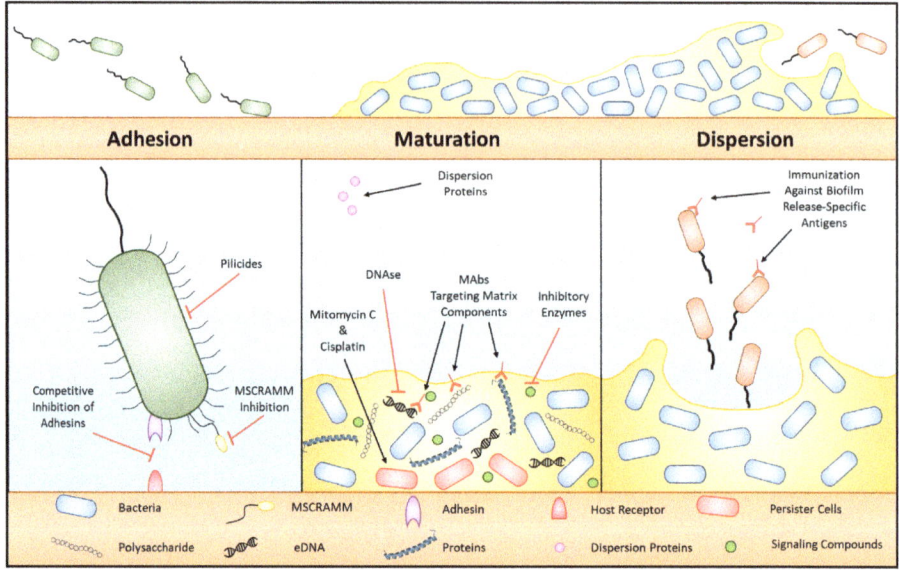

Figure 1. Biofilm formation and therapeutic targets. Schematic drawing of three generalized phases of biofilm formation: bacterial adhesion, biofilm maturation, and dispersion. Characteristics for each phase that represent therapeutic targets or provide opportunities for anti-biofilm strategies are highlighted.

Quorum Sensing During Biofilm Formation

To understand the variety of bacterial phenotypes observed during biofilm formation, it is essential to have an understanding of quorum sensing (QS). In general, this process makes use of a two-component signaling transduction system (TCSTS), which consists of an intercellular response regulator, a membrane-bound histidine kinase sensor, and a signal peptide (i.e., autoinducer (AI)). When AIs accumulate to a threshold concentration, the signaling system will directly or indirectly regulate the transcription of important genes [50,51]. Both Gram-positive and Gram-negative bacteria are known to make use of QS; however, Gram-negative bacteria use luminescence (Lux) I/LuxR-type quorum sensing, which utilizes the signaling molecule acyl-hormoserine lactone (AHL), while Gram-positive pathogens encode for an oligopeptide-two-component-type quorum sensing system. A third QS pathway, distinguished by a *luxS*-encoded autoinducer 2 (AI-2), has also been identified in both Gram-negative and -positive bacteria [52] and has recently been described as the most widespread QS system identified to date [53,54].

The QS pathways have been shown to promote biofilm growth and dispersion through the regulation of essential virulence factors. For example, the expression of *luxS* in immature pneumococcal biofilms has been shown to upregulate the virulence factor *ply* and *lytA* genes [55]. Interestingly however, the upregulation of this pathway has exhibited an inhibitory effect on *Staphylococcus epidermidis*, thus demonstrating the complexity of QS in bacterial biofilms. Other factors for early biofilm development, such as the release of eDNA, have been linked to the expression of the cyclic-peptide-dependent accessory gene regulator (*agr*). Under certain conditions, this QS system regulates the production of autolysin E (AtlE), an enzyme that instigates the release of eDNA and facilitates surface attachment [56].

Another ubiquitous bacterial signaling system utilizing the second messenger signal, cyclic di-GMP (c-di-GMP), has been shown to control the transition from planktonic to biofilm bacteria and vice versa in multiple bacterial species [57], including *P. aeruginosa* [58,59] and *Vibrio cholerae* [60]. Unlike QS, which relies on a small number of signaling cascades to regulate transcription, c-di-GMP signaling requires multiple pathways dependent on the c-di-GMP levels to control a vast number of cellular functions [61]. This variation in molecule concentration is achieved through the use of two classes of enzymes, diguanylate cyclase (DGC) and phosphodiesterase (PDE), capable of producing or degrading c-di-GMP molecules, respectively. The resulting increase or decrease in c-di-GMP concentration is sensed by either riboswitch RNAs or c-di-GMP receptor proteins [62]. An increase in c-di-GMP levels has been linked with biofilm formation, while a decrease in concentration has been shown to result in biofilm dispersion [63]. This trend has been well defined in *P. aeruginosa*, which possesses genes encoding for five DGCs (WspR, SadC, RoeA, SiaD, and YfiN/TpbB) that help control c-di-GMP levels and regulate the transcription of genes for the transition from planktonic to biofilm bacteria and at least three PDEs (DipA (Pch), RbdA, and NbdA) that have been linked to biofilm dispersal [63]. The DGC WspR, for example, regulates the EPS production necessary for biofilm formation [64], while the PDE known as NbdA initiates biofilm dispersion upon exposure to nitric oxide [65].

3. Bacterial Adhesion

As mentioned above, the first critical step in biofilm formation is reversible bacterial adhesion to a surface within an anatomical location (e.g., the nasopharynx), which occurs in response to environmental stimuli, such as changes in nutrient availability and adhesion surface characteristics (i.e., surface roughness and charge) [42,66]. Other factors, such as the deposition of material by non-adhering, or detached, bacteria and the presence of naturally occurring eDNA have also been shown to increase the rate of bacterial adhesion [67,68]. During this process, planktonic bacteria are sequestered to cellular surfaces through the physical forces in the surrounding fluid or through the use of locomotive appendages. These appendages (e.g., flagella), as well as other adhesion structures (pili and curli), define the phenotypes observed during this phase, and adhesion often does not occur without them. For example, one study demonstrated that *Streptococcus pyogenes* cells lacking functional pili were unable to bind to tonsil epithelium or human keratinocytes [45].

Perhaps due to their importance in bacterial survival, both Gram-negative and -positive bacteria express a variety of pili that facilitate adhesion to host cells. The most characterized cell-surface adhesion molecule in Gram-negative bacteria is the type 1 fimbrin D-mannose specific adhesin (FimH), which facilitates bacterial binding to host glycoproteins through the use of surface-exposed terminal mannose residues [69]. Other structures of note include the P-pili, which use the PapG adhesin to bind to host oligosaccharides, and the thin amyloid fibers known as curli. The latter adhesion appendage is found in a fraction of biofilm-forming bacteria, such as clinical isolates of *Escherichia coli*, and lacks specific receptor-ligand affinity [70]. In contrast to Gram-negative bacteria, whose pili are embedded within the outer membrane, Gram-positive bacteria adhesion structures are embedded within their cell wall. Although only two types of Gram-positive pili have been identified to date (sortase assembled pili and type IV pili), these structures have demonstrated mechanisms of adhesion similar to analogous structures in Gram-negative bacteria [71].

Not long after bacteria have accumulated at cellular surfaces, cells begin to form irreversible attachments leading to the initiation of biofilm formation [41,43]. During this critical step, various bacterial genes encoding diverse and vital adhesion surface structures are upregulated, such as those responsible for the expression of surface-anchored proteins that promote adhesion to host receptors [45–47]. The most well studied group of surface proteins, primarily observed in Gram-positive bacteria, are microbial surface components recognizing adhesive matrix molecules (MSCRAMMs) [72]. Examples of these molecules include clumping factor B (ClfB) of *Staphylococcus aureus* [73], pneumococcal adherence and virulence factor B (PavB) of *S. pneumoniae* [74], and the M protein of *S. pyogenes* [75]. Interestingly, there is a large diversity of adhesion proteins which may have arisen as an evolutionary mechanism for evading host immune responses by interfering with the complement system and promoting inflammation. *S. aureus*, for example, expresses 24 different surface adhesion proteins that are implicated in immune evasion [76]. One of these proteins, clumping factor A (ClfA), promotes the destruction of complement factor C3b, which is recognized by receptors on host phagocytes [77–79]. Furthermore, expression of these proteins is dependent on location within the host, thus suggesting that host-pathogen relationships may have driven the evolution of MSCRAMMs [80,81].

Anti-Adhesion Therapies

A better understanding of adhesion phenotypes led to antimicrobial strategies that target bacteria in the early phases of biofilm development. This is most evident in the number of strategies targeting adhesion structures, which often include competitively inhibiting bacterial adhesins and/or host receptors with the use of receptor-like molecules [82,83]. This approach has many advantages as carbohydrate-based inhibitors closely mimic host molecules and therefore are unlikely to be toxic or immunogenic [84]. For example, one study found that synthetic galabinose compounds outcompete the binding of P-fimbrated *E. coli* to galabinose-containing structures expressed on host cell surfaces [22]. In a similar fashion, several mannosides and mannose conjugates have been examined for their ability to inhibit type 1 pili-mediated adhesion, which has led to the identification of a potential therapeutic derived from the mannosidic squaric acid derivative SAMan (p-[N-(4-ethylamino-2,3-dioxocyclobut-1-enyl)amino]phenyl a-D-mannoside) [21]. This compound exhibited a 90% inhibition of *E. coli* attachment to human epithelial cells, making it a strong potential candidate for anti-adhesion therapy. A second popular anti-adhesion strategy is to inhibit the assembly of bacterial pili [85–87]. These molecules, often called pilicides, are small molecule inhibitors designed to dysregulate these adhesion appendages and prevent colonization. For example, Greene et al. engineered a molecule called pilicide ec240 which targets type 1 piliation of uropathogenic *E. coli* (UPEC) by downregulating genes in the *fim* operon, the same operon that encodes for FimH, a fimbrial adhesin associated with surface adhesion [20].

Many studies have also demonstrated the protective capabilities of vaccines composed of pili components [88–91]. Encouraging results have been observed when using pilus component proteins Spy0128 and Spy0130 from Group A Streptococci (GAS), which were able to confer >70% protection in murine models [23]. However, there is evidence that the interaction between pathogen adhesion structures and host immune response could improve bacterial adhesion. It has been found that, when recognized by the host immune system, the FimH adhesion properties are significantly enhanced by the resulting antibodies [92], suggesting that this protein may be ineffective as an antigen target in anti-bacterial vaccines.

The inhibition of MSCRAMMs has also demonstrated potential as a method to prevent bacterial adhesion. To prevent *S. aureus* and other Gram-positive infections, some studies have targeted sortase A (StrA), which enables bacterial adhesion to host cell membranes. Since this protein is not essential for bacterial growth, using StrA inhibitors creates minimal selective pressure that would lead bacteria to develop drug resistance, giving it a strong advantage over some current strategies (i.e., antibiotics) [93]. Interestingly, some promising StrA inhibitors are currently derived from biological sources such as plants and marine invertebrates [94]. For example, a compound found in many Chinese medicinal herbs, known as morin, has shown remarkable capabilities to reduce *Streptococcus mutans* biofilm formation through the inhibition of StrA [24]. Not surprisingly, there has also been interest in developing synthetic small molecule MSCRAMM inhibitors. These include pyrazolethione and pyridazinone compounds, both of which were found to have a significant negative effect on pathogen docking [25].

One cited advantage of anti-adhesion therapy is the belief that bacteria are less likely to identify an evolutionary escape mechanism, as doing so would adversely affect the pathogen's ability to colonize the host [95]. However, many pathogens encode for more than one mechanism of adhesion which allows for host localization even when one mechanism has been blocked [95,96]. Therefore, long-term and effective anti-adhesion strategies must compensate for these diverse biological strategies.

4. Biofilm Maturation

As a biofilm matures, bacteria begin to shift away from adhesion phenotypes by downregulating genes controlling the expression of ahesions and pili and upregulating factors essential to survival in a bacterial community. In fact, as much as 50% of bacterial proteomes within a biofilm can be differentially expressed when compared to planktonic bacteria of the same species [97]. Multiple phenotypes arise within the biofilm during this process due to the presence of microenvironments (i.e., gradients of signaling compounds, nutrients, chemicals, oxygen, and bacterial waste) which can then govern the bacterial function and metabolic state. Therefore, cells in a mature biofilm are not only phenotypically distinct from planktonic and adhering bacteria, they also form phenotypically distinct regions within an individual biofilm [16,98]. This heterogeneity has also been shown to lead to a division of labor in which cells perform specialized tasks to benefit the cellular community [99]. Common examples found within mature biofilms include biofilm matrix producers and persister cells, both of which provide unique challenges as well as promising targets for anti-biofilm strategies.

4.1. Extracellular Matrix Producers

The matrix producing cells within bacterial biofilms are responsible for the production of EPSs (i.e., polysaccharides, nucleic acids, lipids, and proteins) [100]. In some bacterial biofilms, such as *Bacillus subtilis*, this cell type is located primarily in the core of the biofilm in order to maintain its structure and rigidity [98]. Beyond providing structure, the EPS produced enhances biofilm formation by facilitating cell-cell communication and acting as a shield against numerous environmental hazards (i.e., antibiotics). They also serve as an external digestion system by breaking down lysed bacterial cells into nutrients that can be recycled to cells within the biofilm [48]. The most common components of the biofilm matrix are exopolysaccharides, eDNA, and proteins; however, the composition of EPSs is highly dependent on bacterial species and host conditions.

Matrix producing bacteria have been shown to excrete exopolysaccharides, the type of which can also impact bacterial phenotype. For example, during early biofilm formation, *P. aeruginosa* expresses a non-mucoid phenotype. These bacteria primarily produce Pel and Psl as structural exopolysaccharides, which have been found to play roles in increasing biofilm cell density and initial cell attachment, respectively [101–103]. However, over time, this bacterium can switch to the mucoid phenotype, which poses particular problems for cystic fibrosis patients. This switch, due to genetic mutations of the anti-sigma factor MucA, has been attributed to the overexpression of the exopolysaccharide alginate which enhances resistance to antibiotics and host immune cells as well as provides matrix structure [104,105]. As with all EPSs, the type of exopolysaccharide produced varies between bacterial species. However, there is one that is conserved throughout many microbial species, encompassing both Gram-positive and –negative bacteria: poly-β(1-6)-N-acetylglucosamine (PNAG) [102,106]. In bacteria such as *S. aureus*, this polysaccharide provides the main functional component of intracellular adhesion [107].

A second category of EPS, eDNA, which can facilitate adhesion during the early phase of biofilm development, has recently been shown to provide structural support within the biofilm matrix. However, the structural contribution of eDNA varies between bacterial species. For example, while eDNA is only a minor component in *S. epidermidis* biofilms, it is a major structural component in *P. aeruginosa* biofilms. To demonstrate this, an absence of eDNA in *P. aeruginosa* biofilms has been shown to negatively impacts 3-dimensional (3D) biofilm development without impairing individual cell growth, further establishing a role for eDNA in biofilm structure [108]. To build upon this theory, studies have hypothesized that eDNA may be used as scaffolding for the initial 3D structure as the integrity of mature biofilms is only minimally impacted by DNase, an enzyme that can completely dissolve biofilms in their early phases [108]. eDNA is also capable of interacting with other EPSs, such as Psl and Pel, which results in strong biofilm "skeletons" capable of reducing the effectiveness of DNase [109]. The presence of eDNA within the matrix could be the result of passive release from dead cells, active release from physiologically active cells, or bacteriophage infection spurring release [110]. For example, in some cases, eDNA appears to originate from a small subpopulation of autolytic cells, the activation of which are controlled by the *cidA* gene in *S. aureus* [111]. This gene, in turn, is regulated by the LytSR two-component regulatory system [112]. In contrast, nontypeable *Haemophilus influenzae* (NTHI) has recently been shown to secrete chromosomal DNA during biofilm maturation via a two-pore system. It has been shown that this bacteria uses an inner-membrane pore (TraCG) to transport eDNA to the periplasm and ComE to secrete the EPS to the biofilm matrix [113].

Matrix-producing bacteria also excrete matrix proteins. While EPS and eDNA have understood roles in biofilm structure, little is known about the roles proteins play in the biofilm matrix and information regarding the identities of these proteins is scarce. A recent proteomic study sought to characterize the proteins found in the *P. aeruginosa* matrix and found that they were composed largely of outer membrane proteins, secreted proteins, and the contents of lysed cells, including many well-characterized virulence factors [114]. One such protein, cyclic diguanylate-regulated TPS partner A (CdrA), was shown to link cells to the Psl exopolysaccharide, thus reinforcing the biofilm matrix [115]. In addition, DNA binding proteins, like DNA-binding protein HU (PA1804), are also common contributors to EPSs and are thought to alter gene transcription. However, despite their DNA biding properties, it is not yet known if they interact with eDNA [116].

4.2. Persister Cells

During biofilm maturation, microenvironments form that have distinct impacts on bacterial phenotype. These regions can be divided into three generalized categories: (1) an oxygen and substrate rich zone on or near the surface of the biofilm; (2) an intermediate substrate rich and oxygen depleted zone in which cells depend heavily on fermentation; (3) and a substrate and oxygen depleted zone consisting of metabolically dormant near the adhesion surface [16].

Most matrix-producing cells can be found within the first two zones. However, within substrate and oxygen depleted zones of a biofilm a divergent subpopulation of persister cells can be found, which has been a hindrance to the development of effective antimicrobial strategies. These cells exist as a small portion of biofilms that are tolerant to antibiotics while remaining protected from the host immune system. As such, the susceptible cells are killed during an antibiotic regimen, leaving the persister cells to repopulate the biofilms. This not only renders the antimicrobial strategy ineffectual, but can also lead to chronic infections [6]. Like antibiotic resistant bacteria, which obtain resistance through genetic mutations, persister cells are notoriously difficult to treat. However, in contrast to antibiotic resistant cells, persister cells obtain tolerance via transition to a metabolically dormant state that no longer expresses most antimicrobial targets, without undergoing any genetic modifications [117,118].

4.3. Anti-Biofilm Strategies

As bacterial sensing (i.e., QS and c-di-GMP signaling) drives phenotypic variation during biofilm maturation, it is unsurprising that inhibition of these processes can provide effective antimicrobial strategies. A number of methods have been developed that fall under two categories: QS inhibitors and quorum quenchers (QQs) (Figure 2). The first method, QS inhibition, aims to block QS by introducing small-molecule analogs that outcompete signal molecules [119]. Using this strategy, it is possible to alter cellular phenotypes expressed within mature biofilms. For example, the *agr* signaling pathway, despite being implicated in initial cell adhesion under certain conditions, is also capable of inhibiting important biofilm matrix proteins (fibronectin-binding proteins (FnBPs) and Protein A) produced by *S. aureus* [56,120]. To exploit this natural system as an anti-biofilm strategy, it is possible to activate the *arg* signaling system through the addition of autoinducing peptides (AIPs). When combined with serine proteases, AIPs were highly effective at dispersing established, mature biofilms; however, this strategy would be ineffective at targeting *agr* deficient strains [121]. Conversely, quorum quenchers shut down QS via enzyme inhibitors which can be classified as: (1) lactonases; (2) acylases; and (3) oxidoreductases [122]. Most QQ enzymes identified to date fall under the category of lactonases, due to their ability to degrade AHL molecules [123–125]. One such enzyme, *Sso*Pox-W263I, was capable of decreasing the virulence of clinical isolates of *P. aeruginosa* from diabetic foot ulcers by disrupting QS and reducing biofilm formation [26]. Finally, many strategies have attempted to disrupt c-di-GMP signaling due to its large role in regulating the bacterial phenotypes that produce exopolysaccharides and matrix proteins. For example, high levels of c-di-GMP have been linked to increased production of the polysaccharides Pel and Psl and the protein CdrA in *P. aeruginosa* [115,126]. Therefore, degradation of this compound presents an interesting anti-biofilm solution. One PDE of interest, the regulatory enzyme BsmR not only degrades c-di-GMP, but also upregulates genes associated with biofilm dispersal, making it a strong antimicrobial candidate [27].

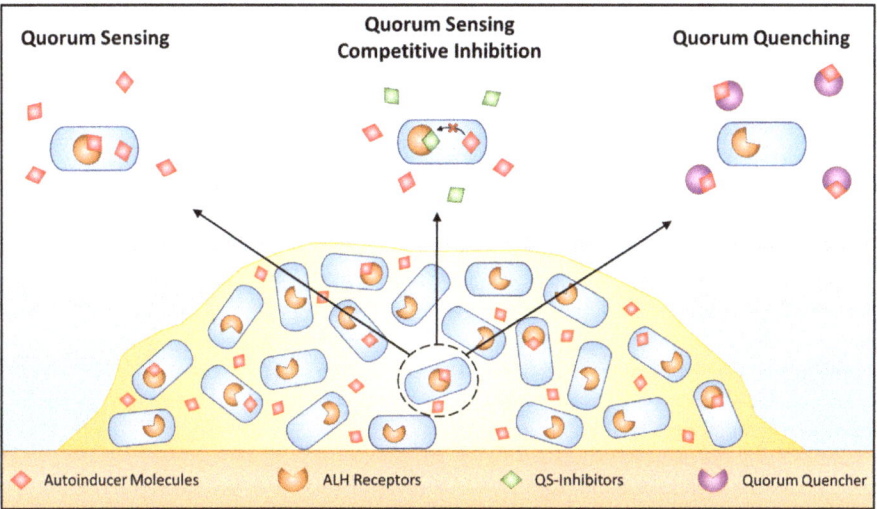

Figure 2. Targeting quorum sensing. Schematic of QS in bacteria as well as methods to block this signaling mechanism. AHL dependent QS within biofilms (left) can be blocked using competitive QS inhibition that outcompete AHL for AHL receptors (middle) or quorum quenching enzymes that inactivate AHL signals (right).

An additional strategy to modify phenotypes within mature biofilms is the transcriptional alteration of essential enzymes. This is possible due to technologies such as CRISPR (clustered regularly interspaced short palindromic repeats), which allows for the alteration of any target gene [127]. One target of particular interest is LuxS, the enzyme that synthesizes AI-2, as it has been shown to influence matrix producing phenotypes. For example, it regulates the production of eDNA through the activation of LytA-dependent autolysis activity in *S. pneumoniae* [128]. As eDNA provides structure to biofilms, inhibition of LuxS could prevent biofilm formation or weaken existing communities. Interestingly, recent studies demonstrated that CRISPR inhibition (i.e., CRISPRi) could knockdown *luxS* which, in turn, prevented metabolically active *E. coli* from developing biofilms, likely due to the prevention of EPS production through AI-2 inhibition [28,29]. These studies appear to be the first attempts to utilize CRISPR in an effort to prevent or eliminate biofilms; however, it may be possible to knockout other genes essential to biofilm maturation.

Instead of targeting various phenotypes, it is also possible to target cellular products in order to weaken or disperse mature biofilms [129,130]. The introduction of dispersion proteins, such as dispersin B of *Aggregatibacter actinomycetemcomitans*, has the ability to inhibit initial biofilm formation, detach existing colonies, and compromise the physical integrity of the matrix in staphylococcal biofilms by attaching to the exopolysaccharide PIA [30,48,49,131,132]. The enzyme DNase may also be effective at dispersing early-staged biofilms and increasing their susceptibility to antibiotics by targeting eDNA within the matrix, thus leading many researchers to analyze its potential as an anti-biofilm therapy [30,133,134]. This strategy has culminated in Genentech's Pulmozyme®, a recombinant human DNase I that targets *P. aeruginosa* infections of cystic fibrosis patients. Antibody-based therapies (i.e., monoclonal antibodies) may also be able to eliminate mature biofilms [135–137]. One antigen of interest is PNAG, an exopolysaccharide that is conserved in many bacterial species, and antibodies targeting this antigen have been shown to prevent and eliminate bacterial biofilms [138]. This success has led to the development of an anti-PNAG monoclonal antibody which has completed a Phase I clinical trial [32,139].

While the strategies detailed above may be effective at targeting the matrix producing phenotypes, resulting dispersion may leave persister cells behind which can repopulate the biofilm. As these cells are metabolically dormant, anti-microbial compounds targeting persister cells must be capable of entering cells without the need for active transport. In addition, their mechanism of action must require no innate cellular machinery [140]. Such compounds exist and include the chemotherapeutic agents mitomycin C and cisplatin [33,141]. Additionally, studies have shown that persister cells can be reawakened, after which they can be targeted with traditional antibiotics. This has been done with *cis*-2-decenoic acid, which revitalized protein synthesis within the previously dormant cells [35].

5. Dispersion

During or after biofilm maturation, a subpopulation of bacteria can disperse from the biofilm matrix to colonize other regions of the host. This population represents a phenotype distinct from both planktonic and biofilm bacteria [141,142]. During this phase, genes for motility and virulence are upregulated in response to environmental cues (i.e., cell density, febrile conditions, bacteriophage infection, changes in nutrient availability) [4,143]. Dispersion can occur as either single motile cells or as multicellular aggregates.

Interestingly, the dispersed single motile cell phenotype has a greater capacity to develop biofilms when compared with planktonic bacteria [19]. However, high density aggregates, which retain similar phenotypes to biofilm bacteria, surpass both planktonic and single dispersed cells in the ability to form biofilms, making them important to disease pathogenesis [144]. As further evidence that biofilm detachment plays a large role in bacterial diseases, there is also increasing evidence that certain methods of dispersal can result in the release bacteria more virulent than their planktonic counterparts [4]. For example, fever-induced biofilm release of pneumococci has been shown to result in bacterial dissemination to the lungs and blood to a greater degree than observed for planktonic bacteria in murine models [36], and it is now apparent that the biofilm colonization phase is essential for disease progression. As the end goal of most anti-biofilm strategies is biofilm dissemination, there is a possibility of inadvertently activating this phenotype; therefore, secondary measures (e.g., antibiotics, vaccines) should be taken to prevent further spread of disease.

In addition, many biofilms are asymptomatic and potentially beneficial to the host (i.e., microbiota) [145]. Therefore, a better understanding of the biofilm-released phase offers the potential for innovative strategies targeting opportunistic pathogens while leaving potentially beneficial bacteria in place. This idea was put into practice during the recent transcriptome analysis of planktonic, biofilm-forming, and biofilm-released cells which identified protein antigens specific to the biofilm-release phase [4]. Two of these proteins, alpha-glycerophosphate oxidase (GlpO) and the bacterocin PncO, were found to be homologous throughout *S. pneumoniae* strains and offered complete protection against this virulent phenotype in murine models when combined into a single vaccine [36,37]. To our knowledge, this is the first strategy to specifically target biofilm-detached bacteria, while leaving the biofilm intact.

6. Conclusions

To develop effective therapeutic strategies against biofilm-forming bacteria, it is essential to understand the phenotypic diversity that is observed within these biofilms. These differences pose many challenges to researchers targeting these colonizing bacteria. However, with a better understanding comes the potential for effective treatment and vaccination strategies such as those mentioned above. While each strategy mentioned in this review has its strengths, few have ever demonstrated the coverage needed to provide full protection against their target pathogen. This is due to the fact that many strategies focus only on one aspect of bacterial diversity. Therefore, combining strategies may provide universal protection against diseases caused by biofilm forming bacteria. For example, as biofilm dispersion therapies may result in virulent biofilm-released bacteria, secondary treatments may be required to prevent the further spread of disease. In summary, this review presents evidence that taking phenotypic differences into account will enable the development of widely effective anti-infective solutions.

Author Contributions: M.B. was responsible for organizing and writing the manuscript, as well as creating the figures. A.H. constructed the tables. A.H., B.A.P. and C.H.J. were responsible for reviewing and editing the manuscript.

Funding: The authors recognize the support from National Institutes of Health (NIH) awards AI088485 and AI117309 (to B.A.P.) and the National Institute of Allergy and Infectious Diseases (NIAID) award R41AI124851 (to C.H.J.).

Conflicts of Interest: C.H.J., A.H. and B.A.P. are co-founders of Abcombi Biosciences Inc., a company focused on vaccine design. M.B. declares that she has no competing interests.

References

1. National Institutes of Health. Available online: https://grants.nih.gov/grants/guide/pa-files/PA-07-288.html (accessed on 3 October 2017).
2. Ribet, D.; Cossart, P. How bacterial pathogens colonize their hosts and invade deeper tissues. *Microbes Infect.* **2015**, *17*, 173–183. [CrossRef] [PubMed]
3. Chao, Y.; Marks, L.R.; Pettigrew, M.M.; Hakansson, A.P. *Streptococcus pneumoniae* biofilm formation and dispersion during colonization and disease. *Front. Cell. Infect. Microbiol.* **2014**, *4*, 194. [CrossRef] [PubMed]
4. Pettigrew, M.M.; Marks, L.R.; Kong, Y.; Gent, J.F.; Roche-Hakansson, H.; Hakansson, A.P. Dynamic changes in the *Streptococcus pneumoniae* transcriptome during transition from biofilm formation to invasive disease upon influenza a virus infection. *Infect. Immun.* **2014**, *82*, 4607–4619. [CrossRef] [PubMed]
5. Lebeaux, D.; Ghigo, J.-M.; Beloin, C. Biofilm-related infections: Bridging the gap between clinical management and fundamental aspects of recalcitrance toward antibiotics. *Microbiol. Mol. Biol. Rev.* **2014**, *78*, 510–543. [CrossRef] [PubMed]
6. Lewis, K. Persister cells, dormancy and infectious disease. *Nat. Rev. Microbiol.* **2007**, *5*, 48–56. [CrossRef] [PubMed]
7. Stewart, P.S.; Costerton, J.W. Antibiotic resistance of bacteria in biofilms. *Lancet* **2001**, *358*, 135–138. [CrossRef]
8. Costerton, J.W.; Stewart, P.S.; Greenberg, E.P. Bacterial biofilms: A common cause of persistent infections. *Science* **1999**, *284*, 1318–1322. [CrossRef] [PubMed]
9. Hoiby, N.; Ciofu, O.; Bjarnsholt, T. *Pseudomonas aeruginosa* biofilms in cystic fibrosis. *Future Microbiol.* **2010**, *5*, 1663–1674. [CrossRef] [PubMed]
10. Rafiei, M.; Kiani, F.; Sayehmiri, F.; Sayehmiri, K.; Sheikhi, A.; Zamanian Azodi, M. Study of *Porphyromonas gingivalis* in periodontal diseases: A systematic review and meta-analysis. *Med. J. Islam. Repub. Iran.* **2017**, *31*, 62. [CrossRef] [PubMed]

11. Rosenthal, V.D.; Bijie, H.; Maki, D.G.; Mehta, Y.; Apisarnthanarak, A.; Medeiros, E.A.; Leblebicioglu, H.; Fisher, D.; Álvarez-Moreno, C.; Khader, I.A. International nosocomial infection control consortium (INICC) report, data summary of 36 countries, for 2004–2009. *Am. J. Infect. Control* **2012**, *40*, 396–407. [CrossRef] [PubMed]
12. Lentino, J.R. Prosthetic joint infections: Bane of orthopedists, challenge for infectious disease specialists. *Clin. Infect. Dis.* **2003**, *36*, 1157–1161. [CrossRef] [PubMed]
13. Balsells, E.; Guillot, L.; Nair, H.; Kyaw, M.H. Serotype distribution of *Streptococcus pneumoniae* causing invasive disease in children in the post-PCV era: A systematic review and meta-analysis. *PLoS ONE* **2017**, *12*, e0177113. [CrossRef] [PubMed]
14. Hanage, W.P. Serotype replacement in invasive pneumococcal disease: Where do we go from here? *J. Infect. Dis.* **2007**, *196*, 1282–1284. [CrossRef] [PubMed]
15. Boles, B.R.; Thoendel, M.; Singh, P.K. Self-generated diversity produces "insurance effects" in biofilm communities. *Proc. Natl. Acad. Sci. USA* **2004**, *101*, 16630–16635. [CrossRef] [PubMed]
16. Stewart, P.S.; Franklin, M.J. Physiological heterogeneity in biofilms. *Nat. Rev. Microbiol.* **2008**, *6*, 199–210. [CrossRef] [PubMed]
17. Elias, S.; Banin, E. Multi-species biofilms: Living with friendly neighbors. *FEMS Microbiol. Rev.* **2012**, *36*, 990–1004. [CrossRef] [PubMed]
18. Marks, L.R.; Davidson, B.A.; Knight, P.R.; Hakansson, A.P. Interkingdom signaling induces *Streptococcus pneumoniae* biofilm dispersion and transition from asymptomatic colonization to disease. *mBio* **2013**, *4*, e00438-13. [CrossRef] [PubMed]
19. Cécile, R.; Laurent, G.; Jean, G. Biofilm-detached cells, a transition from a sessile to a planktonic phenotype: A comparative study of adhesion and physiological characteristics in *Pseudomonas aeruginosa*. *FEMS Microbiol. Lett.* **2008**, *290*, 135–142.
20. Greene, S.E.; Pinkner, J.S.; Chorell, E.; Dodson, K.W.; Shaffer, C.L.; Conover, M.S.; Livny, J.; Hadjifrangiskou, M.; Almqvist, F.; Hultgren, S.J. Pilicide ec240 disrupts virulence circuits in uropathogenic *Escherichia coli*. *mBio* **2014**, *5*, e02038-14. [CrossRef] [PubMed]
21. Hartmann, M.; Papavlassopoulos, H.; Chandrasekaran, V.; Grabosch, C.; Beiroth, F.; Lindhorst, T.K.; Röhl, C. Inhibition of bacterial adhesion to live human cells: Activity and cytotoxicity of synthetic mannosides. *FEBS Lett.* **2012**, *586*, 1459–1465. [CrossRef] [PubMed]
22. Salminen, A.; Loimaranta, V.; Joosten, J.A.; Khan, A.S.; Hacker, J.; Pieters, R.J.; Finne, J. Inhibition of p-fimbriated *Escherichia coli* adhesion by multivalent galabiose derivatives studied by a live-bacteria application of surface plasmon resonance. *J. Antimicrob. Chemother.* **2007**, *60*, 495–501. [CrossRef] [PubMed]
23. Mora, M.; Bensi, G.; Capo, S.; Falugi, F.; Zingaretti, C.; Manetti, A.G.O.; Maggi, T.; Taddei, A.R.; Grandi, G.; Telford, J.L. Group A Streptococcus produce pilus-like structures containing protective antigens and Lancefield T antigens. *Proc. Natl. Acad. Sci. USA* **2005**, *102*, 15641–15646. [CrossRef] [PubMed]
24. Huang, P.; Hu, P.; Zhou, S.Y.; Li, Q.; Chen, W.M. Morin inhibits sortase a and subsequent biofilm formation in *Streptococcus mutans*. *Curr. Microbiol.* **2014**, *68*, 47–52. [CrossRef] [PubMed]
25. Suree, N.; Yi, S.W.; Thieu, W.; Marohn, M.; Damoiseaux, R.; Chan, A.; Jung, M.E.; Clubb, R.T. Discovery and structure–activity relationship analysis of *Staphylococcus aureus* sortase a inhibitors. *Bioorg. Med. Chem.* **2009**, *17*, 7174–7185. [CrossRef] [PubMed]
26. Guendouze, A.; Plener, L.; Bzdrenga, J.; Jacquet, P.; Rémy, B.; Elias, M.; Lavigne, J.-P.; Daudé, D.; Chabrière, E. Effect of quorum quenching lactonase in clinical isolates of *Pseudomonas aeruginosa* and comparison with quorum sensing inhibitors. *Front. Microbiol.* **2017**, *8*, 227. [CrossRef] [PubMed]
27. Liu, W.; Tian, X.-Q.; Wei, J.-W.; Ding, L.-L.; Qian, W.; Liu, Z.; Wang, F.-F. BsmR degrades c-di-GMP to modulate biofilm formation of nosocomial pathogen *Stenotrophomonas maltophilia*. *Sci. Rep.* **2017**, *7*, 4665. [CrossRef] [PubMed]
28. Zuberi, A.; Misba, L.; Khan, A.U. CRISPR interference (crispri) inhibition of luxs gene expression in *E. coli*: An approach to inhibit biofilm. *Front. Cell. Infect. Microbiol.* **2017**, *7*, 214. [CrossRef] [PubMed]
29. Kang, S.; Kim, J.; Hur, J.K.; Lee, S.-S. CRISPR-based genome editing of clinically important *Escherichia coli* SE15 isolated from indwelling urinary catheters of patients. *J. Med. Microbiol.* **2017**, *66*, 18–25. [CrossRef] [PubMed]
30. Kaplan, J.B. Therapeutic potential of biofilm-dispersing enzymes. *IJAO* **2009**, *32*, 545–554. [CrossRef]

31. Shak, S.; Capon, D.J.; Hellmiss, R.; Marsters, S.A.; Baker, C.L. Recombinant human DNAse I reduces the viscosity of cystic fibrosis sputum. *Proc. Natl. Acad. Sci. USA* **1990**, *87*, 9188–9192. [CrossRef] [PubMed]
32. Kelly-Quintos, C.; Cavacini, L.A.; Posner, M.R.; Goldmann, D.; Pier, G.B. Characterization of the opsonic and protective activity against *Staphylococcus aureus* of fully human monoclonal antibodies specific for the bacterial surface polysaccharide poly-n-acetylglucosamine. *Infect. Immun.* **2006**, *74*, 2742–2750. [CrossRef] [PubMed]
33. Kwan, B.W.; Chowdhury, N.; Wood, T.K. Combatting bacterial infections by killing persister cells with mitomycin c. *Environ. Microbiol.* **2015**, *17*, 4406–4414. [CrossRef] [PubMed]
34. Chowdhury, N.; Wood, T.L.; Martinez-Vazquez, M.; Garcia-Contreras, R.; Wood, T.K. DNA-crosslinker cisplatin eradicates bacterial persister cells. *Biotechnol. Bioeng.* **2016**, *113*, 1984–1992. [CrossRef] [PubMed]
35. Marques, C.N.H.; Morozov, A.; Planzos, P.; Zelaya, H.M. The fatty acid signaling molecule cis-2-decenoic acid increases metabolic activity and reverts persister cells to an antimicrobial-susceptible state. *Appl. Environ. Microbiol.* **2014**, *80*, 6976–6991. [CrossRef] [PubMed]
36. Li, Y.; Hill, A.; Beitelshees, M.; Sha, S.; Lovell, J.F.; Davidson, B.A.; Knight, P.R.; Hakansson, A.P.; Pfeifer, B.A.; Jones, C.H. Directed vaccination against pneumococcal disease. *Proc. Natl. Acad. Sci. USA* **2016**, *113*, 6898–6903. [CrossRef] [PubMed]
37. Jones, C.H.; Zhang, G.; Nayerhoda, R.; Beitelshees, M.; Hill, A.; Rostami, P.; Li, Y.; Davidson, B.A.; Knight, P.; Pfeifer, B.A. Comprehensive vaccine design for commensal disease progression. *Sci. Adv.* **2017**, *3*, e1701797. [CrossRef] [PubMed]
38. Roilides, E.; Simitsopoulou, M.; Katragkou, A.; Walsh, T.J. How biofilms evade host defenses. *Microbiol. Spectr.* **2015**, *3*, 3.
39. Thurlow, L.R.; Hanke, M.L.; Fritz, T.; Angle, A.; Aldrich, A.; Williams, S.H.; Engebretsen, I.L.; Bayles, K.W.; Horswill, A.R.; Kielian, T. *Staphylococcus aureus* biofilms prevent macrophage phagocytosis and attenuate inflammation in vivo. *J. Immunol.* **2011**, *186*, 6585–6596. [CrossRef] [PubMed]
40. Medini, D.; Serruto, D.; Parkhill, J.; Relman, D.A.; Donati, C.; Moxon, R.; Falkow, S.; Rappuoli, R. Microbiology in the post-genomic era. *Nat. Rev. Microbiol.* **2008**, *6*, 419–430. [CrossRef] [PubMed]
41. Landini, P.; Antoniani, D.; Burgess, J.G.; Nijland, R. Molecular mechanisms of compounds affecting bacterial biofilm formation and dispersal. *Appl. Microbiol. Biotechnol.* **2010**, *86*, 813–823. [CrossRef] [PubMed]
42. Garrett, T.R.; Bhakoo, M.; Zhang, Z. Bacterial adhesion and biofilms on surfaces. *Prog. Nat. Sci. Mater.* **2008**, *18*, 1049–1056. [CrossRef]
43. O'Toole, G.; Kaplan, H.B.; Kolter, R. Biofilm formation as microbial development. *Annu. Rev. Microbiol.* **2000**, *54*, 49. [CrossRef] [PubMed]
44. Hermansson, M. The DLVO theory in microbial adhesion. *Colloids Surf. B Biointerfaces* **1999**, *14*, 105–119. [CrossRef]
45. Abbot, E.L.; Smith, W.D.; Siou, G.P.; Chiriboga, C.; Smith, R.J.; Wilson, J.A.; Hirst, B.H.; Kehoe, M.A. Pili mediate specific adhesion of *Streptococcus pyogenes* to human tonsil and skin. *Cell. Microbiol.* **2007**, *9*, 1822–1833. [CrossRef] [PubMed]
46. Maisey, H.C.; Hensler, M.; Nizet, V.; Doran, K.S. Group B Streptococcal pilus proteins contribute to adherence to and invasion of brain microvascular endothelial cells. *J. Bacteriol.* **2007**, *189*, 1464–1467. [CrossRef] [PubMed]
47. Manetti, A.G.; Zingaretti, C.; Falugi, F.; Capo, S.; Bombaci, M.; Bagnoli, F.; Gambellini, G.; Bensi, G.; Mora, M.; Edwards, A.M.; et al. *Streptococcus pyogenes* pili promote pharyngeal cell adhesion and biofilm formation. *Mol. Microbiol.* **2007**, *64*, 968–983. [CrossRef] [PubMed]
48. Flemming, H.C.; Wingender, J. The biofilm matrix. *Nat. Rev. Microbiol.* **2010**, *8*, 623–633. [CrossRef] [PubMed]
49. Kaplan, J.B. Biofilm dispersal: Mechanisms, clinical implications, and potential therapeutic uses. *J. Dent. Res.* **2010**, *89*, 205–218. [CrossRef] [PubMed]
50. Cvitkovitch, D.G.; Li, Y.-H.; Ellen, R.P. Quorum sensing and biofilm formation in streptococcal infections. *J. Clin. Investig.* **2003**, *112*, 1626–1632. [CrossRef] [PubMed]
51. Jayaraman, A.; Wood, T.K. Bacterial quorum sensing: Signals, circuits, and implications for biofilms and disease. *Annu. Rev. Biomed. Eng.* **2008**, *10*, 145–167. [CrossRef] [PubMed]
52. Li, Y.H.; Tian, X. Quorum sensing and bacterial social interactions in biofilms. *Sensors (Basel)* **2012**, *12*, 2519–2538. [CrossRef] [PubMed]

53. Chen, X.; Schauder, S.; Potier, N.; Van Dorsselaer, A.; Pelczer, I.; Bassler, B.L.; Hughson, F.M. Structural identification of a bacterial quorum-sensing signal containing boron. *Nature* **2002**, *415*, 545–549. [CrossRef] [PubMed]
54. Xu, L.; Li, H.; Vuong, C.; Vadyvaloo, V.; Wang, J.; Yao, Y.; Otto, M.; Gao, Q. Role of the luxS quorum-sensing system in biofilm formation and virulence of *Staphylococcus epidermidis*. *Infect. Immun.* **2006**, *74*, 488–496. [CrossRef] [PubMed]
55. Vidal, J.E.; Ludewick, H.P.; Kunkel, R.M.; Zahner, D.; Klugman, K.P. The luxS-dependent quorum-sensing system regulates early biofilm formation by *Streptococcus pneumoniae* strain d39. *Infect. Immun.* **2011**, *79*, 4050–4060. [CrossRef] [PubMed]
56. Qin, Z.; Ou, Y.; Yang, L.; Zhu, Y.; Tolker-Nielsen, T.; Molin, S.; Qu, D. Role of autolysin-mediated DNA release in biofilm formation of *Staphylococcus epidermidis*. *Microbiology* **2007**, *153*, 2083–2092. [CrossRef] [PubMed]
57. Cotter, P.A.; Stibitz, S. C-di-GMP-mediated regulation of virulence and biofilm formation. *Curr. Opin. Microbiol.* **2007**, *10*, 17–23. [CrossRef] [PubMed]
58. Simm, R.; Morr, M.; Kader, A.; Nimtz, M.; Romling, U. GGDEF and EAL domains inversely regulate cyclic di-gmp levels and transition from sessility to motility. *Mol. Microbiol.* **2004**, *53*, 1123–1134. [CrossRef] [PubMed]
59. Ha, D.G.; O'Toole, G.A. C-di-GMP and its effects on biofilm formation and dispersion: A *Pseudomonas aeruginosa* review. *Microbiol. Spectr.* **2015**, *3*, 2. [CrossRef] [PubMed]
60. Tischler, A.D.; Camilli, A. Cyclic diguanylate (c-di-GMP) regulates *Vibrio cholerae* biofilm formation. *Mol. Microbiol.* **2004**, *53*, 857–869. [CrossRef] [PubMed]
61. Srivastava, D.; Waters, C.M. A tangled web: Regulatory connections between quorum sensing and cyclic di-GMP. *J. Bacteriol.* **2012**, *194*, 4485–4493. [CrossRef] [PubMed]
62. Hengge, R. Principles of c-di-GMP signalling in bacteria. *Nat. Rev. Microbiol.* **2009**, *7*, 263. [CrossRef] [PubMed]
63. Valentini, M.; Filloux, A. Biofilms and cyclic di-GMP (c-di-GMP) signaling: Lessons from *Pseudomonas aeruginosa* and other bacteria. *J. Biol. Chem.* **2016**, *291*, 12547–12555. [CrossRef] [PubMed]
64. Hickman, J.W.; Tifrea, D.F.; Harwood, C.S. A chemosensory system that regulates biofilm formation through modulation of cyclic diguanylate levels. *Proc. Natl. Acad. Sci. USA* **2005**, *102*, 14422–14427. [CrossRef] [PubMed]
65. Li, Y.; Heine, S.; Entian, M.; Sauer, K.; Frankenberg-Dinkel, N. No-induced biofilm dispersion in *Pseudomonas aeruginosa* is mediated by an MHYT domain-coupled phosphodiesterase. *J. Bacteriol.* **2013**, *195*, 3531–3542. [CrossRef] [PubMed]
66. Yoda, I.; Koseki, H.; Tomita, M.; Shida, T.; Horiuchi, H.; Sakoda, H.; Osaki, M. Effect of surface roughness of biomaterials on *Staphylococcus epidermidis* adhesion. *BMC Microbiol.* **2014**, *14*, 234. [CrossRef] [PubMed]
67. Das, T.; Sharma, P.K.; Busscher, H.J.; van der Mei, H.C.; Krom, B.P. Role of extracellular DNA in initial bacterial adhesion and surface aggregation. *Appl. Environ. Microbiol.* **2010**, *76*, 3405–3408. [CrossRef] [PubMed]
68. Sjollema, J.; van der Mei, H.C.; Hall, C.L.; Peterson, B.W.; de Vries, J.; Song, L.; Jong, E.D.d.; Busscher, H.J.; Swartjes, J.J.T.M. Detachment and successive re-attachment of multiple, reversibly-binding tethers result in irreversible bacterial adhesion to surfaces. *Sci. Rep.* **2017**, *7*, 4369. [CrossRef] [PubMed]
69. Sauer, M.M.; Jakob, R.P.; Eras, J.; Baday, S.; Eriş, D.; Navarra, G.; Bernèche, S.; Ernst, B.; Maier, T.; Glockshuber, R. Catch-bond mechanism of the bacterial adhesin FimH. *Nat. Commun.* **2016**, *7*, 10738. [CrossRef] [PubMed]
70. Kline, K.A.; Fälker, S.; Dahlberg, S.; Normark, S.; Henriques-Normark, B. Bacterial adhesins in host-microbe interactions. *Cell. Host Microbe* **2009**, *5*, 580–592. [CrossRef] [PubMed]
71. Proft, T.; Baker, E.N. Pili in Gram-negative and Gram-positive bacteria—Structure, assembly and their role in disease. *Cell. Mol. Life Sci.* **2009**, *66*, 613–635. [CrossRef] [PubMed]
72. Patti, J.M.; Allen, B.L.; McGavin, M.J.; Hook, M. MSCRAMM-mediated adherence of microorganisms to host tissues. *Annu. Rev. Microbiol.* **1994**, *48*, 585–617. [CrossRef] [PubMed]
73. Walsh, E.J.; Miajlovic, H.; Gorkun, O.V.; Foster, T.J. Identification of the *Staphylococcus aureus* MSCRAMM clumping factor b (ClfB) binding site in the alphac-domain of human fibrinogen. *Microbiology* **2008**, *154*, 550–558. [CrossRef] [PubMed]

74. Jensch, I.; Gamez, G.; Rothe, M.; Ebert, S.; Fulde, M.; Somplatzki, D.; Bergmann, S.; Petruschka, L.; Rohde, M.; Nau, R.; et al. PavB is a surface-exposed adhesin of *Streptococcus pneumoniae* contributing to nasopharyngeal colonization and airways infections. *Mol. Microbiol.* **2010**, *77*, 22–43. [CrossRef] [PubMed]
75. Nobbs, A.H.; Lamont, R.J.; Jenkinson, H.F. Streptococcus adherence and colonization. *Microbiol. Mol. Biol. Rev.* **2009**, *73*, 407–450. [CrossRef] [PubMed]
76. Foster, T.J.; Geoghegan, J.A.; Ganesh, V.K.; Höök, M. Adhesion, invasion and evasion: The many functions of the surface proteins of *Staphylococcus aureus*. *Nat. Rev. Microbiol.* **2014**, *12*, 49–62. [CrossRef] [PubMed]
77. Hair, P.S.; Ward, M.D.; Semmes, O.J.; Foster, T.J.; Cunnion, K.M. *Staphylococcus aureus* clumping factor A binds to complement regulator factor I and increases factor I cleavage of C3b. *J. Infect. Dis.* **2008**, *198*, 125–133. [CrossRef] [PubMed]
78. Hair, P.S.; Echague, C.G.; Sholl, A.M.; Watkins, J.A.; Geoghegan, J.A.; Foster, T.J.; Cunnion, K.M. Clumping factor A interaction with complement factor I increases C3b cleavage on the bacterial surface of *Staphylococcus aureus* and decreases complement-mediated phagocytosis. *Infect. Immun.* **2010**, *78*, 1717–1727. [CrossRef] [PubMed]
79. Sharp, J.A.; Echague, C.G.; Hair, P.S.; Ward, M.D.; Nyalwidhe, J.O.; Geoghegan, J.A.; Foster, T.J.; Cunnion, K.M. *Staphylococcus aureus* surface protein SdrE binds complement regulator factor H as an immune evasion tactic. *PLoS ONE* **2012**, *7*, e38407. [CrossRef] [PubMed]
80. Ghasemian, A.; Najar Peerayeh, S.; Bakhshi, B.; Mirzaee, M. The microbial surface components recognizing adhesive matrix molecules (MSCRAMMs) genes among clinical isolates of *Staphylococcus aureus* from hospitalized children. *Iran. J. Pathol.* **2015**, *10*, 258–264. [PubMed]
81. McCarthy, A.J.; Lindsay, J.A. Genetic variation in *Staphylococcus aureus* surface and immune evasion genes is lineage associated: Implications for vaccine design and host-pathogen interactions. *BMC Microbiol.* **2010**, *10*, 173. [CrossRef] [PubMed]
82. Kato, K.; Ishiwa, A. The role of carbohydrates in infection strategies of enteric pathogens. *Trop. Med. Health* **2015**, *43*, 41–52. [CrossRef] [PubMed]
83. Pieters, R.J. Intervention with bacterial adhesion by multivalent carbohydrates. *Med. Res. Rev.* **2007**, *27*, 796–816. [CrossRef] [PubMed]
84. Cozens, D.; Read, R.C. Anti-adhesion methods as novel therapeutics for bacterial infections. *Expert Rev. Anti-Infect. Ther.* **2012**, *10*, 1457–1468. [CrossRef] [PubMed]
85. Svensson, A.; Larsson, A.; Emtenäs, H.; Hedenström, M.; Fex, T.; Hultgren, S.J.; Pinkner, J.S.; Almqvist, F.; Kihlberg, J. Design and evaluation of pilicides: Potential novel antibacterial agents directed against uropathogenic *Escherichia coli*. *ChemBioChem* **2001**, *2*, 915–918. [CrossRef]
86. Pinkner, J.S.; Remaut, H.; Buelens, F.; Miller, E.; Aberg, V.; Pemberton, N.; Hedenstrom, M.; Larsson, A.; Seed, P.; Waksman, G.; et al. Rationally designed small compounds inhibit pilus biogenesis in uropathogenic bacteria. *Proc. Natl. Acad. Sci. USA* **2006**, *103*, 17897–17902. [CrossRef] [PubMed]
87. Chorell, E.; Pinkner, J.S.; Phan, G.; Edvinsson, S.; Buelens, F.; Remaut, H.; Waksman, G.; Hultgren, S.J.; Almqvist, F. Design and synthesis of C-2 substituted thiazolo and dihydrothiazolo ring-fused 2-pyridones: Pilicides with increased antivirulence activity. *J. Med. Chem.* **2010**, *53*, 5690–5695. [CrossRef] [PubMed]
88. Margarit, I.; Rinaudo, C.D.; Galeotti, C.L.; Maione, D.; Ghezzo, C.; Buttazzoni, E.; Rosini, R.; Runci, Y.; Mora, M.; Buccato, S.; et al. Preventing bacterial infections with pilus-based vaccines: The Group B Streptococcus paradigm. *J. Infect. Dis.* **2009**, *199*, 108–115. [CrossRef] [PubMed]
89. Li, B.; Jiang, L.; Song, Q.; Yang, J.; Chen, Z.; Guo, Z.; Zhou, D.; Du, Z.; Song, Y.; Wang, J.; et al. Protein microarray for profiling antibody responses to *Yersinia pestis* live vaccine. *Infect. Immun.* **2005**, *73*, 3734–3739. [CrossRef] [PubMed]
90. Williamson, E.D.; Flick-Smith, H.C.; LeButt, C.; Rowland, C.A.; Jones, S.M.; Waters, E.L.; Gwyther, R.J.; Miller, J.; Packer, P.J.; Irving, M. Human immune response to a plague vaccine comprising recombinant F1 and V antigens. *Infect. Immun.* **2005**, *73*, 3598–3608. [CrossRef] [PubMed]
91. Strindelius, L.; Filler, M.; Sjoholm, I. Mucosal immunization with purified flagellin from salmonella induces systemic and mucosal immune responses in C3H/HeJ mice. *Vaccine* **2004**, *22*, 3797–3808. [CrossRef] [PubMed]
92. Tchesnokova, V.; Aprikian, P.; Kisiela, D.; Gowey, S.; Korotkova, N.; Thomas, W.; Sokurenko, E. Type 1 fimbrial adhesin FimH elicits an immune response that enhances cell adhesion of *Escherichia coli*. *Infect. Immun.* **2011**, *79*, 3895–3904. [CrossRef] [PubMed]

93. Guo, Y.; Cai, S.; Gu, G.; Guo, Z.; Long, Z. Recent progress in the development of sortase A inhibitors as novel anti-bacterial virulence agents. *RSC Adv.* **2015**, *5*, 49880–49889. [CrossRef]
94. Cascioferro, S.; Cusimano, M.G.; Schillaci, D. Antiadhesion agents against gram-positive pathogens. *Future Microbiol.* **2014**, *9*, 1209–1220. [CrossRef] [PubMed]
95. Ofek, I.; Hasty, D.L.; Sharon, N. Anti-adhesion therapy of bacterial diseases: Prospects and problems. *FEMS Immunol. Med. Microbiol.* **2003**, *38*, 181–191. [CrossRef]
96. Krachler, A.M.; Orth, K. Targeting the bacteria–host interface: Strategies in anti-adhesion therapy. *Virulence* **2013**, *4*, 284–294. [CrossRef] [PubMed]
97. Sauer, K.; Camper, A.K.; Ehrlich, G.D.; Costerton, J.W.; Davies, D.G. *Pseudomonas aeruginosa* displays multiple phenotypes during development as a biofilm. *J. Bacteriol.* **2002**, *184*, 1140–1154. [CrossRef] [PubMed]
98. Vlamakis, H.; Aguilar, C.; Losick, R.; Kolter, R. Control of cell fate by the formation of an architecturally complex bacterial community. *Genes Dev.* **2008**, *22*, 945–953. [CrossRef] [PubMed]
99. Van Gestel, J.; Vlamakis, H.; Kolter, R. Division of labor in biofilms: The ecology of cell differentiation. *Microbiol. Spectr.* **2015**, *3*, MB-0002. [CrossRef] [PubMed]
100. Branda, S.S.; Vik, A.; Friedman, L.; Kolter, R. Biofilms: The matrix revisited. *Trends Microbiol.* **2005**, *13*, 20–26. [CrossRef] [PubMed]
101. Wozniak, D.J.; Wyckoff, T.J.; Starkey, M.; Keyser, R.; Azadi, P.; O'Toole, G.A.; Parsek, M.R. Alginate is not a significant component of the extracellular polysaccharide matrix of PA14 and PAO1 *Pseudomonas aeruginosa* biofilms. *Proc. Natl. Acad. Sci. USA* **2003**, *100*, 7907–7912. [CrossRef] [PubMed]
102. Ghafoor, A.; Hay, I.D.; Rehm, B.H. Role of exopolysaccharides in *Pseudomonas aeruginosa* biofilm formation and architecture. *Appl. Environ. Microbiol.* **2011**, *77*, 5238–5246. [CrossRef] [PubMed]
103. Jackson, K.D.; Starkey, M.; Kremer, S.; Parsek, M.R.; Wozniak, D.J. Identification of Psl, a locus encoding a potential exopolysaccharide that is essential for pseudomonas aeruginosa PAO1 biofilm formation. *J. Bacteriol.* **2004**, *186*, 4466–4475. [CrossRef] [PubMed]
104. Owlia, P.; Nosrati, R.; Alaghehbandan, R.; Lari, A.R. Antimicrobial susceptibility differences among mucoid and non-mucoid *Pseudomonas aeruginosa* isolates. *GMS Hyg. Infect. Control* **2014**, *9*, 2.
105. Cabral, D.A.; Loh, B.A.; Speert, D.P. Mucoid *Pseudomonas aeruginosa* resists nonopsonic phagocytosis by human neutrophils and macrophages. *Pediatr. Res.* **1987**, *22*, 429. [CrossRef] [PubMed]
106. Cywes-Bentley, C.; Skurnik, D.; Zaidi, T.; Roux, D.; DeOliveira, R.B.; Garrett, W.S.; Lu, X.; O'Malley, J.; Kinzel, K.; Zaidi, T.; et al. Antibody to a conserved antigenic target is protective against diverse prokaryotic and eukaryotic pathogens. *Proc. Natl. Acad. Sci. USA* **2013**, *110*, E2209–E2218. [CrossRef] [PubMed]
107. Arciola, C.R.; Campoccia, D.; Ravaioli, S.; Montanaro, L. Polysaccharide intercellular adhesin in biofilm: Structural and regulatory aspects. *Front. Cell. Infect. Microbiol.* **2015**, *5*, 7. [CrossRef] [PubMed]
108. Whitchurch, C.B.; Tolker-Nielsen, T.; Ragas, P.C.; Mattick, J.S. Extracellular DNA required for bacterial biofilm formation. *Science* **2002**, *295*, 1487. [CrossRef] [PubMed]
109. Wang, S.; Liu, X.; Liu, H.; Zhang, L.; Guo, Y.; Yu, S.; Wozniak, D.J.; Ma, L.Z. The exopolysaccharide Psl-eDNA interaction enables the formation of a biofilm skeleton in *Pseudomonas aeruginosa*. *Environ. Microbiol. Rep.* **2015**, *7*, 330–340. [CrossRef] [PubMed]
110. De Aldecoa, A.L.I.; Zafra, O.; González-Pastor, J.E. Mechanisms and regulation of extracellular DNA release and its biological roles in microbial communities. *Front. Microbiol.* **2017**, *8*, 1390. [CrossRef] [PubMed]
111. Rice, K.C.; Mann, E.E.; Endres, J.L.; Weiss, E.C.; Cassat, J.E.; Smeltzer, M.S.; Bayles, K.W. The *cidA* murein hydrolase regulator contributes to DNA release and biofilm development in *Staphylococcus aureus*. *Proc. Natl. Acad. Sci. USA* **2007**, *104*, 8113–8118. [CrossRef] [PubMed]
112. Sharma-Kuinkel, B.K.; Mann, E.E.; Ahn, J.-S.; Kuechenmeister, L.J.; Dunman, P.M.; Bayles, K.W. The *Staphylococcus aureus* LytSR two-component regulatory system affects biofilm formation. *J. Bacteriol.* **2009**, *191*, 4767–4775. [CrossRef] [PubMed]
113. Jurcisek, J.A.; Brockman, K.L.; Novotny, L.A.; Goodman, S.D.; Bakaletz, L.O. Nontypeable *Haemophilus influenzae*; releases DNA and DNABII proteins via a T4SS-like complex and come of the type IV pilus machinery. *Proc. Natl. Acad. Sci. USA* **2017**, *114*, E6632–E6641. [CrossRef] [PubMed]
114. Toyofuku, M.; Roschitzki, B.; Riedel, K.; Eberl, L. Identification of proteins associated with the *Pseudomonas aeruginosa* biofilm extracellular matrix. *J. Proteome Res.* **2012**, *11*, 4906–4915. [CrossRef] [PubMed]

115. Borlee, B.R.; Goldman, A.D.; Murakami, K.; Samudrala, R.; Wozniak, D.J.; Parsek, M.R. *Pseudomonas aeruginosa* uses a cyclic-di-GMP-regulated adhesin to reinforce the biofilm extracellular matrix. *Mol. Microbiol.* **2010**, *75*, 827–842. [CrossRef] [PubMed]
116. Dillon, S.C.; Dorman, C.J. Bacterial nucleoid-associated proteins, nucleoid structure and gene expression. *Nat. Rev. Microbiol.* **2010**, *8*, 185. [CrossRef] [PubMed]
117. Archer, N.K.; Mazaitis, M.J.; Costerton, J.W.; Leid, J.G.; Powers, M.E.; Shirtliff, M.E. *Staphylococcus aureus* biofilms: Properties, regulation, and roles in human disease. *Virulence* **2011**, *2*, 445–459. [CrossRef] [PubMed]
118. Wood, T.K.; Knabel, S.J.; Kwan, B.W. Bacterial persister cell formation and dormancy. *Appl. Environ. Microbiol.* **2013**, *79*, 7116–7121. [CrossRef] [PubMed]
119. Brackman, G.; Coenye, T. Quorum sensing inhibitors as anti-biofilm agents. *Curr. Pharm. Des.* **2015**, *21*, 5–11. [CrossRef] [PubMed]
120. Solano, C.; Echeverz, M.; Lasa, I. Biofilm dispersion and quorum sensing. *Curr. Opin. Microbiol.* **2014**, *18*, 96–104. [CrossRef] [PubMed]
121. Boles, B.R.; Horswill, A.R. Agr-mediated dispersal of *Staphylococcus aureus* biofilms. *PLoS Pathog.* **2008**, *4*, e1000052. [CrossRef] [PubMed]
122. LaSarre, B.; Federle, M.J. Exploiting quorum sensing to confuse bacterial pathogens. *Microbiol. Mol. Biol. Rev.* **2013**, *77*, 73–111. [CrossRef] [PubMed]
123. Dong, Y.-H.; Gusti, A.R.; Zhang, Q.; Xu, J.-L.; Zhang, L.-H. Identification of quorum-quenching N-acyl homoserine lactonases from *Bacillus* species. *Appl. Environ. Microbiol.* **2002**, *68*, 1754–1759. [CrossRef] [PubMed]
124. Lin, Y.H.; Xu, J.L.; Hu, J.; Wang, L.H.; Ong, S.L.; Leadbetter, J.R.; Zhang, L.H. Acyl-homoserine lactone acylase from Ralstonia strain XJ12B represents a novel and potent class of quorum-quenching enzymes. *Mol. Microbiol.* **2003**, *47*, 849–860. [CrossRef] [PubMed]
125. Dong, Y.-H.; Wang, L.-H.; Xu, J.-L.; Zhang, H.-B.; Zhang, X.-F.; Zhang, L.-H. Quenching quorum-sensing-dependent bacterial infection by an n-acyl homoserine lactonase. *Nature* **2001**, *411*, 813–817. [CrossRef] [PubMed]
126. Parsek, M.R. Controlling the connections of cells to the biofilm matrix. *J. Bacteriol.* **2016**, *198*, 12–14. [CrossRef] [PubMed]
127. Doudna, J.A.; Charpentier, E. The new frontier of genome engineering with CRISPR-cas9. *Science* **2014**, *346*, 1258096. [CrossRef] [PubMed]
128. Romao, S.; Memmi, G.; Oggioni, M.R.; Trombe, M.-C. LuxS impacts on LytA-dependent autolysis and on competence in *Streptococcus pneumoniae*. *Microbiology* **2006**, *152*, 333–341. [CrossRef] [PubMed]
129. Verez-Bencomo, V.; Fernández-Santana, V.; Hardy, E.; Toledo, M.E.; Rodríguez, M.C.; Heynngnezz, L.; Rodriguez, A.; Baly, A.; Herrera, L.; Izquierdo, M.; et al. A synthetic conjugate polysaccharide vaccine against *Haemophilus influenzae* type b. *Science* **2004**, *305*, 522–525. [CrossRef] [PubMed]
130. Ramsay, M.E.; Andrews, N.; Kaczmarski, E.B.; Miller, E. Efficacy of meningococcal serogroup C conjugate vaccine in teenagers and toddlers in England. *Lancet* **2001**, *357*, 195. [CrossRef]
131. Jefferson, K. What drives bacteria to produce a biofilm? *FEMS Microbiol. Lett.* **2004**, *236*, 163–173. [CrossRef] [PubMed]
132. Morgan, R.; Kohn, S.; Hwang, S.H.; Hassett, D.J.; Sauer, K. Bdla, a chemotaxis regulator essential for biofilm dispersion in *Pseudomonas aeruginosa*. *J. Bacteriol.* **2006**, *188*, 7335–7343. [CrossRef] [PubMed]
133. Hall-Stoodley, L.; Nistico, L.; Sambanthamoorthy, K.; Dice, B.; Nguyen, D.; Mershon, W.J.; Johnson, C.; Hu, F.Z.; Stoodley, P.; Ehrlich, G.D.; et al. Characterization of biofilm matrix, degradation by DNAse treatment and evidence of capsule downregulation in *Streptococcus pneumoniae* clinical isolates. *BMC Microbiol.* **2008**, *8*, 173. [CrossRef] [PubMed]
134. Tetz, G.V.; Artemenko, N.K.; Tetz, V.V. Effect of DNAse and antibiotics on biofilm characteristics. *Antimicrob. Agents Chemother.* **2009**, *53*, 1204–1209. [CrossRef] [PubMed]
135. Sun, D.; Accavitti, M.A.; Bryers, J.D. Inhibition of biofilm formation by monoclonal antibodies against *Staphylococcus epidermidis* RP62A accumulation-associated protein. *Clin. Diagn. Lab. Immunol.* **2005**, *12*, 93–100. [CrossRef] [PubMed]
136. Novotny, L.A.; Jurcisek, J.A.; Goodman, S.D.; Bakaletz, L.O. Monoclonal antibodies against DNA-binding tips of DNABII proteins disrupt biofilms in vitro and induce bacterial clearance in vivo. *EBioMedicine* **2016**, *10*, 33–44. [CrossRef] [PubMed]

137. Ray, V.A.; Hill, P.J.; Stover, K.C.; Roy, S.; Sen, C.K.; Yu, L.; Wozniak, D.J.; DiGiandomenico, A. Anti-Psl targeting of *Pseudomonas aeruginosa* biofilms for neutrophil-mediated disruption. *Sci. Rep.* **2017**, *7*, 16065. [CrossRef] [PubMed]
138. Skurnik, D.; Davis, J.M.R.; Benedetti, D.; Moravec, K.L.; Cywes-Bentley, C.; Roux, D.; Traficante, D.C.; Walsh, R.L.; Maira-Litràn, T.; Cassidy, S.K.; et al. Targeting pan-resistant bacteria with antibodies to a broadly conserved surface polysaccharide expressed during infection. *J. Infect. Dis.* **2012**, *205*, 1709–1718. [CrossRef] [PubMed]
139. Skurnik, D.; Cywes-Bentley, C.; Pier, G.B. The exceptionally broad-based potential of active and passive vaccination targeting the conserved microbial surface polysaccharide PNAG. *Expert Rev. Vaccines* **2016**, *15*, 1041–1053. [CrossRef] [PubMed]
140. Wood Thomas, K. Strategies for combating persister cell and biofilm infections. *Microb. Biotechnol.* **2017**, *10*, 1054–1056. [CrossRef] [PubMed]
141. Chua, S.L.; Liu, Y.; Yam, J.K.H.; Chen, Y.; Vejborg, R.M.; Tan, B.G.C.; Kjelleberg, S.; Tolker-Nielsen, T.; Givskov, M.; Yang, L. Dispersed cells represent a distinct stage in the transition from bacterial biofilm to planktonic lifestyles. *Nat. Commun.* **2014**, *5*, 4462. [CrossRef] [PubMed]
142. Uppuluri, P.; Lopez-Ribot, J.L. Go forth and colonize: Dispersal from clinically important microbial biofilms. *PLoS Pathog.* **2016**, *12*, e1005397. [CrossRef] [PubMed]
143. Sauer, K.; Cullen, M.C.; Rickard, A.H.; Zeef, L.A.H.; Davies, D.G.; Gilbert, P. Characterization of nutrient-induced dispersion in *Pseudomonas aeruginosa* PAO1 biofilm. *J. Bacteriol.* **2004**, *186*, 7312–7326. [CrossRef] [PubMed]
144. Kragh, K.N.; Hutchison, J.B.; Melaugh, G.; Rodesney, C.; Roberts, A.E.L.; Irie, Y.; Jensen, P.Ø.; Diggle, S.P.; Allen, R.J.; Gordon, V.; et al. Role of multicellular aggregates in biofilm formation. *mBio* **2016**, *7*, e00237-16. [CrossRef] [PubMed]
145. Jandhyala, S.M.; Talukdar, R.; Subramanyam, C.; Vuyyuru, H.; Sasikala, M.; Reddy, D.N. Role of the normal gut microbiota. *World J. Gastroenterol.* **2015**, *21*, 8787–8803. [CrossRef] [PubMed]

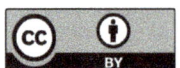

© 2018 by the authors. Licensee MDPI, Basel, Switzerland. This article is an open access article distributed under the terms and conditions of the Creative Commons Attribution (CC BY) license (http://creativecommons.org/licenses/by/4.0/).

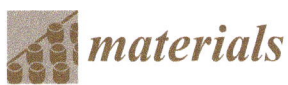

Article

Candida auris Dry Surface Biofilm (DSB) for Disinfectant Efficacy Testing

Katarzyna Ledwoch and Jean-Yves Maillard *

School of Pharmacy and Pharmaceutical Sciences, Cardiff University, Cardiff CF10 3NB, UK; LedwochK@cardiff.ac.uk
* Correspondence: MaillardJ@cardiff.ac.uk; Tel.: +44(0)-292-0879-088

Received: 20 November 2018; Accepted: 14 December 2018; Published: 21 December 2018

Abstract: *Candida auris* is an emerging pathogen that needs to be controlled effectively due to its association with a high mortality rate. The presence of biofilms on dry surfaces has been shown to be widespread in healthcare settings. We produced a *C. auris* dry surface biofilm (DSB) on stainless steel surfaces following sequential hydration and desiccation cycles for 12 days. The ASTM2967-15 was used to measure the reduction in viability of 12 commercially wipe-based disinfectants and sodium hypochlorite (1000 ppm) against *C. auris* DSB. We also evaluated *C. auris* transferability and biofilm regrowth post-treatment. A peracetic acid (3500 ppm) product and two chlorine-based products (1000 ppm available chlorine) were successful in reducing *C. auris* viability and delaying DSB regrowth. However, 50% of the products tested failed to decrease *C. auris* viability, 58% failed to prevent its transferability, and 75% did not delay biofilm regrowth. Using three different parameters to measure product efficacy provided a practical evaluation of product effectiveness against *C. auris* DSB. Although $\log_{10}$ reduction in viability is traditionally measured, transferability is an important factor to consider from an infection control and prevention point of view as it allows for determination of whether the surface is safe to touch by patients and hospital staff post-treatment.

Keywords: *Candida auris*; dry-biofilm; disinfection; peracetic acid; sodium hypochlorite; chlorine dioxide; sodium dichloroisocyanurate; transferability; regrowth

---

1. Introduction

Candida auris was first isolated and identified in Japan in 2009 [1]. *C. auris* is an emerging pathogen responsible for many life-threating infections and it can be associated with high mortality rates [2]. *C. auris* infections are difficult to treat mostly due to the unpredictable resistance profile of the yeast to anti-fungal agents, frequent misidentification, non-aggregative phenotype, and its ability to form biofilm [3]. Higher risk of candidemia occurs in immunocompromised patients, patients that have undergone antibiotic or anti-fungal therapy, patients after surgeries, and patients with central venous catheters [4].

Contaminated surfaces in healthcare settings contribute to the transmission of infectious diseases [5–7]. Vickery and colleagues [8] showed that pathogens embedded in dry surface biofilms (DSB) remain on hospital surfaces despite rigorous surface decontamination. The widespread presence of dry surface biofilms on healthcare surfaces has now been established [9,10]. *C. auris* can persist on surfaces for weeks [11,12] and transmission of *C. auris* in healthcare settings have been reported [2,4,13,14]. The elimination of *C. auris* from surfaces is therefore important to consider. However, not many studies have investigated the effectiveness of disinfectants against *C. auris* [15]. Public Health England guidance [16] for the management and infection prevention and control of *C. auris* recommends using hypochlorite at 1000 ppm available chlorine to terminally clean room or bed space after the discharge of a *C. auris* infected or colonized patient. Not surprisingly, the majority of efficacy studies against *C. auris* relates to chlorine-releasing agents [14,17–19], although other biocides have been considered, such as quaternary ammonium compounds [14,18], acetic acid [18], peracetic acid [19], and hydrogen peroxide [17]. All these studies but one studied planktonic (suspension of) *C. auris* [20]. None of these studies investigated the transferability of *C. auris* to other surfaces post-treatment. Here, we investigated the efficacy of 12 commercially available products and sodium hypochlorite 1000 ppm against *C. auris* DSB using a modified product efficacy test protocol ASTM2967-15 [21] to measure decreases in viability, transferability, and biofilm regrowth post-treatment. The evaluation of three different parameters provides a better and more practical understanding of product efficacy against this pathogen.

2. Materials and Methods

C. auris Growth and Maintenance

C. auris (DSM 21092) was propagated overnight in malt extract broth (MEB, Oxoid, Thermo Scientific™, Loughborough, UK) at 25 °C and the pellet was re-suspended in MEB following centrifugation at $1200\times g$. The yeast suspension was adjusted to 1×10^6 CFU/mL.

C. auris Organic Load (OL) Dry-Biofilm Model

The *C. auris* DSB model is based on a recently developed *Staphylococcus aureus* DSB protocol [22]. Briefly, dry-biofilm formation consists of alternating hydration and desiccation phases in the presence of an organic load (OL). Stainless steel AISI 430 discs (0.7 ± 0.07 mm thickness; 10 ± 0.5 mm diameter, Goodfellow Cambridge Limited, Huntington, UK) were used as support. Sterile discs were placed in wells of a Corning™ Costar™ flat-bottom cell culture plates (Fisher Scientific™, Loughborough, UK), containing 1 mL of MEB with 5% anhydrous D-glucose (Fisher Scientific, Loughborough, UK), 3 g/L bovine serum albumin (BSA; Sigma® Life Science, Dorset, UK), and 10^6 CFU/mL washed *C. auris* suspension. Yeasts were first allowed to attach and form a biofilm on the disc surface for 2 days at 25 °C under gentle agitation using an Orbit P4 plate rocker (Labnet International, Edison, NJ, USA). The suspension was then drained from the wells, and plates were incubated at 25 °C for 48 h. Following this dry phase, 1 mL of MEB with 3 g/L BSA was added to each well, and a new hydrated phase began for 48 h. Hydrated and dry phases alternated every 48 h for a period of 12 days, ending with biofilm in a dry phase.

Scanning Electron Microscopy (SEM) Imaging

C. auris DSB samples were prepared by overnight incubation of discs in a 2.5% glutaraldehyde solution (ACROS Organics™, Fisher Scientific, Loughborough, UK) followed by immersion in successive concentrations of 10%, 25%, 50%, 70%, 90%, and 100% ethanol (Honeywell, Fisher Scientific Ltd., Loughborough, UK) for 10 min each. Prior to scanning electron microscopy (SEM, Carl Zeiss Ltd., Cambridge, UK) scanning, samples were coated with 20 nm of AuPd coating with a sputter coater (SC500, Biorad, UK). Secondary electron images were acquired with a beam energy of 5 kV using an in-lens detector on a Sigma HD Field Emission Gun Scanning Electron Microscope (Carl Zeiss Ltd., Cambridge, UK) at $\times 2000$ and $\times 10,000$ magnification and a 5 mm working distance. SEM images were false-colored to help visualization and contrast using GNU Image manipulation program (GIMP 2.8) software. Images were not otherwise altered.

Product Tested

The effectiveness of four commercially available wipes and eight commercially available liquid disinfectants was tested against *C. auris* OL dry-biofilm (Table 1). Disinfectants were prepared according to manufacturers' instructions and combined with Rubbermaid® HYGEN™ disposable microfiber cloth (Rubbermaid Products, Surrey, UK), allowing 2.5 mL of disinfectant per 1 g of wipe. Wipes were cut into 3×3 cm^2 squares prior to testing.

Table 1. Disinfectants tested.

Abbreviation	Main Active Ingredient [1]	Excipients (from MSDS) [1]	Concentration of the Main Active Ingredient [4]	pH [5]	Mechanism of Disinfectant Action [6]	Wipe Material
BZK	Benzalkonium chloride, polyhexamethylene biguanide (PHMB)	Didecyl dimethyl ammonium chloride	< 0.5% (<5000 ppm)	5.41	Membrane active agents; damage cytoplasmic membrane and increase permeability [23]	Non-Woven Wipe [7]
ClO_2-1	Chlorine dioxide	Sodium chlorite, sodium dodecyl sulphate, sodium carbonate, citric acid, sodium dichloroisocyanurate	300 ppm	5.05	Affect membrane permeability of the membrane and inhibits cellular respiration [23]	Microfiber cloth [8]
ClO_2-2	Chlorine dioxide	Not mentioned	1000 ppm	4.31		Microfiber cloth [8]
NaDCC-1	Sodium dichloroisocyanurate	Adipic acid, arylsulfonates, sodium fatty acid sarcosides	1000 ppm	6.31		Microfiber cloth [8]
NaDCC-2	Sodium dichloroisocyanurate	Adipic acid, sodium toluene sulphonate, sodium n-lauroylsarcosinate	1000 ppm	5.93	Permeabilization of the cytoplasmic membrane [24], progressive oxidation of thiol groups to disulphides [25] and deleterious effects on DNA synthesis [26]	Microfiber cloth [8]
NaDCC-3	Sodium dichloroisocyanurate	Sulfonic acid	10,000 ppm	5.77		Non-woven wipe [9]
NaDCC-4	Sodium dichloroisocyanurate	Adipic acid, sodium carbonate	1000 ppm	5.86		Microfiber cloth [8]
NaDCC-5	Sodium dichloroisocyanurate	Adipic acid, sodium toluenesulphonate, sodium N-lauroyl sarcosinate	1000 ppm	5.64		Microfiber cloth [8]
NaOCl-Ref	Sodium hypochlorite	N/A	1000 ppm	11.31		Microfiber cloth [8]
NaOCl-2	Sodium hypochlorite	Sodium hydroxide, sodium chloride	500 ppm	8.68	Biosynthetic alterations in cellular metabolism [27], phospholipid degradation, irreversible enzymatic inactivation in bacteria, lipid and fatty acid degradation [28]	Non-woven wipe [7]
NaOCl-3	Sodium hypochlorite	phosphoric acid (trisodium salt, dodecahydrate), sodium hydroxide, phosphoric acid	1000 ppm	13.13		Non-woven wipe [7]
PAA-1	Peracetic acid	sodium percarbonate, citric acid	3500 ppm	8.82	Rupture or dislocation of cell wall, disruption of biochemical processes intercellularly [29] and impairment of DNA replication [30]	Non-woven wipe [9]
PAA-2	Peracetic acid	Not mentioned	250 ppm	7.74		Microfibre cloth [8]
Water [3]	N/A	N/A	N/A	6.99	N/A	Microfibre cloth [8]

[1]: Main active ingredient and excipients mentioned in the MSDS information of the commercial products used in this study. [2]: Unformulated sodium hypochlorite (1000 ppm), used as reference. [3]: Sterile deionized water. [4]: Concentration of available chlorine/peracetic acid concentration was measured with Pocket Colorimeter™ (HACH®, Manchester, UK) (regardless of the product claim on label) via the N, N-diethyl-p-phenylenediamine (DPD) method. [5]: pH was measured by bench top pH meter (HANNA® Instruments, Leighton Buzzard, UK). [6]: Reported mechanisms of action, mainly from studies of bacteria. [7]: Wipe originally moisturized with disinfectant by the manufacturer. [8]: Disinfectant prepared according to manufacturer's instruction and then placed on Rubbermaid® HYGEN™ disposable microfibre cloth (2.5 mL of liquid per 1 g of cloth). [9]: Dry non-woven wipe impregnated with powder particles—needs to be wetted according to manufacturer instructions prior to use.

ASTM E2967-15 Test

Disinfection tests were performed according to a modified ASTM E2967-15 test [21]. Briefly, DSB were wiped with the Wiperator (Filtaflex Ltd., Almonte, Ontario, Canada) from both sides for 10 s under 500 g pressure, left for 2 min at 25 °C, and then neutralized in Dey-Engley neutralizing (DE) broth (Neogen® Corporation, Ayr, UK). Transfer of viable yeasts from used wipes to clean sterile disc was not performed.

Reduction in Viability for Yeasts Embedded in Dry Biofilms

Following wiping, samples were incubated for 1 h at 25 °C in 2 mL DE with 100 µg/mL proteinase K (Fisher Bioreagents™, Fisher Scientific, Loughborough, UK) and 1 g of glass beads (Fisher Scientific, Loughborough, UK). After incubation, samples were vortexed for 2 min and then serially diluted, and 3 × 10 µL^2 drops of each dilution was plated onto tryptone soya agar (TSA; Oxoid, Thermo Fisher Scientific, Newport, UK). Reduction in yeast viability, expressed as a $\log_{10}$ reduction, was calculated as the difference between the number of yeasts recovered from untreated (control) and treated samples.

Transferability Test

Following wiping, discs were pressed 36 separate times with 100 g pressure on the surface of DE agar. Following the transfer test, DE agar was incubated at 25 °C for a up to 5 days until colonies appeared. Positive growth/adpression was recorded, and transferability was calculated as the number of positive contact/number of adpressions.

Dry-Biofilm Regrowth

Following wiping, discs were placed in 30 mL capacity flat bottom glass bottle with 2 mL of DE broth. The number of days for turbidity change, which is indicative of growth, was recorded. Samples were plated on TSA to confirm yeast growth and purity.

Statistical Analysis

The statistical significance of data sets was evaluated with GraphPad PRISM® (version 7.04, GraphPad Software, San Diego, CA, USA) using two- and one-way Analysis of Variance (ANOVA). All experiments were performed in triplicates in three independent biological replicates unless otherwise stated. The sample standard deviation was evaluated with Bassel's correction.

3. Results

SEM Analysis of C. auris Dry Surface Biofilm

C. auris formed a thin biofilm that was evenly scattered throughout the stainless-steel disc surface with no evidence of extracellular polymeric substances (Figure 1). There was no statistically significant difference (two-way ANOVA, $p = 0.06$) in viable count of yeasts ($\log_{10}$ CFU/mL = 7.8 ± 0.3) recovered from each disc between four independent biofilm batches.

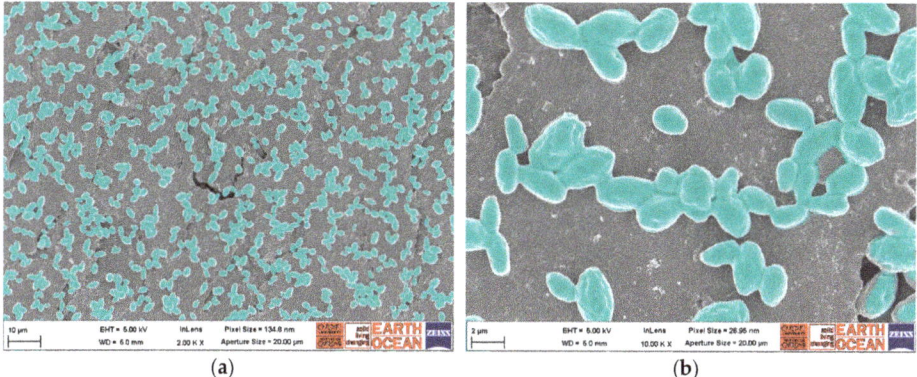

Figure 1. Scanning electron microscope images of *C. auris* organic load (OL) dry surface biofilm: (**a**) ×2000 magnification; (**b**) ×10,000 magnification. The images presented are representative for the whole disc surface. Observations were made on three independent triplicates of *C. auris* dry-biofilm, and whole disc surface (~0.8 cm^2) was investigated each time with ×500 magnification. Images of dry surface biofilm (DSB) were colored in green to help visualization and contrast using GNU Image manipulation program (GIMP 2.8) software. Images were not otherwise altered.

Product Efficacy

The most effective treatments including PAA-1 (3500 ppm), NaDCC-5 (1000 ppm), NaOCl-Ref (1000 ppm), and NaOCl-3 (1000 ppm) removed or killed more than 7 log$_{10}$ of *C. auris* embedded in DSB (Figure 2). Peracetic acid at 3500 ppm combined with a non-woven wipe was significantly (one-way ANOVA, $p < 0.05$) more effective in biofilm eradication than PAA at 250 ppm combined with a microfiber cloth (0.84 ± 0.11 log$_{10}$ reduction). NaDCC-5 was the most effective (two-way ANOVA, $p < 0.05$) in killing or removing *C. auris* DSB compared to the other NaDCC-based products that all failed to produce a 4 log$_{10}$ reduction in viability (Figure 2). Chlorine-dioxide-based products overall did not perform very well, achieving less than 2.5 log$_{10}$ reduction even with ClO$_2$-2 containing a higher concentration (1000 ppm) of available chlorine (Figure 2). There was no difference (one-way ANOVA, $p = 0.22$) in activity between ClO$_2$-1 and ClO$_2$-2. Overall, half of the products tested (ClO$_2$-1, NaDCC-2, and NaOCl-2) showed either a similar performance (one-way ANOVA, $p > 0.05$) to water combined with the microfiber cloth or performed worse (one-way ANOVA, $p < 0.05$) than water combined with the microfiber cloth (ClO$_2$-2, NaDCC-3, and PAA-2).

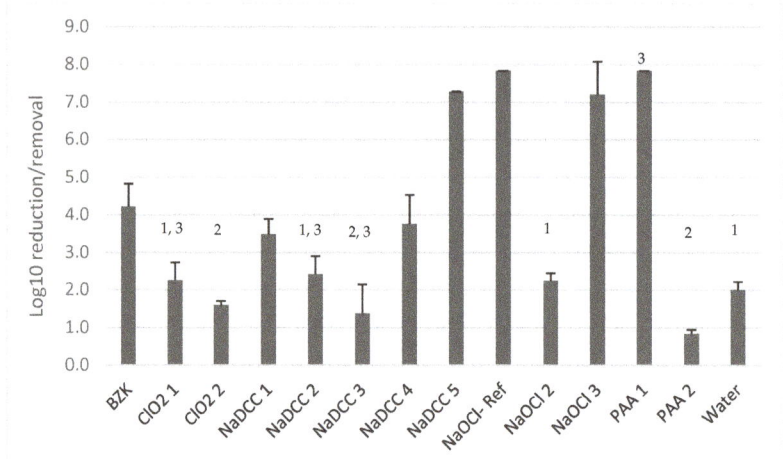

Figure 2. Product efficacy in killing/removing *C. auris* embedded in a DSB. 1: indicates no statistical difference (one-way ANOVA, $p > 0.05$) in $\log_{10}$ reduction/removal from surfaces; 2: $\log_{10}$ reduction/removal lower than wiping with water (one-way ANOVA, $p < 0.05$); and 3: indicates that only two biological replicates were performed.

Only two products, PAA-1 and NaOCl-3, prevented *C. auris* transfer after treatment (Figure 3). Seven out of 12 commercially available disinfectants were not effective in lowering the transferability of *C. auris* from DSB post-wiping. For four product/materials combinations (ClO$_2$-2, NaDCC-2, NaDCC-3, and NaOCl-1), there was no statistically significant difference (one-way ANOVA, for each pair $p > 0.05$) between their performance and that of water (Figure 3). The remaining three treatments (NaDCC-4, NaOCl-2 and PAA-2) were even less effective than wiping with water (one-way ANOVA, for each pair $p < 0.05$).

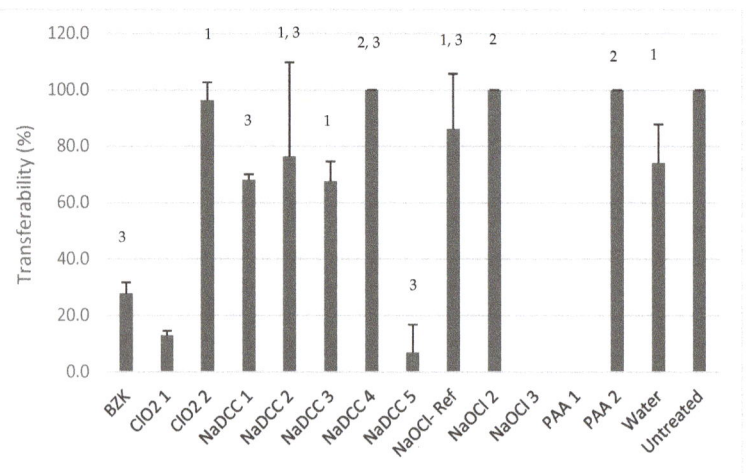

Figure 3. Product efficacy in preventing *C. auris* transferability post-wiping. 1: indicates no statistical difference (one-way ANOVA, for each pair $p > 0.05$) in transferability; 2: higher transferability (one-way ANOVA, for each pair $p < 0.05$) than with water control; and 3: indicates that only two biological replicates were performed.

The best commercial products, NaDCC-3, NaDCC-5, and PAA-1, delayed the recovery of biofilm post-treatment for more than 4 days (5.0 ± 0.0, 4.7 ± 1.2 and 6.5 ± 2.1 days, respectively; Figure 4). Such activity was similar (two-way ANOVA, $p = 0.53$) to NaOCl-Ref which delayed regrowth by 4.5 ± 0.7 days. Nine out of 12 commercial treatments failed to prevent the regrowth of *C. auris* DSB for more than 2 days (Figure 4).

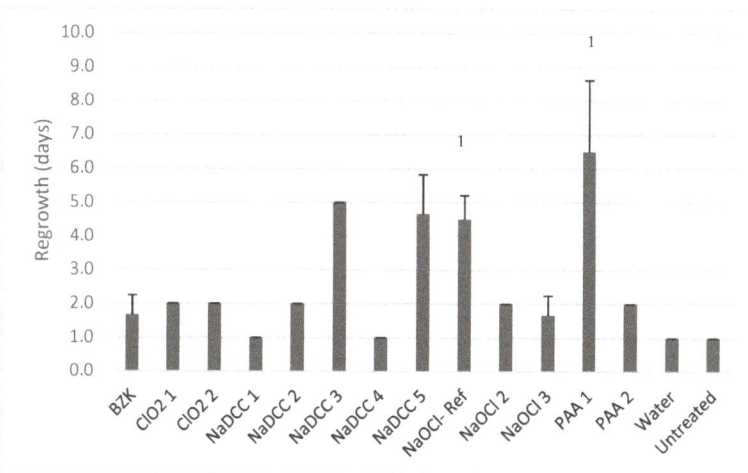

Figure 4. Efficacy of products in preventing regrowth post-wiping. 1: indicates that only two biological replicates were performed.

The less-reactive chemistry (as compared to the oxidizing chemistries) based on a quaternary ammonium compound produced a 4 $\log_{10}$ reduction in *C. auris* on surfaces and reduced transferability post-wiping to 20%.

4. Discussion

Environmental surfaces play an important role in the transmission of infection [5,6]. Infection control regimens include the combination of cleaning and disinfection processes [16] and are often based on the use of a disinfectant or cleaner combined with diverse materials [31]. Performance of biocidal products still relies, however, on testing the efficacy of the formulation and not the combination of formulation and material [22]. A number of US-based protocols to test wipe activity have been described, but all had severe limitations in their setting or performance [31]. Recently, the ASTM2967-15 and the EN16615-15 protocols [32] have been recommended for evaluating the efficacy of antimicrobial wipes, although EN16615-15 has recently been shown to lack stringency [33]. Both tests evaluate the reduction in microbial number from the test surface and the transfer of micro-organisms during wiping. Attaining a > 5$\log_{10}$ reduction in microbial inoculum following treatment has been, until now, deemed to provide enough assurance that all micro-organisms would be killed on surfaces in practice. Although this might be the case where surfaces are contaminated with a low number of microorganisms, this might not be correct with surfaces contaminated with a high number of microorganisms or when dry surface biofilms are present. Hence, the evaluation of microbial transferability post-treatment is important to take into consideration to provide reassurance that a surface would be safe to touch. The presence of DSB on healthcare surfaces has been established [8–10], and the resilience of DSB to disinfection has been described [8]. The presence of *C. auris* DSB has not been yet established in healthcare settings, although its persistence in healthcare settings has been described [11,12].

Here, we have successfully produced reproducible dry surface biofilms of *C. auris* on stainless steel surfaces, for which appearance and characteristics are not dissimilar to artificial DSB of *Staphylococcus* aureus (Ledwoch, Said and Maillard, unpublished results) or DSB isolated from endoscopes [34]. These dry surface biofilms of *C. auris* provided a platform for testing the efficacy of commercially available wipe-based products or formulation combined with a microfiber cloth. Here, we observed that the majority of commercially available chlorine-releasing agents widely used by hospitals do not effectively eradicate a *C. auris* DSB or lower its transferability. The ability of *C. auris* to form dry surface biofilm on surfaces contribute somewhat to its resistance against disinfection. We showed that *C. auris* inactivation was product dependent. NaOCl-containing products are widely used in healthcare settings, although the efficacy of NaOCl against *C. auris* dried on surfaces differs in the literature. While only 2.5–3 $\log_{10}$ of *C. auris* were killed by NaOCl (1000 ppm) within 5 min [20], a 3000 ppm NaOCl solution resulted in reducing *C. auris* dried on surfaces for 2 h by 6 $\log_{10}$ in 1 min [18]. An 8000 ppm NaOCl solution, however, produced a 6 $\log_{10}$ reduction in 10 min for *C. auris* dried on surfaces for 1 h [14]. Here, NaOCl-Ref (1000 ppm) and NaOCl-3 (1000 ppm) produced a 7 $\log_{10}$ reduction in number within 2 min following wiping.

The microfiber cloth loaded with sterile water enabled the removal of *C. auris* (2 $\log_{10}$ reduction) but failed to prevent transfer or biofilm re-growth post wiping. Interestingly, a number of products performed similarly to water, indicating either that the combination with the Rubbermaid® HYGEN™ disposable microfiber cloth was incompatible with the product formulation, or that the product activity was caused by the material only. Wesgate et al. [33] recently showed that the type of material might have a small impact on the formulation presumably because the concentration of the active ingredient was high. In this study, it was interesting to observe that lower concentration and, possibly, the type of material affected the efficacy of peracetic acid and NaOCl. It has also been reported that the formulation itself impacts activity [35]. Here, different NaOCl formulations produced different results. While the use of unformulated NaOCl (NaOCl-Ref) was effective in reducing counts of *C. auris* on surfaces and prolonged biofilm regrowth, it failed to prevent *C. auris* transfer. The formulated NaOCl product (NaOCl-3) containing the same concentration of available chlorine produced a high reduction in count, thus preventing transfer but was less efficacious in delaying biofilm regrowth. NaOCl-2 containing a lower concentration of available chlorine was not effective in reducing *C. auris* count, preventing transfer, or delaying regrowth. The impact of formulation is also evident with NaDCC-based products. Overall, the peracetic acid wipe product containing 3500 ppm of PAA performed the best against *C. auris* DSB.

5. Conclusions

We successfully developed a dry surface biofilm in vitro model of *C. auris*. Although *C. auris* has not yet been isolated from environmental DSB, its presence on surfaces and associated high pathogenicity highlights the need to select an efficient infection control regimen. The use of a product efficacy test such as ASTM2967-15 is essential to evaluate the efficacy of formulated products. The additional evaluation of transferability of microorganisms post-wiping provides important information on a product's overall efficacy as well as reassurance that surfaces are safe to touch post-treatment. Here, we observed that measuring $\log_{10}$ reduction in viability was not enough to discriminate between product efficacy. Importantly, we observed that a number of commercially-available formulations combined with a microfiber cloth, or products, failed to control dry surface biofilms of *C. auris*. It was also clear that high concentration and an appropriate formulation of the active ingredient was key for efficacy, with the PAA-based product performing better.

Author Contributions: Conceptualization, J.-Y.M.; Data Curation, K.L.; Formal Analysis, K.L.; Funding Acquisition, J.-Y.M.; Investigation, K.L. and J.-Y.M.; Methodology, K.L.; Project Administration, J.-Y.M.; Supervision, J.-Y.M.; Writing–Original Draft, K.L.; Writing–Review & Editing, J.-Y.M.

Funding: This research was funded by GAMA Healthcare Ltd.

Acknowledgments: The authors wish to acknowledge D.D. Duncan for his help with SEM imaging

Conflicts of Interest: K. Ledwoch is partially funded by GAMA Healthcare Ltd.

References

1. Satoh, K.; Makimura, K.; Hasumi, Y.; Nishiyama, Y.; Uchida, K.; Yamaguchi, H. *Candida auris* sp. nov., a novel ascomycetous yeast isolated from the external ear canal of an inpatient in a Japanese hospital. *Microbiol. Immunol.* **2009**, *53*, 41–44. [CrossRef]
2. Araúz, A.B.; Caceres, D.H.; Santiago, E.; Armstrong, P.; Arosemena, S.; Ramos, C.; Espinosa-Bode, A.; Borace, J.; Hayer, L.; Cedeño, I.; et al. Isolation of Candida auris from 9 patients in Central America: Importance of accurate diagnosis and susceptibility testing. *Mycoses* **2018**, *61*, 44–47. [CrossRef]
3. Morales-López, S.E.; Parra-Giraldo, C.M.; Ceballos-Garzón, A.; Martínez, H.P.; Rodríguez, G.J.; Álvarez-Moreno, C.A.; Rodríguez, J.Y. Invasive Infections with Multidrug-Resistant Yeast Candida auris, Colombia. *Emerg. Infect. Dis.* **2017**, *23*, 162. [CrossRef]
4. Calvo, B.; Melo, A.S.A.; Perozo-Mena, A.; Hernandez, M.; Francisco, E.C.; Hagen, F.; Meis, J.F.; Colombo, A.L. First report of *Candida auris* in America: Clinical and microbiological aspects of 18 episodes of candidemia. *J. Infect.* **2016**, *73*, 369–374. [CrossRef]
5. Weber, D.J.; Rutala, W.A.; Miller, M.B.; Huslage, K.; Sickbert-Bennett, E. Role of hospital surfaces in the transmission of emerging healthcare associated pathogens: Norovirus, *Clostridium difficile*, and *Acinetobacter* species. *Am. J. Infect. Control* **2010**, *38*, S25–S33. [CrossRef] [PubMed]
6. Weber, D.J.; Anderson, D.; Rutala, W.A. The role of the surface environment in healthcare-associated infections. *Curr. Opin. Infect. Dis.* **2013**, *26*, 338–344. [CrossRef]
7. Otter, J.A.; Yezli, S.; Salkeld, J.A.G.; French, G.L. Evidence that contaminated surfaces contribute to the transmission of hospital pathogens and an overview of strategies to address contaminated surfaces in hospital settings. *Am. J. Infect. Control* **2013**, *41*, S6–S11. [CrossRef] [PubMed]
8. Vickery, K.; Deva, A.; Jacombs, A.; Allan, J.; Valente, P.; Gosbell, I.B. Presence of biofilm containing viable multiresistant organisms despite terminal cleaning on clinical surfaces in an intensive care unit. *J. Hosp. Infect.* **2012**, *80*, 52–55. [CrossRef] [PubMed]
9. Hu, H.; Johani, K.; Gosbell, I.B.; Jacombs, A.S.W.; Almatroudi, A.; Whiteley, G.S.; Deva, A.K.; Jensen, S.; Vickery, K. Intensive care unit environmental surfaces are contaminated by multidrug-resistant bacteria in biofilms: Combined results of conventional culture, pyrosequencing, scanning electron microscopy, and confocal laser microscopy. *J. Hosp. Infect.* **2015**, *91*, 35–44. [CrossRef]
10. Ledwoch, K.; Dancer, S.J.; Otter, J.A.; Kerr, K.; Roposte, D.; Rushton, L.; Weiser, R.; Mahenthiralingam, E.; Muir, D.D.; Maillard, J.-Y. Beware biofilm! Dry biofilms containing bacterial pathogens on multiple healthcare surfaces; a multi-centre study. *J. Hosp. Infect.* **2018**, *100*, 47–56. [CrossRef]
11. Piedrahita, C.T.; Cadnum, J.L.; Jencson, A.L.; Shaikh, A.A.; Ghannoum, M.A.; Donskey, C.J. Environmental surfaces in healthcare facilities are a potential source for transmission of *Candida auris* and other *Candida* species. *Infect. Control Hosp. Epidemiol.* **2017**, *38*, 1107–1109. [CrossRef] [PubMed]
12. Welsh, R.M.; Bentz, M.L.; Shams, A.; Houston, H.; Lyons, A.; Rose, L.; Litvintseva, A.P. Survival, persistence, and isolation of the emerging multidrug-resistant pathogenic yeast *Candida auris* on a plastic health care surface. *J. Clin. Microbiol.* **2017**, *55*, 2996–3005. [CrossRef] [PubMed]
13. Vallabhaneni, S.; Kallen, A.; Tsay, S.; Chow, N.; Welsh, R.; Kerins, J.; Kemble, S.K.; Pacilli, M.; Black, S.R.; Landon, E.; et al. Investigation of the first seven reported cases of *Candida auris*, a globally emerging invasive, multidrug-resistant fungus-United States, May 2013–August 2016. *Am. J. Transplant.* **2017**, *17*, 296–299. [CrossRef] [PubMed]
14. Biswal, M.; Rudramurthy, S.M.; Jain, N.; Shamanth, A.S.; Sharma, D.; Jain, K.; Yaddanapudi, L.N.; Chakrabarti, A. Controlling a possible outbreak of *Candida auris* infection: Lessons learnt from multiple interventions. *J. Hosp. Infect.* **2017**, *97*, 363–370. [CrossRef] [PubMed]
15. Ku, T.S.N.; Walraven, C.J.; Lee, S.A. *Candida auris*: Disinfectants and implications for infection control. *Front. Microbiol.* **2018**, *9*, 1–12. [CrossRef] [PubMed]
16. *Guidance for the Laboratory Investigation, Management and Infection Prevention and Control for Cases of Candida auris (August 2017 v2.0)*; Public Health England: London, UK, 2016; PHE publications gateway number: 2016122.
17. Abdolrasouli, A.; Armstrong-James, D.; Ryan, L.; Schelenz, S. In vitro efficacy of disinfectants utilised for skin decolonization and environmental decontamination during a hospital outbreak with *Candida auris*. *Mycoses* **2017**, *60*, 758–763. [CrossRef] [PubMed]

18. Cadnum, J.L.; Shaikh, A.A.; Piedrahita, C.T.; Sankar, T.; Jencson, A.L.; Larkin, E.L.; Ghannoum, M.A.; Donskey, C.J. Effectiveness of disinfectants against *Candida auris* and other *Candida* species. *Infect. Control Hosp. Epidemiol.* **2017**, *38*, 1240–1243. [CrossRef] [PubMed]
19. Moore, G.; Schelenz, S.; Borman, A.M.; Johnson, E.M.; Brown, C.S. Yeasticidal activity of chemical disinfectants and antiseptics against *Candida auris*. *J. Hosp. Infect.* **2017**, *97*, 371–375. [CrossRef]
20. Kean, R.; Sherry, L.; Townsend, E.; McKloud, E.; Short, B.; Akinbobola, A.; Mackay, W.G.; Williams, C.; Jones, B.L.; Ramage, G. Surface disinfection challenges for *Candida auris*: An in vitro study. *J. Hosp. Infect.* **2018**, *98*, 433–436. [CrossRef]
21. *ASTM E2967-15 Standard Test Method for Assessing the Ability of Pre-wetted Towelettes to Remove and Transfer Bacterial Contamination on Hard, Non-Porous Environmental Surfaces Using the Wiperator*; ASTM: West Conshohocken, PA, USA, 2015.
22. Ledwoch, K.; Said, J.; Maillard, J.-Y. Artificial dry-biofilm models for disinfectant efficacy testing. *Lett. Appl. Microbiol.* **2018**, under review.
23. Maris, P. Modes of action of disinfectants. *Rev. Sci. Tech.* **1995**, *14*, 47–55. [CrossRef]
24. Virto, R.; Mañas, P.; Álvarez, I.; Condon, S.; Raso, J. Membrane damage and microbial inactivation by chlorine in the absence and presence of a chlorine-demanding substrate. *Appl. Environ. Microbiol.* **2005**, *71*, 5022–5028. [CrossRef] [PubMed]
25. Russell, A.D. Microbial sensitivity and resistance to chemical and physical agents. In *Topley and Wilson's Microbiology and Microbial Infections*, 9th ed.; Edward Arnold: London, UK, 1998; pp. 149–184.
26. McDonnell, G.; Russell, A.D. Antiseptics and disinfectants: Activity, action and resistance. *Clin. Microbiol. Rev.* **1999**, *12*, 147–179. [CrossRef] [PubMed]
27. Estrela, C.; Estrela, C.R.A.; Barbin, E.L.; Spanó, J.C.E.; Marchesan, M.A.; Pécora, J.D. Mechanism of action of sodium hypochlorite. *Braz. Dent. J.* **2002**, *13*, 113–117. [CrossRef] [PubMed]
28. Block, S.S. *Disinfection, Sterilization and Preservation*, 4th ed.; Lea & Febiger Press: Philadelphia, PA, USA, 1991.
29. Kitis, M. Disinfection of wastewater with peracetic acid: A review. *Environ. Int.* **2004**, *30*, 47–54. [CrossRef]
30. Tutumi, M.; Imamura, K.; Hatano, S.; Watanabe, T. Antimicrobial action of peracetic acid. *J. Food Hyg. Soc. Jpn.* **1973**, *14*, 443–447. [CrossRef]
31. Sattar, S.A.; Maillard, J.Y. The crucial role of wiping in decontamination of high-touch environmental surfaces: Review of current status and directions for the future. *Am. J. Infect. Control* **2013**, *41*, S97–S104. [CrossRef]
32. *Chemical Disinfectants and Antiseptics-Quantitative Test Method for The Evaluation of Bactericidal and Yeasticidal Activity on Non-Porous Surfaces with Mechanical Action Employing Wipes in the Medical Area (4-Field Test)*; British Standards Institute: London, UK, 2015.
33. Wesgate, R.; Robertson, A.; Barrell, M.; Tesca, P.; Maillard, J.-Y. Impact of test protocols and material binding on antimicrobial wipes efficacy. *J. Hosp. Infect.* **2018**, in press. [CrossRef]
34. Pajkos, A.; Vickery, K.; Cossart, Y. Is biofilm accumulation on endoscope tubing a contributor to the failure of cleaning and decontamination? *J. Hosp. Infect.* **2004**, *58*, 224–229. [CrossRef]
35. Forbes, S.; Cowley, N.; Humphreys, G.; Mistry, H.; Amézquita, A.; McBain, A.J. Formulation of biocides increases antimicrobial potency and mitigates the enrichment of nonsusceptible bacteria in multispecies biofilms. *Appl. Environ. Microbiol.* **2017**, *83*, AEM.03054-16. [CrossRef]

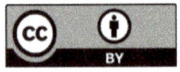

© 2018 by the authors. Licensee MDPI, Basel, Switzerland. This article is an open access article distributed under the terms and conditions of the Creative Commons Attribution (CC BY) license (http://creativecommons.org/licenses/by/4.0/).

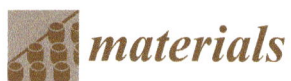

Review

Targeting the Bacterial Protective Armour; Challenges and Novel Strategies in the Treatment of Microbial Biofilm

Nor Fadhilah Kamaruzzaman [1,*], Li Peng Tan [1], Khairun Anisa Mat Yazid [1], Shamsaldeen Ibrahim Saeed [1], Ruhil Hayati Hamdan [1], Siew Shean Choong [1], Weng Kin Wong [2], Alexandru Chivu [3] and Amanda Jane Gibson [4]

1. Faculty of Veterinary Medicine, Universiti Malaysia Kelantan, Pengkalan Chepa 16100, Kelantan, Malaysia; li.peng@umk.edu.my (L.P.T.); anisa932@gmail.com (K.A.M.Y.); Shams88ns@gmail.com (S.I.S.); ruhil@umk.edu.my (R.H.H.); shean.cs@umk.edu.my (S.S.C.)
2. School of Health Sciences, Universiti Sains Malaysia, Kubang Kerian 16150, Kelantan, Malaysia; wengkinwong@usm.my
3. UCL Centre for Nanotechnology and Regenerative Medicine, Division of Surgery & Interventional Science, University College London, London NW3 2PF, UK; a.chivu.14@ucl.ac.uk
4. Royal Veterinary College, Pathobiology and Population Sciences, Hawkshead Lane, North Mymms, Hatfield AL9 7TA, UK; ajgibson@rvc.ac.uk
* Correspondence: norfadhilah@umk.edu.my

Received: 1 August 2018; Accepted: 9 September 2018; Published: 13 September 2018

Abstract: Infectious disease caused by pathogenic bacteria continues to be the primary challenge to humanity. Antimicrobial resistance and microbial biofilm formation in part, lead to treatment failures. The formation of biofilms by nosocomial pathogens such as *Staphylococcus aureus* (*S. aureus*), *Pseudomonas aeruginosa* (*P. aeruginosa*), and *Klebsiella pneumoniae* (*K. pneumoniae*) on medical devices and on the surfaces of infected sites bring additional hurdles to existing therapies. In this review, we discuss the challenges encountered by conventional treatment strategies in the clinic. We also provide updates on current on-going research related to the development of novel anti-biofilm technologies. We intend for this review to provide understanding to readers on the current problem in health-care settings and propose new ideas for new intervention strategies to reduce the burden related to microbial infections.

Keywords: biofilms; anti-biofilms; nosocomial pathogens; *Staphylococcus aureus*; *Pseudomonas aeruginosa*; *Klebsiella* pneumoniae

1. Microbial Biofilms and the Challenges in Infectious Disease

Bacterial infections remain a threat to human health despite the progress made in improving the quality of health care, and continuous development of antibiotics and vaccines to control disease. Bacterial infections can occur at any stage in human life and can often be controlled by a healthy immune system of the host. During hospitalization, patients are exposed to pathogen sources within the environment including medical equipment, other infected patients, and healthcare staff and are thus susceptible to hospital-acquired infections (HAI) [1]. Immunocompromised patients, the elderly or patients with existing chronic disease such as diabetes, cancer, cardiovascular diseases, or breakage of skin barrier such occurs with wounds, are reported to face a higher risk of nosocomial infection [2]. The typical medical device associated with HAI are related to central line bloodstream infections, ventilator pneumonia, and catheter urinary infections [1].

The increasing trend of nosocomial bacterial infections in immunocompromised hospitalized patients is worrying as HAI are the primary cause of morbidity in the health-care setting [3,4]. In the

United States alone, it was estimated that a total of 1.7 million HAI occurred in the year 2002 alone, with 4.5 cases occurring for every 100 admissions, resulting in almost 99,000 deaths [5]. At the European level, more than 2 million patients contracted HAI, with 175,000 deaths per year [6]. The incidence of HAI are substantially lower at 7.1% and 4.5% in Europe and USA, respectively, compared to the low and middle-income countries (LMICs), where the average prevalence of HAI is 15.5% [7]. Among the leading bacteria that cause the HAI is *Staphylococcus aureus* (*S. aureus*), *Pseudomonas aeruginosa* (*P. aeruginosa*), *Escherichia coli* (*E. coli*), *Klebsiella pneumoniae* (*K. pneumoniae*), *Acinetobacter baumanii*, *Clostridium difficile*, and *Enterococci* [8,9]. The ability of these bacteria to form biofilms at the infected site or on medical devices has been increasingly recognized as one of the factors causing failure in the treatment of HAI, with biofilms estimated to contribute to approximately half of HAI [8,10]. Figure 1 shows the common site of infections related to the formation of bacterial biofilms.

1.1. Methicillin-Resistant *Staphylococcus aureus* (MRSA)

Staphylococcus aureus is a Gram-positive cocci-shaped bacterium that forms part of the normal flora on the body and is frequently isolated from the skin, respiratory tract, and female lower reproductive tract [11,12]. Infections by *S. aureus* were once treatable by penicillin. However, increasing resistance towards penicillin led to the introduction of methicillin for the treatment in 1960 [13]. However, soon after that, *S. aureus* acquired resistance towards methicillin, giving rise to methicillin-resistant *S. aureus* (MRSA) clones [12,13]. Currently, the Center for Disease Control (CDC) reported that infections by MRSA are the second most common cause of HAI in the USA [14]. The most common route of MRSA transmission is through direct contact. The ability of the organism to form biofilms on tissues such as the skin and inert indwelling device surfaces such as intravenous catheters and surgical implants further expose susceptible individuals [15]. Development of worldwide antibiotic resistance towards first-line therapies such as vancomycin and teicoplanin continues to hinder and restrict the successful treatment of MRSA infection [15]. Additionally, *S. aureus* also can invade host cells and evade the antimicrobial effects of administered therapies [16]. Together, these characteristics allow this organism to remain an important pathogen.

1.2. Pseudomonas aeruginosa

P. aeruginosa is a Gram-negative, rod-shaped, facultative anaerobe ubiquitous in the environment and forms part of the normal gut flora. Increasing resistance towards the multiple antibiotics, e.g., cephalosporins and carbapenem further compounds the problem due to the emergence of extremely drug-resistant (XDR) *P. aeruginosa* infections [17,18]. The last available treatment resort is colistin, a polymyxin antibiotic which was avoided for the past three decades as it may cause both neuro- and nephrotoxicity [19–21]. Patients dependent on breathing machines or fitted with an invasive device such as a catheter, are at risk of severe and life-threatening illness from *P. aeruginosa* capable of forming biofilms on medical device surfaces [22–25]. *P. aeruginosa* biofilms were reported to cause endocardial valve infection through endocardial tubes, ventilator-associated pneumonia (VAP), and catheter-associated urinary tract infections (CAUTI). Additionally, *P. aeruginosa* has also been reported to be able to grow in intravenous fluid and could enter the bloodstream and cause sepsis [26–28].

1.3. Klebsiella pneumoniae

Klebsiella pneumoniae (*K. pneumoniae*) is a non-fastidious, Gram-negative bacillus, and is usually encapsulated. The bacterium is one of the normal flora present in the mouth, skin, and intestine, yet it has been reported to cause pneumonia, urinary tract infections, and bacteremia in patients from hospitals, nursing homes, and other healthcare facilities [18]. *K. pneumoniae* is known as a remarkably resilient pathogen as it can evade and survive rather than actively suppress many components of the immune system of the infected host [29]. The bacteria have developed resistance towards almost all available antibiotics; fluoroquinolones, third-generation cephalosporins and aminoglycosides [30]. Recently, the emergence of the carbapenem-resistant *K. pnemoniae* strains which currently circulating across the globe has forced the administration of colistin, an old and considered the last available antibiotic [31]. Additionally, resistance towards colistin was recently reported, showed that the bacteria are capable of evading all types of available antibiotics, leaving no drugs left for the treatment [32]. Compounding the problem, this organism can survive and grow within the intravenous fluid and form biofilm on medical devices such as the urinary catheter, leading to detrimental septicemia in patients [26,33–35].

2. The Physiology of Biofilms

2.1. Definition and the Structure of the Biofilm

Biofilms have been described in environmental and technical microbiology for more than 90 years. However, the importance of microbial biofilms in medicine has only been recognized since the early 1980s [36]. A microbial biofilm is defined as a structured consortium of microbial cells surrounded by the self-produced matrix [37]. The rough structure can be described as polymicrobial aggregates that resemble mats, flocs, or sludge that accumulate at interfaces. Because of the soft and fragile structure, it is difficult to physically characterize the structure from the infected or adhered surfaces in-vivo. Thus, characterizations of biofilm were mostly performed using in-vitro cultured biofilm cells. The thickness of biofilms can vary depending on the species of the bacteria, the duration and the method used to grow the biofilm. In-vitro, the biofilms of *P. aeruginosa* can reach 209 µm; *S. aureus*, 8.0 µm; and *K. pneumoniae*, 231 µm [33,38,39]. Figure 2 shows the three-dimensional structure of *S. aureus* biofilms visualized with a confocal microscope with the thickness of approximately 8.0 µm.

Biofilms are built of planktonic (individual) bacterial cells 'glued' together with self-released extra-polymeric substances (EPS) which consists of lipopolysaccharides, proteins, lipids, glycolipids, and nucleic acids [40]. The type of polysaccharides found within the biofilm depends on the bacteria species, *S. aureus* and *S. epidermidis* produce poly-ß(1,6)-N-acetyl-D-glucosamine (PNAG) [41], while *P. aeruginosa* produces Pel (a cationic exopolysaccharide composed of 1–4 linked galactosamine and glucosamine sugars) and Psl (a penta-saccharide composed of D-glucose, D-mannose and L-rhamnose) [42,43]. The nucleic acid found in EPS is known as extracellular DNA (eDNA), generated by lysis of a subpopulation of the same bacteria under the control of quorum sensing, a mode of communication between cells. The role of EPS is to promote adhesion and aggregation of bacteria to the surfaces and provides stability to the biofilm structure. Direct interaction of eDNA with extracellular calcium (Ca^{2+}) within the biofilm induces bacterial aggregation via cationic bridging. The positive charge of the extracellular Ca^{2+} modifies the bacterial cell surface charge by neutralizing the electrostatic repulsion between negatively charged biofilm components, thus assisting cellular aggregation and adherence of bacteria to material and tissue surface [44,45]. Once the biofilm is established, negatively charged eDNA acts as a biofilm defence mechanism by chelating the cationic antimicrobial peptides from the host immune system. eDNA also chelates divalent cations triggering the bacterial transcription of genes responsible for increasing pathogenicity and resistance to antimicrobials [46].

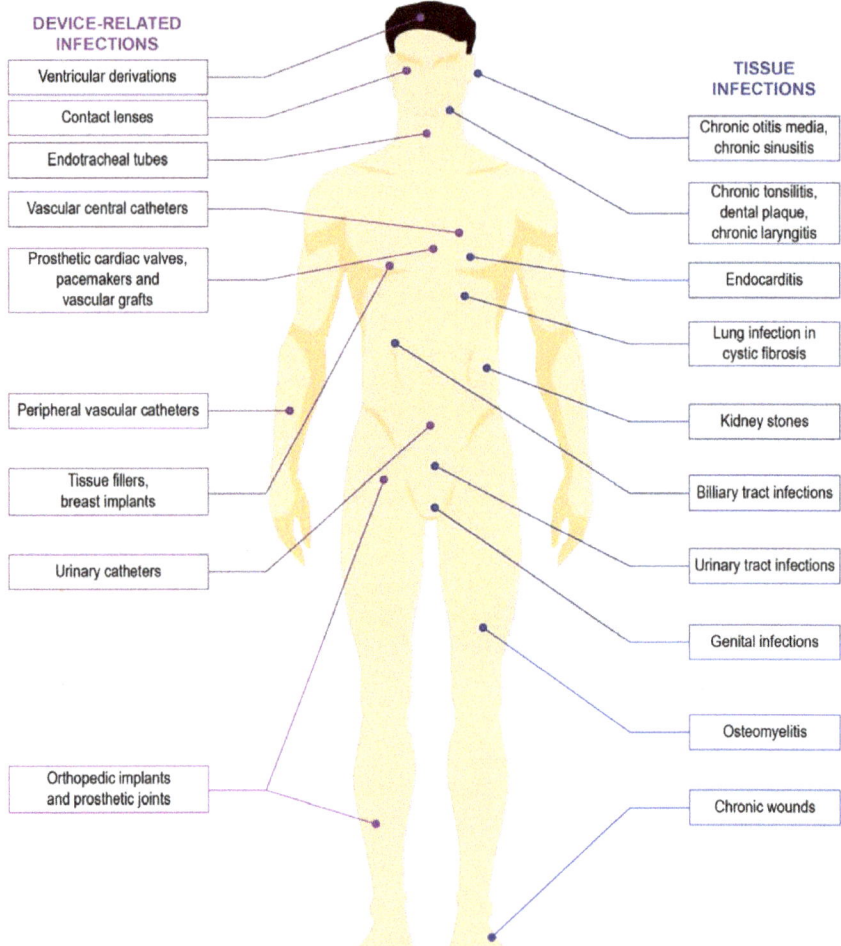

Figure 1. Common site of infections related to the formation of bacterial biofilms.

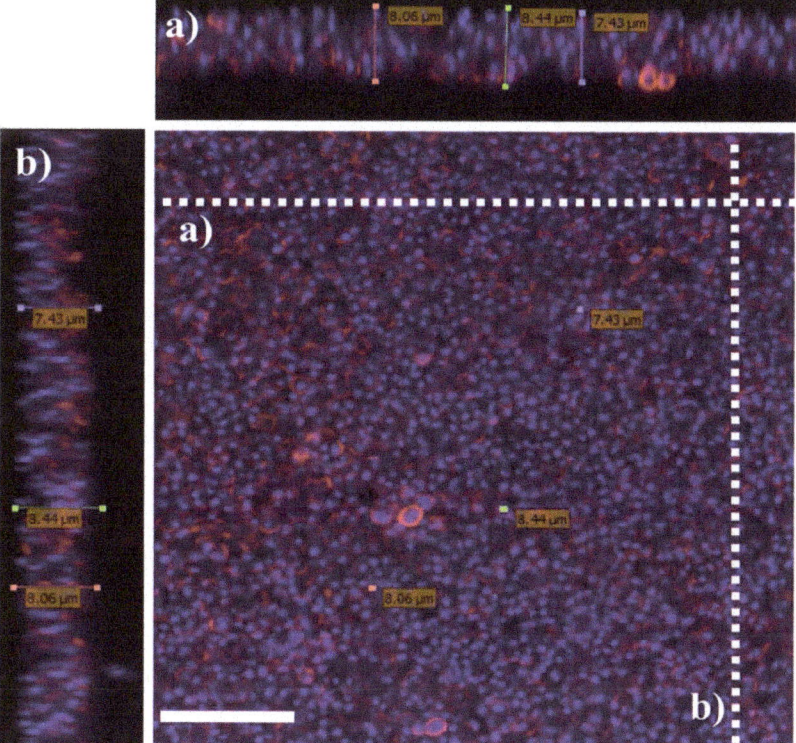

Figure 2. The three-dimensional structure of *S. aureus* biofilms visualized with a confocal microscope.

S. aureus biofilms were cultured in tryptic soy broth for 48 hours, fixed with 4% paraformaldehyde and treated with wheat germ agglutinin (WGA, red) to stain n-acetylglucoseamine component of polysaccharide and DAPI (blue) to stain the bacteria nuclear material, followed by confocal microscopy z-stack projection that moved through 111 slices across the cell. (a) Horizontal cross-section of biofilms and (b) Vertical cross-section of biofilms. White scale bar is 7.5 µm. The approximate thickness of the biofilms was 7.9 ± 0.5 µm. Image adapted from Kamaruzzaman et al., 2017 [39].

2.2. Development of Biofilms

Development of biofilms generally involves several stages, represented schematically in Figure 3. (1) Attachment of cells to surfaces: In this step, bacteria use eDNA and organelles and proteins (such as flagella, pili, fimbriae, and outer membrane proteins) that can assist in sensing and attaching to surfaces [47]; (2) Adhesion between cells and surfaces: Here, the EPS components consisting of DNA, lipoproteins, and lipids secreted by the bacteria encourages cell to cell and cell to surface adhesion; (3) Replication of cell and formation of microcolonies: In this stage, the bacteria become encapsulated in a layer of hydrogel, which functions as a physical barrier between the community and the extracellular environment. The bacteria within the community communicate with each other through quorum sensing (QS), a chemical communication chemical signal that modulates cellular functions, including pathogenesis, nutrient acquisition, conjugation, motility, and production of secondary metabolites [48,49]. Within this stage, the biofilm will mature as cells replicate and EPS accumulates; (4) Cell detachment from biofilms: The final stage involves the detachment of bacterial cells from the microcolonies. Cells are then capable of forming a new biofilm colony at another location [50,51].

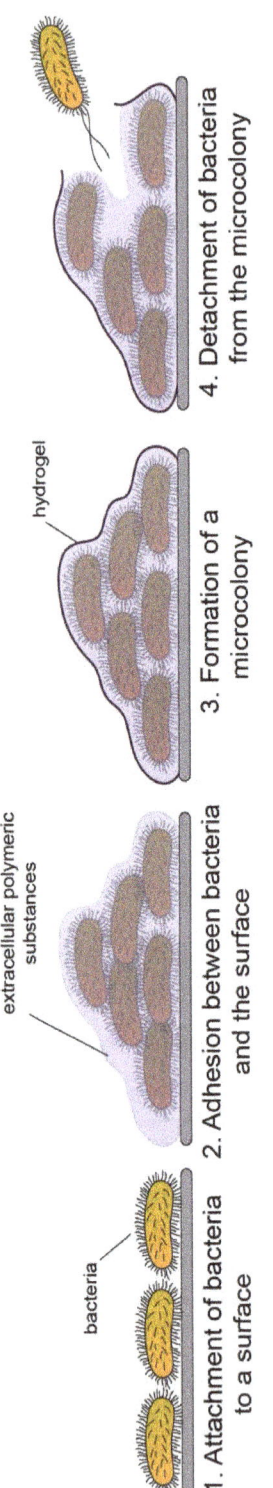

Figure 3. Stages in biofilm information The image is adapted from [50].

2.3. Mechanism of Antibiotic Resistance in Microbial Biofilms

Bacterial cells existing as biofilms can be 10–1000 times more resistant to antibiotics [52–54]. This condition is attributed by several factors and briefly summarised in Table 1. An excellent review on detailed mechanism of biofilm mediated antimicrobial resistance and tolerance was recently published by Hall & Mah (2017), thus readers are invited to refer to this article for detailed information [55].

Table 1. Mechanism of biofilm-mediated antimicrobial resistance.

Physiology of Biofilm	Mechanism of Antimicrobial Resistance	References
Component of the biofilm matrix		
• Thick biofilm matrix	• Reduced permeation of antimicrobials across biofilm matrix	[52,54,56,57]
• Expression of polysaccharide subunits in biofilm matrix	• Expression of PsI polysaccharides in *P. aeruginosa* sequesters antimicrobials in the biofilm matrix via electrostatic interaction	[42]
• Expression of antimicrobial modifying enzymes in the biofilm matrix	• Beta lactamases produced by *Klebsiella pneumoniae* biofilm degrade beta lactam antibiotics	[58]
• Expression of eDNA	• eDNA interacts with antimicrobials and prevent further penetration of the agent across the biofilm matrix to reach cellular targets	[59]
Nutritional factors		
• Oxygen deprived environment	• Deeper layer of the biofilm is oxygen deprived (hypoxic). Hypoxic conditions reduce outer membrane potential of bacteria, diminishing intracellular transport of antibiotics into the bacterial cells • Hypoxia induces increased (or is new expression?) expression of bacterial membrane efflux pumps, potentially reducing antimicrobial accumulation in the cell	[60–62]
• Amino acid deprived environment	• Amino acid starvation activates a stringent response in bacteria within biofilm increasing antimicrobial tolerance	[57]
Physiology of bacteria		
• Small colony variants and persister cells	• Surviving bacteria within the biofilm may change into small colony variants and persister cells. These variants present different phenotypes compared to the wild type planktonic cells including greater tolerance towards antimicrobials	[63]

Table adapted from Hall & Mah (2017) [55].

2.4. Immune Evasion of Biofilms

Bacteria within the biofilm can evade recognition by the innate immune system and thus avoid being eliminated or controlled by the immune system. While the purpose of this article is not to provide a comprehensive review of immune evasion of biofilms, there are aspects worth comment in the context of novel therapies and control strategies. We direct the reader to reviews by Roilides et al., Le et al., and Gunn et al. for more extensive information [64–66]. Despite a clear shortage of studies concerning biofilm recognition by the immune system compared to planktonic cells, several common evasion mechanisms have been described. Biofilms evade the natural antimicrobial properties of innate immune cells by thwarting pathogen recognition, phagocytosis, and cellular activation [67]. In some cases, the cells of the innate immune system assist the process of biofilm growth and maturation [68].

Biofilms modulate leukocyte function by reducing phagocytosis, despite active migration of cells towards the biofilm. Phagocytosis rates of biofilm material are thought to be diminished through a lack of microbial recognition by pattern recognition receptors due to concealed or obscured bacterial ligands such as lipoproteins, lipopolysaccharides, and nucleic acids (i.e., though EPS protection) [69].

EPS protection also retains bacterial content within the biofilm, resulting in large complexes which leukocytes are incapable of engulfing. Detached or homogenised (via sonication) bacteria from biofilms are readily phagocytosed suggesting that leukocyte modulation is temporary [67]. Leukocyte antimicrobial function and killing via oxidative burst (production of reactive oxygen species and nitric oxide) is generally considered to be greatly reduced when considering responses against biofilms [70]. Oxidative burst is readily linked to reduced receptor mediated recognition, further highlighting the role of the protective function of the biofilm matrix in immune evasion.

Experimental investigations with relevant HAI associated biofilms such as those of *S. aureus* and *P. aeruginosa* continue to enhance the knowledge surrounding immune recognition in the context of biofilms. Neutrophils are attracted to and migrate towards both *S. aureus* and *P. aeruginosa* biofilms upon which a reduced phagocytic behaviour is observed along with decreased microbial killing [67]. Lack of *S. aureus* recognition by pattern recognition receptors known as Toll-like Receptors (TLR) is likely due to ligand inaccessibility within the biofilm [69]. TLR binding and subsequent activation potentiates phagocytosis and antimicrobial activity through oxidative burst mechanisms, thus the arrangement of biofilms within a protective matrix serves to conceal internal components. Disruption of *P. aeruginosa* biofilms to homogenised individual cells exhibited an increase in phagocytosis demonstrating the importance of the protective nature of the biofilm matrix [67].

Understanding fundamental interactions between biofilms and the immune system presents opportunities for novel control strategies. Glycolipids involved in quorum sensing produced by *P. aeruginosa*, rhamnolipids, protects against neutrophil activity by inducing lytic necrosis [71]. Disruption of this protection via mutation or quorum inhibitors increases phagocytosis rates, thus targeting active evasion mechanisms offers a route for innovative biofilm treatment strategies.

3. Guideline for Management of Biofilm Associated Infection

Tackling the central issue of HAI biofilms requires that diagnosis and treatment be collectively examined (in a concerted manner) and selected to avoid senseless efforts and increase chances for effective therapy. Several guidelines and recommendations are available for diagnosis and treatment of biofilm infection [72,73] and are summarised in Table 2.

Table 2. Summary of guidelines for diagnosis and treatment of biofilm infections.

Steps	Detail Action
Biofilm diagnosis	1. Sampling on tissue biopsy or device/prosthesis (foreign bodies). 2. Microbial cultivation and identification. 3. Antibiotic susceptibilities test.
Reporting of biofilm associated infections	Biofilm associated infections may be reported using descriptive terms. 1. Detected e.g., 'Microscopy shows Gram-negative rods in biofilm-like structures' 2. Suspected e.g., 'Growth of/PCR-detected microorganisms possibly from a biofilm infection'
Treatment of biofilm related infections 1. Removal sources of infections	1. Debridement of tissues 2. Removal of foreign bodies
2. Administration of topical antiseptics	1. Empiric therapy to prevent biofilm formation after debridement of tissues 2. Pre-emptive therapy to prevent possible biofilm reformation when specific bacteria is detected from the debride tissue
3. Administration of antibiotics	1. Selection of antibiotics suitable for biofilm associated infections 2. Administration of antibiotics 3. Optimization of dosage
Monitoring	1. Assessment of wounds 2. Appropriate/maintenance debridement 3. Re-evaluation of antiseptics/antibiotics efficacy

Table 2. Cont.

Steps	Detail Action
Standard care	1. Set-up the advance therapies 2. Incorporation of novel techniques

Diagnosis and treatment of biofilm can be achieved by various methods, approaches in diagnosing and treating biofilm infections will be further discussed in the following sections.

4. Diagnosis of Biofilm Mediated Infections

The diagnosis of biofilm-related infections is complex and should combine different approaches and a multidisciplinary perspective from clinical and laboratory diagnosis [74]. The European Society for Clinical Microbiology and Infectious Disease (ESCMID) has provided a detailed guideline to aid clinicians in the diagnosis of biofilm related infections. Briefly the guideline emphasizes the combination of clinical and laboratory diagnosis to facilitate clinicians in providing an effective therapy to patients [73]. Generally, the clinical diagnosis may include clinical signs, case history, failure of antibiotic therapy and persistent infection. For laboratory diagnosis, the following techniques have demonstrated high efficacy, successfully discriminating between planktonic and biofilm mediated infections.

4.1. Sonication

Sonication is a process that uses acoustic energy to agitate particles in a solution. This method is useful and recommended to be applied to remove microbial biofilms from the biomaterial surface [75]. The suspected source of infection (e.g., implant) is removed from the patient and subjected for sonication. The process disrupts strongly adhered biomass and releases the biofilm into the solution allowing further analysis to further identify the microbial species [76]. Sonication has been shown to be useful in removing biofilms from urinary catheters, cardiac implantable electronic devices, and prosthetic implants [75–77].

4.2. Polymerase Chain Reaction (PCR)

PCR is one of the common methods used for detection of pathogens directly from clinical specimens. The method is based on the amplification of specific conserved regions within the targeted organism, providing high specificity and sensitivity in discriminating species of bacteria. Due to the robustness of the method, PCR-based diagnostic tests have been used for detecting a range of pathogens including bacteria, viruses, parasites, and fungi [78–81]. In biofilm diagnosis, PCR has been applied to detect the microbial species that forms biofilms on tissues or biomaterials following the sonication process. For example, PCR was used to detect coagulase negative staphylococci, *S. aureus*, *Cutibacterium* species, *Enterococci*, and *Candida* spp. following sonication of implants in the case of orthopedic hardware associated infections [77].

4.3. Matrix-Assisted Laser Desorption Ionization Time-of-Flight Mass Spectrometry (MALDI-TOF MS)

In recent years, matrix-assisted laser desorption ionization time-of-flight mass spectrometry (MALDI-TOF MS) devices have become widely available, changing laboratory workflows for identification of pathogens in most clinical microbiology laboratories [82]. The bacterial protein profiles obtained from intact or cell extracts can be compared to a database of bacterial reference mass spectra for rapid identification at the genus, species, and subspecies level [83]. Also, the method allows for differentiation between planktonic and biofilm cells, as these two populations display different spectra. The method has been tested in different species of Gram-positive and negative bacteria [84].

4.4. Fluorescence In Situ Hybridization (FISH)

FISH is a method that involves binding of short (between 18–25 base pairs), fluorescently labeled oligonucleotides that can bind to the specific ribosomal RNA of the target organism (bacteria, protozoa, and yeast). Analysis involves visualization of targeted ribosomal RNA by fluorescence microscopy [85]. This method can be applied directly on intact specimen fragments, without the need for time consuming sub-culture. Identification of biofilms using FISH is further enhanced by the ability to easily detect bacterial aggregation. The method has been successfully applied to detect biofilm of the following bacteria: *Streptoccous* spp.; *S. aureus*; *Gardnerella vaginalis*; and *Atopobium vaginae* in vaginal biofilms [85–88].

4.5. Microscopy

Microscopy is commonly used following the sonication or FISH to visualize the bacterial aggregates in the specimen. Bacterial growth within biofilms are commonly found as aggregates compared to individual dispersed cells observed during the growth of planktonic cells [85]. The most common microscopy technique used to visualize microbial biofilms are scanning electron microscopy (SEM), transmission electron microscopy (TEM), and scanning confocal laser microscopy (SCLM). The high resolution provided by these techniques allows for depth analysis within the biofilm structure and thus assists the diagnosis of infection mediated by microbial biofilm [89–91]. Table 3 summarizes the common laboratory techniques employed to assist the diagnosis of biofilm mediated infections.

Table 3. The common laboratory techniques applied for laboratory diagnosis of biofilm mediated infections.

Biofilm Mediated Infections	Bacterial Species	Techniques	References
Chronic otitis media	*S. pneumoniae, M. catarrhalis, P. aeruginosa, S. aureus*, and *K. pneumoniae*	PCR and SEM	[92]
Periprosthetic Infection	Coagulase-negative *Staphylococci, Propionibacterium* spp., *Streptococci* and *Enterococci*	Sonication & PCR	[93]
Chronic wound	*P. aeruginosa* and *S. aureus*	TEM & FISH	[93]
Catheter-associated infection	*E. coli*	Sonication & SEM	[76]
Chronic rhinosinusitis	*S. aureus* and *P. acnes*	FISH	[94]
Cystic fibrosis	*P. aeruginosa*	FISH and light microscope	[93]

5. The Potency of Existing Therapies against Microbial Biofilm

Existing antibiotics are useful resources for the treatment of infections with potential formation of biofilm and are summarized in Table 4. Application of suitable antibiotics that are effective against biofilm can improve the outcome, reduce relapse, and improve recovery of the patients. Effective eradication of biofilms could be achieved with high doses of antibiotics, combined with drugs that weaken the biofilm. Efficient treatment of biofilm infections demands a well-established multidisciplinary collaboration which includes: removal of the infected foreign bodies, selection of biofilm-active and -penetrating antibiotics, systemic or topical antibiotic administration in high dosage combinations, and administration of anti-quorum sensing or biofilm dispersal agents [72]. Specifically, treatment of biofilms requires effective and well-penetrating antibiotics to ensure a sufficient concentration of effective antibiotic at the site of biofilm infection. In general, macrolides, lincosamides, tetracyclines, rifamycins, quinolones, fusidic acid, nitroimidazole, sulfonamides, and oxazolidinones penetrate better in tissues and cells than beta-lactam (including penicillins, cephalosporins, and carbapenems), aminoglycosides, glycopeptide, and polymyxin [72]. Antimicrobial agents such as meropenem, colistin, and azithromycin are good candidates for combination strategies which maintain their activity under conditions of reduced oxygen tension and low metabolic activity as found in deeper layers of biofilms. Some of the widely used antibiotics such as azithromycin, ceftazidime, and ciprofloxacin have Quorum Sensing Inhibitor (QSI) activity in addition to their conventional antibiotic activity. An example of a drug that can be included in combination approaches for *P. aeruginosa* biofilm infection is azithromycin. The drug has been shown to inhibit or reduce the production of several of the virulence factors (elastase and rhamnolipids) of *P. aeruginosa*, as well as the matrix component alginate as well as inhibiting quorum sensing. More drugs like azithromycin are required, ideally with higher potency [95].

Table 4. Summary of existing antibiotic regimens according to the specific microbial species.

Bacteria	Biofilm Site of Infection	Antibiotic Regimen	Duration	Route of Administration	References
P. aeruginosa	Lung infection in cystic fibrosis (CF)	0.5–2 MU colistin, twice daily	Continuous	Inhalation	[96]
		300 mg tobramycin, twice daily	28 days on/off cycles		
		75 mg aztreonam, three times daily	28 days on/off cycles		
		32.5 mg or 65 mg ciprofloxacin, once daily	28 days		
	Lung infection in non-CF bronchiestasis	1 MU colistin, twice daily	Continuous	Inhalation	[97]
		32.5 mg ciprofloxacin, twice daily	28 days	Inhalation	[98]
P. aeruginosa and/or S. aureus	Rhinosinusitis	3 drops ofloxacin 0.3%, three times daily	28 days	Nasal drops	[99]
S. aureus	Wounds	Mupirocin 2% ointment	-	Cutaneous	[100]
S. aureus	Catheters	50 mg/mL daptomycin	24 h	Catheter lumen	[101]
		10 mg/mL tigecycline			
		10 mg/mL rifampicin			
		10 mg/mL cotrimoxazole + 2500 U/mL heparin	12–24 h	Catheter lumen	[102]
		Minocycline-rifampin	-	Coating	[28]
K. pneumoniae	Catheters	doripenem and tobramycin	-	Catheter lumen	[103]
P. aeruginosa	Orthopedic procedures	1 g tobramycin + 12 or 24 MU colistin + 40 g polymethylmethacrylate	-	Intraoperative (PMMA beads)	[104]
S. aureus	Orthopedic procedures	40 mg/mL tobramycin + 1 g vancomycin + 10 mL packet of calcium sulfate	-	Intraoperative (calcium sulfate beads)	[104]
		2 mg/mL gentamicin aqueous solution	-	Intraoperative (injection)	[105]

The current combination regimen recommended for the treatment of carbapenem-resistant *K. pneumoniae* (CR-KP) includes high-dose carbapenem therapy (first-line antibiotic), which is combined with colistin and or tigecycline, gentamicin, or fosfomycin (second-line antibiotics). Synergistic interactions between the first-line and second-line antibiotics minimize the use of extremely high doses and the emergence of resistance, as well as potentiate the effectiveness of individual agents. Rifampicin is also occasionally considered for inclusion in combination regimens because of its ability to penetrate intracellular sites and biofilms, which could be important in the treatment of CR-KP infections involving prosthetic material. A new antimicrobial with activity against CR-KP, ceftolozone, is a potent new cephalosporin that is not degraded by current AmpC cephalosporinases or affected by known porin mutations and efflux pumps circulating in CR-KP strains. When tested in combination with tazobactam, the drug has demonstrated promising activity in-vitro against multi-drug resistant Gram-negative isolates, including CR-KP [72].

6. Promising Novel Therapies for Prevention and Treatment of Biofilm Associated Infections

6.1. Nanoparticles

Nanoparticles are particles that have an internal structural measurement or external dimensions within the nanometers size and can be acquired from metallic, metal oxide, semiconductor, polymer, or carbon-based materials [16,106]. There are two major groups of nanoparticles, organic (e.g., micelles, dendrimers, liposomes, hybrid, and compact polymer) and inorganic nanoparticles (e.g., fullerenes, quantum dots, silica, gold, and graphene) [107]. Nanoparticle-mediated antibacterial activities depend on the composition, surface modification, intrinsic properties, and the bacterial species [108]. The reported mechanisms of antibacterial activities include disruption of the bacterial membrane, condensation of the bacterial genome and induction of reactive oxygen species that can be harmful to the physiology of the bacteria [109–111]. Graphene, one of the recently discovered nanoparticles, exhibits antibacterial activity through direct interaction of the compound with the bacterial membrane, causing stress to the membrane, releasing the intracellular contents and bacterial cell death [107].

Additionally, nanoparticles are reported to have anti-biofilm activities by effectively removing and preventing formation of biofilm on surfaces. Table 5 summaries nanoparticles with anti-biofilm activities. The mechanisms of nanoparticle anti-biofilm activity have only been partially understood. For example, silver nanoparticles mediate anti-biofilm activity by suppressing the polysaccharide intercellular adhesion (PIA) synthesis, thus preventing bacterial adhesion to surfaces [112]. On the other hand, zinc oxide (ZnO) prevents biofilm formation by inhibiting microbial growth and prevents biofilm to reach a steady state [113]. Additionally, Yadav et al. demonstrated that graphene oxide coated on surfaces reduced attachment of bacteria, thus preventing biofilm formation [107].

Application of nanoparticles as an antibacterial provides several advantages compared to conventional antibiotics. Nanoparticles have multiple modes of action and range of bacterial targets which would require several bacterial mutations to resist antimicrobial activity. As such nanoparticles present a considerable advantage over conventional antibiotics as they offer an option where there is a reduced likelihood to develop resistance based on intrinsic properties [114]. This is especially important when there is an increase of bacteria resistance of new strains against most potent antibiotics.

Table 5. Examples of nanoparticles with anti-biofilm activities.

Type of Nanoparticles	Microbial Biofilm	References
Silver (immobilized on titanium)	*S. intermedius*	[112]
Silver	*P. aeruginosa, Shigella flexneri, S. aureus* and *S. pneumonia*	[115]
Titanium dioxide	*S. aureus* and *P. putida*	[116]
Selenium and selenium dioxide	*S. aureus, P. aeruginosa* and *Proteus mirabilis*	[117]
Zinc oxide and combination of zinc oxide and hydroxyapatite	*Streptococcus* sp.	[113]
Graphene oxide	*E. coli* and *S. aureus*	[107]

6.2. Diterpenoids

Diterpenoids are a group of plant-derived metabolites composed of two terpene units with molecular formula $C_{20}H_{32}$. Based on number of rings present in the molecular structure, diterpenoids were classified into acyclic (e.g., phytanes), monocyclic (e.g., Cembrene A), bicyclic (e.g., labdanes, halimanes, and clerodanes), tricyclic (e.g., pimaranes, abietanes, cassanes, and dehydroabietic acid), tetracyclic (e.g., trachylobanes and kauranes,), and macrocyclic diterpenes (e.g., taxanes, cembranes) [118]. These metabolites have shown potential values to substitute antibiotics for the treatment of antibiotic-resistant and biofilm forming microbes such as *S. aureus*. Abietane-type diterpenoids extracted from the root of *Salvia sclarea*, a medicinal plant used for easing stomach ache, diarrhoea, sore throat swelling, and headaches, revealed microbicidal and microbiostatic activity against *S. aureus* as well as acanthamoeba, a free-living amoeba. The active compound, salvipisone, showed potential anti-biofilm activity against the antibiotic-resistant Staphylococci, greater than most reported antibiotics [16]. Dehydroabietic acid (DA), an abietane-type diterpenoid found in the resin of coniferous trees, is effective in the inhibition of *S. aureus* biofilm formation in the low molar range, while the effective dose that reduced the viability and biomass of the formation of a biofilm was just two to four-fold higher than the inhibitory dose [119]. Hybrids of DA and selected amino acids resulted in potent fast-acting disassembly of biofilms and weakened the integrity of the bacterial membrane. Also, the DA-amino acid hybrids are potentially more resistant against proteolysis as compared to DA alone. The concentration of bactericidal dose is only three to six folds higher than the bactericidal dose [120]. 8-hydroxyserrulat-14-en-19-oic acid, a plant-derived serrulatane diterpenoid (extracted from the Australian medicinal plant *Eremophila neglecta*) showed anti-biofilm formation activity against Gram-positive bacterial but not Gram-negative bacteria by inhibiting the macromolecular biosynthesis of the bacterial membrane [121]. Table 6 summarises examples of diterpenoids with anti-biofilm activities

Table 6. Examples of diterpenoids with anti-biofilm activities.

Type of Diterpenoids	Microbial Biofilm	Mechanism of Action (Hypothetical)	References
Abietane (natural) • salvipisone • aethiopinone	*S. aureus, S. epidermidis*	NA	[14]
Abietane (synthetic) • dehydroabietic acid scaffold with different amino acids	*S. aureus, S. epidermidis*	Bacterial membrane or the peptidoglycan (PG) layer	[81]
Diterpene • serrulatane compound 8-hydroxyserrulat-14-en-19-oic acid (EN4)	*S. aureus* (methicillin-susceptible and methicillin-resistant), *S. epidermidis*	Membranolytic properties as well as a general inhibition of macromolecular biosynthesis	[83]

6.3. Biomacromolecules

Biomacromolecules such as polysaccharides, naturally secreted polymers, aliphatic, cyclic, and aromatic organic acids were studied for their potential in preventing and constraining biofilm formation or resolving the formed biofilm. Distinct from antibiotics, these macromolecules do not target specific intracellular molecules within the microbes. Instead, with their amphiphilic characteristics, the cationic group of the molecules facilitates microbial targeting and water solubility; while the hydrophobic group induces membrane lysis; being attracted to the microbial membrane via interaction between their cationic groups and the anionic membrane's surface. Upon physical interaction, the hydrophobic group penetrates the microbial membrane leading to membrane destabilization and cytoplasmic content leakage. Antimicrobial agents with physical membrane disruption mechanisms are less likely to be targeted by antimicrobial resistance [122]. Polysaccharides produced by a bacterium may affect biofilm formation of other species through competition and cooperation phenomena [123]. For instance, *K. pneumoniae* capsular polysaccharide was suggested to restrict biofilm formation in several clinically important Gram-positive and Gram-negative bacterial species such as *S. epidermidis*, *S. aureus*, *E. coli*, and *Enterobacter aerogenes* [124,125]. Extracellular polymeric substances such as natural high molecular weight polymers secreted by bacteria have also been suggested to be anti-biofilm candidates [126]. Interruption of bacterial signaling systems such as quorum sensing affects bacterial biofilm formation. In case of a mixed culture, acyl-homoserine lactonase produced by *Bacillus cereus* showed inhibition and settlement of *Vibrio cholera* biofilm [127]. On the other hand, commercial organic acid products usually used in food industry showed the ability to reduce *Salmonella enterica* viable count and biofilm post-treatment, but not total elimination of the bacterium [128].

Incorporating macromolecules with anti-biofilm properties onto the surface of biomaterials has gained increasing interest, especially in implant-associated medical devices such as intravascular catheters, urinary catheters, and orthopedic implants [129]. Coating of biomaterial surface with natural or modified polysaccharide polymers such as hyaluronic acid, heparin, and chitosan revealed promising findings in battling implant-associated biofilm infections [130]. Table 7 summarises examples of examples of biomacromolecules with anti-biofilm activities.

Table 7. Examples of biomacromolecules with anti-biofilm activities.

Type of Macromolecule	Microbial Biofilm	Mechanism of Action (Hypothetical)	References
Polyether ether ketone–octafluoropentyl methacrylate surface	-	Reduced protein adsorption	[91]
AHL lactonase (AiiA), a metallo-beta-lactamase produced by *Bacillus* spp.	*Vibrio cholerae*	blocks quorum sensing in Gram-negative bacteria by hydrolyzing N-acyl-homoserine lactones (AHLs)	[89]
Chitosan-based surface coating	*S. aureus*, *S. epidermidis*	anti-adhesive and bactericidal via contact membrane disruption	[92]
K. pneumoniae capsular polysaccharide	*S. aureus*, *S. epidermidis*, *E. coli*	NA	[87]
Commercially available organic acid water additives	*Salmonella Typhimurium* biofilms	Interference to intracellular pH homeostasis, membrane structure, osmolality and macromolecule synthesis	[90]
Synthetic PDMEA MeI polymers	*S. epidermidis*, *S. aureus*, *E. coli* and *P. aeruginosa*, *Candida albicans*	Membrane disruption	[84]

6.4. Honey

Honey, an ancient wound remedy has gathered renewed interest in its clinical potential for inhibiting a wide range of infectious agents and promoting rapid wound healing [131]. The availability of medical grade honey with laboratory proven effects at the cellular and molecular level against certain microorganisms is not uncommon [131–134]. Mechanisms of bacterial inhibition within biofilm formation attributed to honey is a particular focus due to the increasing multidrug resistance of biofilm-associated organisms. Fortunately, there is accumulating evidence to show honey displays activity in both preventing the formation of a biofilm either through interfering with adherence to host cells or interfering with quorum sensing and disrupting an established biofilm. Several types of honey have been shown to exhibit anti-biofilm activity in-vitro (Table 8).

Besides being used alone, honey also exhibits synergistic activity in combination therapy with certain antibiotics for planktonic cells [135–137]. Although promising, the application of honey as an antibacterial, anti-biofilm, and wound healing promoting alternative is still primarily confined to in-vitro testing. This is mainly due to the varying reports describing different sources of honey, the strain of bacteria, biofilm stage, optimum dosage used, and wound/biotic conditions that might influence the effectiveness of honey when being applied. A few in-vivo model using merino sheep and albino mice demonstrated that anti-biofilm activity was found in honey used, but advised that optimal clinical application should be titrated carefully as tissue toxicity and rejection of the necrosed area from the epidermis was also found with increasing concentration [138,139]. However, care also should be taken on the biofilm-enhancing action of low doses (<MIC) of honey that could be due to a stress response, which has been observed when bacteria in biofilms are exposed to sub-inhibitory concentrations of antibiotics [140].

Table 8. Examples of honey with anti-biofilm activity.

Type of Honey	Microbial Biofilm	Source
Manuka	• *P. aeruginosa*, *Streptococcus pyogenes*, *S. aureus*, *Klebsiella* spp., *Proteus mirabilis* *, *E. coli*, *Acinetobacter baumannii*, *Clostridium difficile*	[141–148]
Clover	• *P. aeruginosa*, *S. aureus*, *Klebsiella* spp., *Proteus mirabilis*	[141,149]
Pumpkin	• *Bacillus subtilis* (*B. subtilis*)	[150]
Chestnut and thyme	• *B. subtilis*, *S. aureus*	[150]
Euphorbia	• *B. subtilis*, *S. aureus*, *P. aeruginosa*, *E. coli*	[150,151]
Chaste	• *B. subtilis*, *S. aureus*, *S. epidermis*	[150]
Multifloral	• *B. subtilis*, *S. aureus*, *S. epidermis* • *Staphylococcus mutans* • *Listeria monocytogenes*	[150]
Eucalyptus	• *B. subtilis*, *S. aureus*	[150]
Honeydew	• *B. subtilis*, *S. aureus*, *S. epidermis*, *S. aureus*, *S. agalactiae*, *P. aeruginosa*, *E. faecalis* *	[145,150]
Lavender, strawberry and citrus	• *P. aeruginosa*, *S. aureus* & MRSA	[152]
Sidr	• *P. aeruginosa*, *S. aureus*, *E. coli*	[151]

* With a certain degree of resistance.

6.5. Antimicrobial Peptides

Antimicrobial peptides (AMPs) are peptides molecules which are produced by many tissues and cell types in a variety of invertebrate, plant, and animal species. The natural peptides are generally made up of 10–50 amino acid residues, positively charged (+2 to +9), with around 50% of hydrophobic properties and diverse sequences and structures [153]. The antimicrobial activities of these peptides are attributed by the amino acid composition, ampipathicy, cationic charge, and size that allow them to attach and insert themselves into the bacterial membrane bilayers to form pores and thus, kill the bacteria [154]. Other than working effectively against planktonic bacterial cells, AMP has also been shown to be effective against biofilms. Mataraci, 2012 evaluated the anti-biofilm activities of two AMPs, indolicin and CAMA: cecropin (1–7)-melittin A (2–9) amide which was found to inhibit MRSA biofilms formation [9]. Additionally other AMPs are currently highlighted as a promising approach to prevent biofilm formation or to treat established biofilms, for instance, LL-37, HBD3, hep-20, IDR-1018 are able to inhibit several species of biofilm formation by either down-regulating the genes essential for biofilm development or up-regulate the expression of genes resulting in a marked attenuation of biofilm production and even by altering the architecture and reducing the amount of extracellular matrix [155–157]. AMPs also are known as host defense peptides are essential components of innate immunity in higher organisms, contributing to the first line of defense against infections [158]. While investigating possible anti-biofilm peptides from natural resources, synthetic peptides produced either by de novo synthesis or by modification gained increased interest based on their improved biological functions and reduced size, which in turn reduces production costs [159,160]. A curated list of useful AMP along with their antimicrobial properties has been documented by de Luca and held within a database called BaAMP accessed via www.baamps.it [161].

Several comprehensive works reviewing various aspects of AMPs have been performed [155–157]. Success of AMPs in both antimicrobial and anti-biofilm activities are collectively due to several characteristics namely: (i) rapid bactericidal effects; (ii) high plasticity in different microenvironments; (iii) good penetration into the matrix of extracellular polymeric substances (EPS); (iv) anti-quorum sensing; (v) host response modulator; and (vi) synergistic effects with other conventional and unconventional antimicrobial compounds [155]. The mechanisms exhibited by AMPs are illustrated in a different state in Figure 4.

6.6. Antimicrobial Polymer

Antimicrobial polymers are synthetic polymers covalently linked with functional groups with high antimicrobial activity such as amino, hydroxyl, and carboxyl groups [162]. Antimicrobial polymers are effective against a range of bacteria including the bacteria commonly associated with HAIs [163]. Due to the long and repeating chain of active and charged functional groups, the common mechanism of antimicrobial activity is through disruption of the cell wall or cytoplasmic membranes. Takahashi et al. demonstrated that cationic homopolymer PE0 and copolymer PE31 containing 31% of ethyl methacrylate was effective in removing biofilm of *Staphylococcus mutans* (*S. mutans*) compared to chlorohexidine and the cationic surfactant that was tested at the same concentration [162]. Another study by Li et al. showed that cationic monomer, methacryloxylethylcetyl dimethyl ammonium chloride (DMAE-CB) was also effective in the removal of a biofilm of *S. mutans*, the common bacteria associated dental problems [164]. Peng et al. modified the polyurethane compound, the main compound for catheter by copolymerization of an amine functionalized N-substituted diol to give a cationic polyurethane (Tecoflex-NH3), and showed that the cationic polyurethane shown contact killing of *E. coli* and prevent build-up of biofilm on the surfaces, thus, reducing the chances of CAUTI, one of the main causes of the nosocomial infections [165]. Another example of an antimicrobial polymer is Polyhexamethlene biguanide (PHMB), a cationic polymer that has been used in the clinic for over than 40 years with no sign of bacterial resistance [166]. PHMB mediates antibacterial activities through disruption of the cell wall and condensation of the bacterial chromosome [111], and recent discovery demonstrate PHMB efficacy in killing intracellular bacteria [16,167]. PHMB is also effective against biofilms from a range of bacterial species and thus effective when applied for the treatment of wound infections [39,168,169]. Though there are increasing findings for polymer mediated anti-biofilm activities, the complete mechanism of the activities is not fully understood. The anti-biofilm activities posed by the polymers could possibly be due to the interaction of the charged group on the polymer structure with the eDNA or Ca^{2+}, thus disrupting the biofilm structure and cause destabilization.

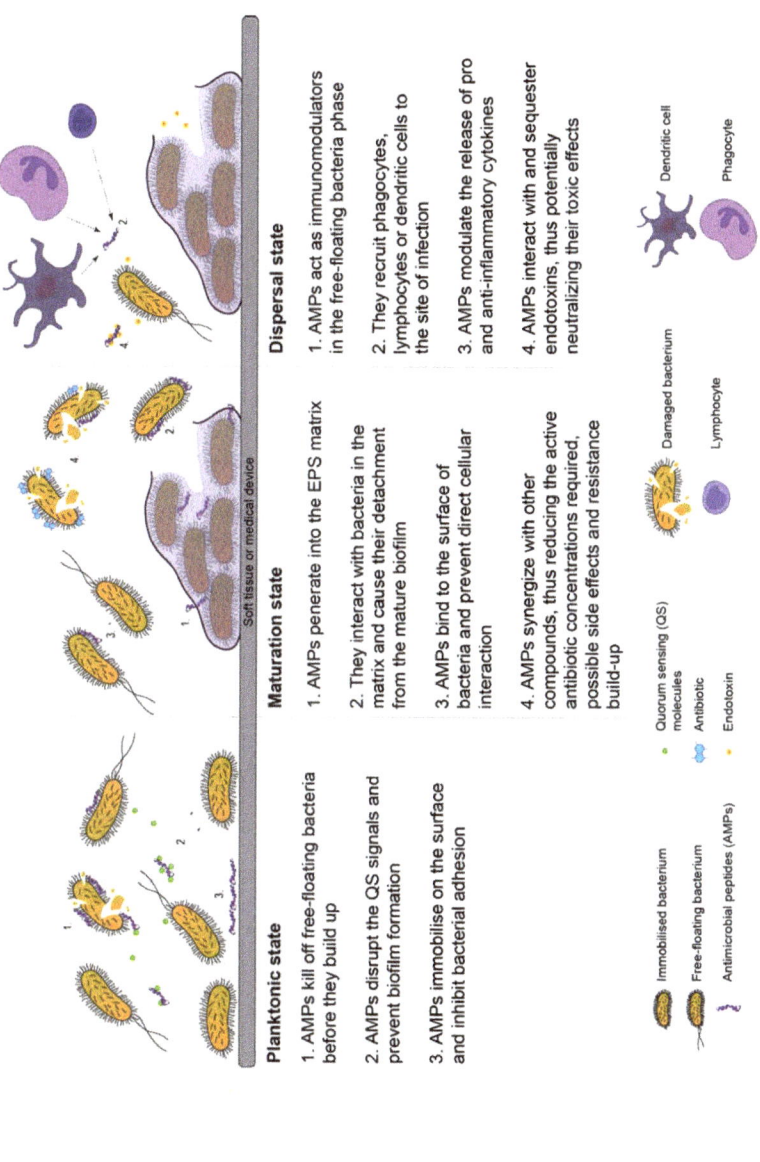

Figure 4. The three main steps of the biofilm life-cycle (attachment to a surface, maturation, and dispersal) and the mechanisms exhibited by Antimicrobial peptides (AMPs) in every step.

7. Summary and Outlook

Biofilms, a form of protective armour for the bacteria, are generally more resistant to the treatment. Biofilms will remain a challenge for the prevention and control of infection; thus it is critical that we continue to explore and understand the physiology and structure of biofilms to develop an improved, innovative, and novel targeted therapies. Based on promising in-vitro studies and reports investigating the use of nanoparticles, AMPs, diterpenoids, and biomacromolecules; we propose that these compounds should be the focus of future novel biofilm control strategies. Further studies focusing on the efficacy and tolerability in-vivo are required to ascertain the level of translation of in-vitro results to clinical resolution of infections caused by biofilms. Together with the increased understanding of the fundamental biology of biofilms, the application of novel or repurposed compounds will undoubtedly improve the prospect of treating and resolving biofilm infection within clinical settings.

Funding: This research received no external funding

Acknowledgments: Khairun Anisa Mat Yazid is funded by UMK Zamalah Scheme, Shamsaldeen Ibrahim Saeed is funded by Universiti of Nyala, Sudan, Alexandru Chivu is funded by UCL LiDO scheme, and Amanda Jane Gibson is funded by BBSRC.

Conflicts of Interest: The authors declare no conflicts of interest

References

1. Khan, H.A.; Baig, F.K.; Mehboob, R. Nosocomial infections: Epidemiology, prevention, control and surveillance. *Asian Pac. J. Trop. Biomed.* **2017**, *7*, 478–482. [CrossRef]
2. Bjarnsholt, T. The role of bacterial biofilms in chronic infections. *Apmis* **2013**, *121*, 1–58. [CrossRef] [PubMed]
3. Jiang, W.; Hu, X.; Hu, Z.; Tang, Z.; Wu, H.; Chen, L. Morbidity and mortality of nosocomial infection after cardiovascular surgery: A report of 1606 cases. *Curr. Med. Sci.* **2018**, *38*, 329–335. [CrossRef] [PubMed]
4. Barrasa-Villar, J.I.; Aibar-Remón, C.; Prieto-Andrés, P.; Mareca-Doñate, R.; Moliner-Lahoz, J. Impact on morbidity, mortality and length of stay of hospital acquired infections by resistant microorganisms. *Clin. Infect. Dis.* **2017**, *65*, 644–652. [CrossRef] [PubMed]
5. Klevens, R.M.; Edwards, J.R.; Richards, C.; Horan, T.C.; Gaynes, R.P.; Pollock, D.A.; Cardo, D.M. Estimating Health Care-Associated Infections and Deaths in U.S. Hospitals, 2002. *Public Health Rep.* **2007**, *122*, 160–166. [CrossRef] [PubMed]
6. Chopra, I.; Schofield, C.; Everett, M.; O'Neill, A.; Miller, K.; Wilcox, M.; Frere, J.M.; Dawson, M.; Czaplewski, L.; Urleb, U.; et al. Treatment of health-care-associated infections caused by Gram-negative bacteria: A consensus statement. *Lancet Infect. Dis.* **2008**, *8*, 133–139. [CrossRef]
7. Allegranzi, B.; Nejad, S.B.; Combescure, C.; Graafmans, W.; Attar, H.; Donaldson, L.; Pittet, D. Burden of endemic health-care-associated infection in developing countries: Systematic review and meta-analysis. *Lancet* **2011**, *377*, 228–241. [CrossRef]
8. Herman-Bausier, P.; Dufrene, Y.F. Force matters in hospital-acquired infections. *Science* **2018**, *359*, 1464–1465. [CrossRef] [PubMed]
9. Mataraci, E.; Dosler, S. In vitro activities of antibiotics and antimicrobial cationic peptides alone and in combination against methicillin-resistant *Staphylococcus aureus* biofilms. *Antimicrob. Agents Chemother.* **2012**, *56*, 6366–6371. [CrossRef] [PubMed]
10. Percival, S.L.; Suleman, L.; Donelli, G. Healthcare-Associated infections, medical devices and biofilms: Risk, tolerance and control. *J. Med. Microbiol.* **2015**, *64*, 323–334. [CrossRef] [PubMed]
11. Al-Talib, H.; Yean, C.; Al-Jashamy, K.; Hasan, H. Methicillin-resistant *Staphylococcus aureus* nosocomial infection trends in Hospital Universiti Sains Malaysia during 2002–2007. *Ann. Saudi Med.* **2010**, *30*, 358–363. [CrossRef] [PubMed]
12. Macmorran, E.; Harch, S.; Athan, E.; Lane, S.; Tong, S.; Crawford, L.; Krishnaswamy, S.; Hewagama, S. The rise of methicillin resistant *Staphylococcus aureus*: Now the dominant cause of skin and soft tissue infection in Central Australia. *Epidemiol. Infect.* **2017**, *145*, 2817–2826. [CrossRef] [PubMed]

13. Enright, M.C.; Robinson, D.A.; Randle, G.; Feil, E.J.; Grundmann, H.; Spratt, B.G. The evolutionary history of methicillin-resistant *Staphylococcus aureus* (MRSA). *Proc. Natl. Acad. Sci. USA* **2002**, *99*, 7687–7692. [CrossRef] [PubMed]
14. Malani, P.N. National burden of invasive methicillin-resistant *Staphylococcus aureus* infection. *JAMA* **2014**, *311*, 1438–1439. [CrossRef] [PubMed]
15. Sisirak, M.; Zvizdic, A.; Hukic, M. Methicillin-resistant *Staphylococcus aureus* (MRSA) as a cause of nosocomial wound infections. *Bosn. J. Basic Med. Sci.* **2010**, *10*, 32–37. [CrossRef] [PubMed]
16. Kamaruzzaman, N.F.; Firdessa, R.; Good, L. Bactericidal effects of polyhexamethylene biguanide against intracellualar *Staphylococcus aureus* EMRSA-15 and USA 300. *J. Antimicrob. Chemother.* **2016**, *71*, 1252–1259. [CrossRef] [PubMed]
17. Zhou, Y.; Li, G. Diagnosis and management of complicated intra-abdominal infection in adults and children: Guidelines by the surgical infection society and the infectious diseases society of America. *Chin. J. Infect. Chemother.* **2010**, *10*, 241–247. [CrossRef]
18. Codjoe, F.; Donkor, E. Carbapenem Resistance: A Review. *Med. Sci.* **2017**, *6*, 1. [CrossRef] [PubMed]
19. Johansen, H.K.; Moskowitz, S.M.; Ciofu, O.; Pressler, T.; Høiby, N. Spread of colistin resistant non-mucoid *Pseudomonas aeruginosa* among chronically infected Danish cystic fibrosis patients. *J. Cyst. Fibros.* **2008**, *7*, 391–397. [CrossRef] [PubMed]
20. Criss, A.K.; Katz, B.Z.; Seifert, H.S. Resistance of Neisseria gonorrhoeae to non-oxidative killing by adherent human polymorphonuclear leucocytes. *Cell. Microbiol.* **2009**, *11*, 1074–1087. [CrossRef] [PubMed]
21. Fiaccadori, E.; Antonucci, E.; Morabito, S.; d'Avolio, A.; Maggiore, U.; Regolisti, G. Colistin Use in Patients With Reduced Kidney Function. *Am. J. Kidney Dis.* **2016**, *68*, 296–306. [CrossRef] [PubMed]
22. Chatterjee, M.; Anju, C.P.; Biswas, L.; Anil Kumar, V.; Gopi Mohan, C.; Biswas, R. Antibiotic resistance in *Pseudomonas aeruginosa* and alternative therapeutic options. *Int. J. Med. Microbiol.* **2016**, *306*, 48–58. [CrossRef] [PubMed]
23. Cornejo-Juárez, P.; Vilar-Compte, D.; Pérez-Jiménez, C.; Ñamendys-Silva, S.A.; Sandoval-Hernández, S.; Volkow-Fernández, P. The impact of hospital-acquired infections with multidrug-resistant bacteria in an oncology intensive care unit. *Int. J. Infect. Dis.* **2015**, *31*, 31–34. [CrossRef] [PubMed]
24. Golan, Y. Empiric therapy for hospital-acquired, Gram-negative complicated intra-abdominal infection and complicated urinary tract infections: A systematic literature review of current and emerging treatment options. *BMC Infect. Dis.* **2015**, *15*, 1–7. [CrossRef] [PubMed]
25. Yayan, J.; Ghebremedhin, B.; Rasche, K. Antibiotic resistance of *Pseudomonas aeruginosa* in pneumonia at a single university hospital center in Germany over a 10-Year Period. *PLoS ONE* **2015**, *10*, 1–20. [CrossRef] [PubMed]
26. Jamal, M.; Ahmad, W.; Andleeb, S.; Jalil, F.; Imran, M.; Nawaz, M.A.; Hussain, T.; Ali, M.; Rafiq, M.; Kamil, M.A. Bacterial biofilm and associated infections. *J. Chin. Med. Assoc.* **2018**, *81*, 7–11. [CrossRef] [PubMed]
27. Mcguffie, B.A.; Vallet-gely, I.; Dove, S.L. σ factor and anti-σ factor that control swarming motility and biofilm formation in *Pseudomonas aeruginosa*. *J. Bacteriol.* **2016**, *198*, 755–765. [CrossRef] [PubMed]
28. Chaftari, A.M.; Zakhem, A.E.; Jamal, M.A.; Jiang, Y.; Hachem, R.; Raad, I. The use of minocycline-rifampin coated central venous catheters for exchange of catheters in the setting of *Staphylococcus aureus* central line associated bloodstream infections. *BMC Infect. Dis.* **2014**, *14*, 1–5. [CrossRef] [PubMed]
29. Paczosa, M.K.; Mecsas, J. *Klebsiella pneumoniae*: Going on the offense with a strong defense. *Microbiol. Mol. Biol. Rev.* **2016**, *80*, 629–661. [CrossRef] [PubMed]
30. *Surveillance of Antimicrobial Resistance in Europe 2016*; Annual report of the European Antimicrobial REsistance Surveillance Network (EARS-Net); European Centre for Disease Prevention and Control: Solna, Sweden, 2017; ISBN 9789294980991.
31. Livermore, D.M.; Maya, J.J.; Nordmann, P.; Wang, H.; Woodford, N.; Quinn, J.P. Clinical epidemiology of the global expansion of *Klebsiella pneumoniae* carbapenemases. *Lancet Infect. Dis.* **2013**, *13*, 785–796. [CrossRef]
32. Otter, J.A.; Doumith, M.; Davies, F.; Mookerjee, S.; Dyakova, E.; Gilchrist, M.; Brannigan, E.T.; Bamford, K.; Galletly, T.; Donaldson, H.; et al. Emergence and clonal spread of colistin resistance due to multiple mutational mechanisms in carbapenemase-producing *Klebsiella pneumoniae* in London. *Sci. Rep.* **2017**, *7*, 1–8. [CrossRef] [PubMed]

33. Singla, S.; Harjai, K.; Chhibber, S. Artificial *Klebsiella pneumoniae* biofilm model mimicking in vivo system: Altered morphological characteristics and antibiotic resistance. *J. Antibiot.* **2014**, *67*, 305–309. [CrossRef] [PubMed]
34. Chung, P.Y. The emerging problems of *Klebsiella pneumoniae* infections: Carbapenem resistance and biofilm formation. *FEMS Microbiol. Lett.* **2016**, *363*, 1–6. [CrossRef] [PubMed]
35. Anderl, J.N.; Franklin, M.J.; Stewart, P.S. Role of antibiotic penetration limitation in *Klebsiella pneumoniae* biofilm resistance to ampicillin and ciprofloxacin. *Antimicrob. Agents Chemother.* **2000**, *44*, 1818–1824. [CrossRef] [PubMed]
36. Jendresen, M.D.; Glantz, P.O. Clinical adhesiveness of selected dental materials: An in-vivo study. *Acta Odontol. Scand.* **1981**, *39*, 39–45. [CrossRef] [PubMed]
37. Høiby, N. A personal history of research on microbial biofilms and biofilm infections. *Pathog. Dis.* **2014**, *70*, 205–211. [CrossRef] [PubMed]
38. Werner, E.; Roe, F.; Bugnicourt, A.; Michael, J.; Heydorn, A.; Molin, S.; Pitts, B.; Stewart, P.S.; Franklin, M.J. Stratified growth in *Pseudomonas aeruginosa* biofilms stratified growth in *Pseudomonas aeruginosa* biofilms. *Appl. Environ. Microbiol.* **2004**, *70*, 6188–6196. [CrossRef] [PubMed]
39. Kamaruzzaman, N.F.; Chong, S.Q.Y.; Edmondson-Brown, K.M.; Ntow-Boahene, W.; Bardiau, M.; Good, L. Bactericidal and anti-biofilm effects of polyhexamethylene Biguanide in models of intracellular and biofilm of *Staphylococcus aureus* isolated from bovine mastitis. *Front. Microbiol.* **2017**, *8*, 1–10. [CrossRef] [PubMed]
40. Czaczyk, K.; Myszka, K. Biosynthesis of extracellular polymeric substances (EPS) and its role in microbial biofilm formation. *Pol. J. Environ. Stud.* **2007**, *16*, 799–806.
41. Izano, E.A.; Amarante, M.A.; Kher, W.B.; Kaplan, J.B. Differential roles of poly-N-acetylglucosamine surface polysaccharide and extracellular DNA in *Staphylococcus aureus* and *Staphylococcus epidermidis* biofilms. *Appl. Environ. Microbiol.* **2008**, *74*, 470–476. [CrossRef] [PubMed]
42. Billings, N.; Ramirez Millan, M.; Caldara, M.; Rusconi, R.; Tarasova, Y.; Stocker, R.; Ribbeck, K. The extracellular matrix component Psl provides fast-acting antibiotic defense in *Pseudomonas aeruginosa* biofilms. *PLoS Pathog.* **2013**, *9*, e1003526. [CrossRef] [PubMed]
43. Jennings, L.K.; Storek, K.M.; Ledvina, H.E.; Coulon, C.; Marmont, L.S.; Sadovskaya, I.; Secor, P.R.; Tseng, B.S.; Scian, M.; Filloux, A.; et al. Pel is a cationic exopolysaccharide that cross-links extracellular DNA in the *Pseudomonas aeruginosa* biofilm matrix. *Proc. Natl. Acad. Sci. USA* **2015**, *112*, 11353–11358. [CrossRef] [PubMed]
44. Das, T.; Sehar, S.; Koop, L.; Wong, Y.K.; Ahmed, S.; Siddiqui, K.S.; Manefield, M. Influence of calcium in extracellular DNA mediated bacterial aggregation and biofilm formation. *PLoS ONE* **2014**, *9*, 1–11. [CrossRef] [PubMed]
45. Bos, R.; Van Der Mei, H.C.; Busscher, H.J. Physico-chemistry of initial microbial adhesive interactions-its mechanisms and methods for study. *FEMS Microbiol. Rev.* **1999**, *23*, 179–229. [CrossRef] [PubMed]
46. Okshevsky, M.; Meyer, R.L. The role of extracellular DNA in the establishment, maintenance and perpetuation of bacterial biofilms. *Crit. Rev. Microbiol.* **2013**, *41*, 1–11. [CrossRef] [PubMed]
47. Montanaro, L.; Poggi, A.; Visai, L.; Ravaioli, S.; Campoccia, D.; Speziale, P.; Arciola, C.R. Extracellular DNA in biofilms. *Int. J. Artif. Organs* **2011**, *34*, 824–831. [CrossRef] [PubMed]
48. Davies, D.G.; Parsek, M.R.; Pearson, J.P.; Iglewski, B.H.; Costerton, J.W.; Greenberg, E.P. The involvement of cell-to-cell signals in the development of a bacterial biofilm. *Science* **1998**, *280*, 295–298. [CrossRef] [PubMed]
49. Braga, R.M.; Dourado, M.N.; Araújo, W.L. Microbial interactions: Ecology in a molecular perspective. *Braz. J. Microbiol.* **2016**, *47*, 86–98. [CrossRef] [PubMed]
50. Costerton, A.J.W.; Stewart, P.S.; Greenberg, E.P. Bacterial Biofilms: A Common Cause of Persistent Infections. *Science* **2011**, *284*, 1318–1322. [CrossRef]
51. Stewart, P.S.; Franklin, M.J. Physiological heterogeneity in biofilms. *Nat. Rev. Microbiol.* **2008**, *6*, 199–210. [CrossRef] [PubMed]
52. Mah, T.C.; Toole, G.A.O. Mechanisms of biofilm resistance to antimicrobial agents. *Trends Microbiol.* **2001**, *9*, 34–39. [CrossRef]
53. La, B.; Prosser, T.; Taylor, D.; Dix, B.A.; Cleeland, R.O.Y. Method of evaluating effects of antibiotics on bacterial biofilm. *Antimicrob. Agents Chemother.* **1987**, *31*, 1502–1506.

54. Nickel, J.C.; Ruseska, I.; Wright, J.B.; Costerton, J.W. Tobramycin resistance of cells of *Pseudomonas aeruginosa* growing as biofilm on urinary catheter material. *Antimicrob. Agents Chemother.* **1985**, *27*, 619–624. [CrossRef] [PubMed]
55. Hall, C.W.; Mah, T.F. Molecular mechanisms of biofilm-based antibiotic resistance and tolerance in pathogenic bacteria. *FEMS Microbiol. Rev.* **2017**, *41*, 276–301. [CrossRef] [PubMed]
56. Singh, R.; Sahore, S.; Kaur, P.; Rani, A.; Ray, P. Penetration barrier contributes to bacterial biofilm-associated resistance against only select antibiotics, and exhibits genus-, strain- and antibiotic-specific differences. *Pathog. Dis.* **2016**, *74*, 1–6. [CrossRef] [PubMed]
57. Nguyen, D.; Joshi-Datar, A.; Lepine, F.; Bauerle, E.; Olakanmi, O.; Beer, K.; McKay, G.; Siehnel, R.; Schafhauser, J.; Wang, Y.; et al. Active starvation responses mediate antibiotic tolerance in biofilms and nutrient-limited bacteria. *Science* **2011**, *334*, 982–986. [CrossRef] [PubMed]
58. Bowler, L.L.; Zhanel, G.G.; Ball, T.B.; Saward, L.L. Mature *Pseudomonas aeruginosa* biofilms prevail compared to young biofilms in the presence of ceftazidime. *Antimicrob. Agents Chemother.* **2012**, *56*, 4976–4979. [CrossRef] [PubMed]
59. Johnson, L.; Horsman, S.R.; Charron-Mazenod, L.; Turnbull, A.L.; Mulcahy, H.; Surette, M.G.; Lewenza, S. Extracellular DNA-induced antimicrobial peptide resistance in *Salmonella enterica* serovar Typhimurium. *BMC Microbiol.* **2013**, *13*, 115. [CrossRef] [PubMed]
60. Walters, M.C.; Roe, F.; Bugnicourt, A.; Franklin, M.J.; Stewart, P.S. Contributions of Antibiotic Penetration, Oxygen Limitation. *Antimicrob. Agents Chemother.* **2003**, *47*, 317–323. [CrossRef] [PubMed]
61. Borriello, G.; Werner, E.; Roe, F.; Kim, A.M.; Ehrlich, G.D.; Stewart, P.S. Oxygen limitation contributes to antibiotic tolerance of *Pseudomonas aeruginosa* in biofilms oxygen limitation contributes to antibiotic tolerance of *Pseudomonas aeruginosa* in biofilms. *Antimicrob. Agents Chemother.* **2004**, *48*, 2659–2664. [CrossRef] [PubMed]
62. Stewart, P.S.; Franklin, M.J.; Williamson, K.S.; Folsom, J.P.; Boegli, L.; James, G.A. Contribution of stress responses to antibiotic tolerance in *Pseudomonas aeruginosa* biofilms. *Antimicrob. Agents Chemother.* **2015**, *59*, 3838–3847. [CrossRef] [PubMed]
63. Waters, E.M.; Rowe, S.E.; O'Gara, J.P.; Conlon, B.P. Convergence of *Staphylococcus aureus* persister and biofilm research: Can biofilms be defined as communities of adherent persister cells? *PLoS Pathog.* **2016**, *12*, 2–6. [CrossRef] [PubMed]
64. Le, K.Y.; Park, M.D.; Otto, M. Immune evasion mechanisms of *Staphylococcus epidermidis* biofilm infection. *Front. Microbiol.* **2018**, *9*, 1–8. [CrossRef] [PubMed]
65. Gunn, J.S.; Bakaletz, L.O.; Wozniak, D.J. What's on the outside matters: The role of the extracellular polymeric substance of gram-negative biofilms in evading host immunity and as a target for therapeutic intervention. *J. Biol. Chem.* **2016**, *291*, 12538–12546. [CrossRef] [PubMed]
66. Roilides, E.; Simitsopoulou, M.; Katragkou, A.; Walsh, T.J. How Biofilms Evade Host Defenses. In *Microbial Biofilms*, 2nd ed.; American Society for Microbiology: Washington, DC, USA, 2015; pp. 287–300. ISBN1 978-1-55581-745-9. ISBN2 978-1-55581-746-6.
67. Leid, J.G.; Shirtliff, M.E.; Costerton, J.W.; Stoodley, P. Human leukocytes adhere to, penetrate, and respond to *Staphylococcus aureus* biofilms. *Infect. Immun.* **2002**, *70*, 6339–6345. [CrossRef] [PubMed]
68. Walker, T.S.; Tomlin, K.L.; Worthen, G.S.; Poch, R.; Lieber, J.G.; Saavedra, M.T.; Michael, B.; Malcolm, K.C.; Vasil, M.L.; Jerry, A.N.; et al. Enhanced *Pseudomonas aeruginosa* biofilm development mediated by human neutrophils enhanced *Pseudomonas aeruginosa* biofilm development mediated by human neutrophils. *Infect. Immun.* **2005**, *73*, 3693–3701. [CrossRef] [PubMed]
69. Thurlow, L.R.; Hanke, M.L.; Fritz, T.; Angle, A.; Aldrich, A.; Williams, S.H.; Engebretsen, I.L.; Bayles, K.W.; Horswill, A.R.; Kielian, T. *Staphylococcus aureus* biofilms prevent macrophage phagocytosis and attenuate inflammation in vivo. *J. Immunol.* **2011**, *186*, 6585–6596. [CrossRef] [PubMed]
70. Jesaitis, A.J.; Franklin, M.J.; Berglund, D.; Sasaki, M.; Lord, C.I.; Bleazard, J.B.; Duffy, J.E.; Beyenal, H.; Lewandowski, Z. Compromised host defense on *Pseudomonas aeruginosa* biofilms: Characterization of neutrophil and biofilm interactions. *J. Immunol.* **2003**, *171*, 4329–4339. [CrossRef] [PubMed]
71. Jensen, E.T.; Kharazmi, A.; Lam, K.; Costerton, J.W.; Hoiby, N. Human polymorphonuclear leukocyte response to *Pseudomonas aeruginosa* grown in biofilms. *Infect. Immun.* **1990**, *58*, 2383–2385. [PubMed]
72. Wu, H.; Moser, C.; Wang, H.Z.; Høiby, N.; Song, Z.J. Strategies for combating bacterial biofilm infections. *Int. J. Oral. Sci.* **2015**, *7*, 1–7. [CrossRef] [PubMed]

73. Høiby, N.; Bjarnsholt, T.; Moser, C.; Bassi, G.L.; Coenye, T.; Donelli, G.; Hall-Stoodley, L.; Holá, V.; Imbert, C.; Kirketerp-Møller, K.; et al. ESCMID* guideline for the diagnosis and treatment of biofilm infections 2014. *Clin. Microbiol. Infect.* **2015**, *21*, S1–S25. [CrossRef] [PubMed]
74. Macià, M.D.; del Pozo, J.L.; Díez-Aguilar, M.; Guinea, J. Microbiological diagnosis of biofilm-related infections. *Enferm. Infecc. Microbiol. Clin.* **2018**, *36*, 375–381. [CrossRef] [PubMed]
75. Almani, S.A.; Naseer, A.; Maheshwari, S.K.; Maroof, P. Detection of biofilm-associated implant pathogens in cardiac device infections: High sensitivity of sonication fluid culture even in the presence of antimicrobials. *J. Glob. Infect. Dis.* **2017**, *9*, 135–138. [CrossRef] [PubMed]
76. Mandakhalikar, K.D.; Rahmat, J.N.; Chiong, E.; Neoh, K.G.; Shen, L.; Tambyah, P.A. Extraction and quantification of biofilm bacteria: Method optimized for urinary catheters. *Sci. Rep.* **2018**, *8*, 1–9. [CrossRef] [PubMed]
77. Renz, N.; Cabric, S.; Morgenstern, C.; Schuetz, M.A.; Trampuz, A. Value of PCR in sonication fluid for the diagnosis of orthopedic hardware-associated infections: Has the molecular era arrived? *Injury* **2018**, *49*, 806–811. [CrossRef] [PubMed]
78. Schuurs, T.A.; Koelewijn, R.; Brienen, E.A.T.; Kortbeek, T.; Mank, T.G.; Mulder, B.; Stelma, F.F.; Van Lieshout, L.; Van Hellemond, J.J. Harmonization of PCR-based detection of intestinal pathogens: Experiences from the Dutch external quality assessment scheme on molecular diagnosis of protozoa in stool samples. *Clin. Chem. Lab. Med.* **2018**, 1–6. [CrossRef] [PubMed]
79. Stavnsbjerg, C.; Frimodt-Møller, N.; Moser, C.; Bjarnsholt, T. Comparison of two commercial broad-range PCR and sequencing assays for identification of bacteria in culture-negative clinical samples. *BMC Infect. Dis.* **2017**, *17*, 1–7. [CrossRef] [PubMed]
80. Morio, F.; Dannaoui, E.; Chouaki, T.; Cateau, E.; Malard, O.; Bonfils, P.; Page, C.; Dufour, X.; Cottrel, C.; Erwan, T.; et al. PCR-based detection of Aspergillus fumigatus and absence of azole resistance due to TR34/L98H in a french multicenter cohort of 137 patients with fungal rhinosinusitis. *Mycoses* **2018**, *61*, 30–34. [CrossRef] [PubMed]
81. Davis, L.E.; Tyler, K.L. *Molecular Diagnosis of CNS Viral Infections*; Elsevier Inc.: New York, NY, USA, 2005; Voluem 76, ISBN 9780128138069.
82. Bizzini, A.; Greub, G.; Greub, G. Matrix-assisted laser desorption ionization time-of-flight mass spectrometry, a revolution in clinical microbial identification. *Clin. Microbiol. Infect.* **2010**, *16*, 1614–1619. [CrossRef] [PubMed]
83. Kliem, M.; Sauer, S. The essence on mass spectrometry based microbial diagnostics. *Curr. Opin. Microbiol.* **2012**, *15*, 397–402. [CrossRef] [PubMed]
84. Gaudreau, A.M.; Labrie, J.; Goetz, C.; Dufour, S.; Jacques, M. Evaluation of MALDI-TOF mass spectrometry for the identification of bacteria growing as biofilms. *J. Microbiol. Methods* **2018**, *145*, 79–81. [CrossRef] [PubMed]
85. Frickmann, H.; Zautner, A.E.; Moter, A.; Kikhney, J.; Hagen, R.M.; Stender, H.; Poppert, S. Fluorescence in situ hybridization (FISH) in the microbiological diagnostic routine laboratory: A review. *Crit. Rev. Microbiol.* **2017**, *43*, 263–293. [CrossRef] [PubMed]
86. Schrøder, S.A.; Eickhardt, S.; Bjarnsholt, T.; Nørgaard, T.; Homøe, P. Morphological evidence of biofilm in chronic obstructive sialadenitis. *J. Laryngol. Otol.* **2018**, *132*, 1–4. [CrossRef] [PubMed]
87. Al-Ahmad, A.; Wunder, A.; Auschill, T.M.; Follo, M.; Braun, G.; Hellwig, E.; Arweiler, N.B. The in vivo dynamics of *Streptococcus* spp., *Actinomyces naeslundii*, *Fusobacterium nucleatum* and *Veillonella* spp. in dental plaque biofilm as analysed by five-colour multiplex fluorescence in situ hybridization. *J. Med. Microbiol.* **2007**, *56*, 681–687. [CrossRef] [PubMed]
88. Hardy, L.; Jespers, V.; Dahchour, N.; Mwambarangwe, L.; Musengamana, V.; Vaneechoutte, M.; Crucitti, T. Unravelling the bacterial vaginosis-associated biofilm: A multiplex *Gardnerella vaginalis* and *Atopobium vaginae* fluorescence in situ hybridization assay using peptide nucleic acid probes. *PLoS ONE* **2015**, *10*, 1–16. [CrossRef] [PubMed]
89. Hu, H.; Johani, K.; Gosbell, I.B.; Jacombs, A.S.W.; Almatroudi, A.; Whiteley, G.S.; Deva, A.K.; Jensen, S.; Vickery, K. Intensive care unit environmental surfaces are contaminated by multidrug-resistant bacteria in biofilms: Combined results of conventional culture, pyrosequencing, scanning electron microscopy, and confocal laser microscopy. *J. Hosp. Infect.* **2015**, *91*, 35–44. [CrossRef] [PubMed]

90. Mohmmed, S.A.; Vianna, M.E.; Penny, M.R.; Hilton, S.T.; Mordan, N.; Knowles, J.C. Confocal laser scanning, scanning electron, and transmission electron microscopy investigation of *Enterococcus faecalis* biofilm degradation using passive and active sodium hypochlorite irrigation within a simulated root canal model. *Microbiologyopen* **2017**, *6*, 1–9. [CrossRef] [PubMed]
91. Tani, S.; Lepetsos, P.; Stylianakis, A.; Vlamis, J.; Birbas, K.; Kaklamanos, I. Superiority of the sonication method against conventional periprosthetic tissue cultures for diagnosis of prosthetic joint infections. *Eur. J. Orthop. Surg. Traumatol.* **2018**, *28*, 51–57. [CrossRef] [PubMed]
92. Hayes, J.; Forbes, M.; Greenberg, D.P.; Dice, B.; Burrows, A.; Wackym, P.A.; Kerschner, J.E. Direct Detection of Bacterial Biofilms on the Middle-Ear Mucosa of Children. *JAMA* **2006**, *296*, 202–211.
93. Renz, N.; Feihl, S.; Cabric, S.; Trampuz, A. Performance of automated multiplex PCR using sonication fluid for diagnosis of periprosthetic joint infection: A prospective cohort. *Infection* **2017**, *45*, 877–884. [CrossRef] [PubMed]
94. Boase, S.; Foreman, A.; Cleland, E.; Tan, L.; Melton-Kreft, R.; Pant, H.; Hu, F.Z.; Ehrlich, G.D.; Wormald, P.J. The microbiome of chronic rhinosinusitis: Culture, molecular diagnostics and biofilm detection. *BMC Infect. Dis.* **2013**, *13*, 1–9. [CrossRef] [PubMed]
95. Bjarnsholt, T.; Ciofu, O.; Molin, S.; Givskov, M.; Høiby, N. Applying insights from biofilm biology to drug development-can a new approach be developed? *Nat. Rev. Drug Discov.* **2013**, *12*, 791–808. [CrossRef] [PubMed]
96. Cantón, R.; Máiz, L.; Escribano, A.; Olveira, C.; Oliver, A.; Asensio, O.; Gartner, S.; Roma, E.; Quintana-Gallego, E.; Salcedo, A.; et al. Spanish Consensus on the Prevention and Treatment of *Pseudomonas aeruginosa* Bronchial Infections in Cystic Fibrosis Patients. *Arch. Bronconeumol.* **2015**, *51*, 140–150. [CrossRef] [PubMed]
97. Haworth, C.S.; Foweraker, J.E.; Wilkinson, P.; Kenyon, R.F.; Bilton, D. Inhaled colistin in patients with bronchiectasis and chronic *Pseudomonas aeruginosa* infection. *Am. J. Respir. Crit. Care Med.* **2014**, *189*, 975–982. [CrossRef] [PubMed]
98. Wilson, R.; Welte, T.; Polverino, E.; De Soyza, A.; Greville, H.; O'Donnell, A.; Alder, J.; Reimnitz, P.; Hampel, B. Ciprofloxacin dry powder for inhalation in non-cystic fibrosis bronchiectasis: A phase II randomised study. *Eur. Respir. J.* **2013**, *41*, 1107–1115. [CrossRef] [PubMed]
99. Ezzat, W.F.; Fawaz, S.A.; Rabie, H.; Hamdy, T.A.; Shokry, Y.A. Effect of topical ofloxacin on bacterial biofilms in refractory post-sinus surgery rhino-sinusitis. *Eur. Arch. Oto-Rhino-Laryngol.* **2015**, *272*, 2355–2361. [CrossRef] [PubMed]
100. Kaiser, M.; Gil, J.; Treu, R.; Valdes, J.; Davis, S. An in vitro analysis of the effects of various topical antimicrobial agents on methicillin-resistant and methicillin-sensitive strains of *Staphylococcus aureus*. *Ostomy Wound Manag.* **2014**, *60*, 18–28.
101. Hogan, S.; Zapotoczna, M.; Stevens, N.T.; Humphreys, H.; O'Gara, J.P.; O'Neill, E. In vitro approach for identification of the most effective agents for antimicrobial lock therapy in the treatment of intravascular catheter-related infections caused by *Staphylococcus aureus*. *Antimicrob. Agents Chemother.* **2016**, *60*, 2923–2931. [CrossRef] [PubMed]
102. Moghaddas, A.; Abbasi, M.R.; Gharekhani, A.; Dashti-Khavidaki, S.; Razeghi, E.; Jafari, A.; Khalili, H. Prevention of hemodialysis catheter-related blood stream infections using a cotrimoxazole-lock technique. *Future Microbiol.* **2015**, *10*, 169–178. [CrossRef] [PubMed]
103. Mataraci Kara, E.; Ozbek Celik, B. Investigation of the effects of various antibiotics against *Klebsiella pneumoniae* biofilms on in vitro catheter model. *J. Chemother.* **2018**, *30*, 82–88. [CrossRef] [PubMed]
104. Krajewski, J.; Bode-Boger, S.M.; Tröger, U.; Martens-Lobenhoffer, J.; Mulrooney, T.; Mittelstädt, H.; Russlies, M.; Kirchner, R.; Knobloch, J.K.M. Successful treatment of extensively drug-resistant *Pseudomonas aeruginosa* osteomyelitis using a colistin- and tobramycin-impregnated PMMA spacer. *Int. J. Antimicrob. Agents* **2014**, *44*, 363–366. [CrossRef] [PubMed]
105. Cancienne, J.M.; Tyrrell Burrus, M.; Weiss, D.B.; Yarboro, S.R. Applications of Local Antibiotics in Orthopedic Trauma. *Orthop. Clin. N. Am.* **2015**, *46*, 495–510. [CrossRef] [PubMed]
106. Subbenaik, S.C. *Plant Nanotechnology: Principles and Practices*; Khodakovskaya, C.K.S.K.V., Ed.; Springer International Publishing: Basel, Switzerland, 2016; ISBN 9783319421544.

107. Yadav, N.; Dubey, A.; Shukla, S.; Saini, C.P.; Gupta, G.; Priyadarshini, R.; Lochab, B. Graphene oxide-coated surface: Inhibition of bacterial biofilm formation due to specific surface-interface interactions. *ACS Omega* **2017**, *2*, 3070–3082. [CrossRef] [PubMed]
108. Hajipour, M.J.; Fromm, K.M.; Akbar Ashkarran, A.; Jimenez de Aberasturi, D.; De Larramendi, I.R.; Rojo, T.; Serpooshan, V.; Parak, W.J.; Mahmoudi, M. Antibacterial properties of nanoparticles. *Trends Biotechnol.* **2012**, *30*, 499–511. [CrossRef] [PubMed]
109. Aditya, A.; Chattopadhyay, S.; Jha, D.; Gautam, H.K.; Maiti, S.; Ganguli, M. Zinc Oxide nanoparticles dispersed in ionic liquids show high antimicrobial efficacy to skin-specific bacteria. *ACS Appl. Mater. Interfaces* **2018**, *10*, 15401–15411. [CrossRef] [PubMed]
110. Van Acker, H.; Coenye, T. The Role of Reactive Oxygen species in antibiotic-mediated killing of bacteria. *Trends Microbiol.* **2017**, *25*, 456–466. [CrossRef] [PubMed]
111. Chindera, K.; Mahato, M.; Kumar Sharma, A.; Horsley, H.; Kloc-Muniak, K.; Kamaruzzaman, N.F.; Kumar, S.; McFarlane, A.; Stach, J.; Bentin, T.; et al. The antimicrobial polymer PHMB enters cells and selectively condenses bacterial chromosomes. *Sci. Rep.* **2016**, *6*, 23121. [CrossRef] [PubMed]
112. Qin, H.; Cao, H.; Zhao, Y.; Zhu, C.; Cheng, T.; Wang, Q.; Peng, X.; Cheng, M.; Wang, J.; Jin, G.; et al. In vitro and in vivo anti-biofilm effects of silver nanoparticles immobilized on titanium. *Biomaterials* **2014**, *35*, 9114–9125. [CrossRef] [PubMed]
113. Abdulkareem, E.H.; Memarzadeh, K.; Allaker, R.P.; Huang, J.; Pratten, J.; Spratt, D. Anti-biofilm activity of zinc oxide and hydroxyapatite nanoparticles as dental implant coating materials. *J. Dent.* **2015**, *43*, 1462–1469. [CrossRef] [PubMed]
114. Allaker, R.P. Critical review in oral biology & medicine: The use of nanoparticles to control oral biofilm formation. *J. Dent. Res.* **2010**, *89*, 1175–1186. [CrossRef] [PubMed]
115. Gurunathan, S.; Han, J.W.; Kwon, D.N.; Kim, J.H. Enhanced antibacterial and anti-biofilm activities of silver nanoparticles against Gram-negative and Gram-positive bacteria. *Nanoscale Res. Lett.* **2014**, *9*, 1–17. [CrossRef] [PubMed]
116. Jalvo, B.; Faraldos, M.; Bahamonde, A.; Rosal, R. Antimicrobial and antibiofilm efficacy of self-cleaning surfaces functionalized by TiO_2 photocatalytic nanoparticles against *Staphylococcus aureus* and Pseudomonas putida. *J. Hazard. Mater.* **2017**, *340*, 160–170. [CrossRef] [PubMed]
117. Shakibaie, M.; Forootanfar, H.; Golkari, Y.; Mohammadi-Khorsand, T.; Shakibaie, M.R. Anti-biofilm activity of biogenic selenium nanoparticles and selenium dioxide against clinical isolates of Staphylococcus aureus, *Pseudomonas aeruginosa*, and Proteus mirabilis. *J. Trace Elem. Med. Biol.* **2015**, *29*, 235–241. [CrossRef] [PubMed]
118. Tchimene, M.K.; Okunji, C.O.; Iwu, M.M.; Kuete, V. Monoterpenes and Related Compounds from the Medicinal Plants of Africa. In *Medicinal Plant Research in Africa*; Elsevier: New York, NY, USA, 2013; pp. 261–300. ISBN 9780124059276.
119. Manner, S.; Vahermo, M.; Skogman, M.E.; Krogerus, S.; Vuorela, P.M.; Yli-Kauhaluoma, J.; Fallarero, A.; Moreira, V.M. New derivatives of dehydroabietic acid target planktonic and biofilm bacteria in *Staphylococcus aureus* and effectively disrupt bacterial membrane integrity. *Eur. J. Med. Chem.* **2015**, *102*, 68–79. [CrossRef] [PubMed]
120. Kuźma, Ł.; Różalski, M.; Walencka, E.; Różalska, B.; Wysokińska, H. Antimicrobial activity of diterpenoids from hairy roots of *Salvia sclarea* L.: Salvipisone as a potential anti-biofilm agent active against antibiotic resistant Staphylococci. *Phytomedicine* **2007**, *14*, 31–35. [CrossRef] [PubMed]
121. Nowakowska, J.; Griesser, H.J.; Textor, M.; Landmann, R.; Khanna, N. Antimicrobial properties of 8-hydroxyserrulat-14-en-19-oic acid for treatment of implant-associated infections. *Antimicrob. Agents Chemother.* **2013**, *57*, 333–342. [CrossRef] [PubMed]
122. Tan, J.P.K.; Coady, D.J.; Sardon, H.; Yuen, A.; Gao, S.; Lim, S.W.; Liang, Z.C.; Tan, E.W.; Venkataraman, S.; Engler, A.C.; et al. Broad Spectrum Macromolecular Antimicrobials with Biofilm Disruption Capability and In Vivo Efficacy. *Adv. Healthc. Mater.* **2017**, *6*, 1–9. [CrossRef]
123. Nadell, C.D.; Drescher, K.; Foster, K.R. Spatial structure, cooperation and competition in biofilms. *Nat. Rev. Microbiol.* **2016**, *14*, 589–600. [CrossRef] [PubMed]
124. Donlan, R.M. Biofilms and device-associated infections. *Emerg. Infect. Dis.* **2001**, *7*, 277–281. [CrossRef] [PubMed]

125. Dos Santos Goncalves, M.; Delattre, C.; Balestrino, D.; Charbonnel, N.; Elboutachfaiti, R.; Wadouachi, A.; Badel, S.; Bernardi, T.; Michaud, P.; Forestier, C. Anti-biofilm activity: A function of *Klebsiella pneumoniae* capsular polysaccharide. *PLoS ONE* **2014**, *9*, e99995. [CrossRef]
126. Brian-Jaisson, F.; Molmeret, M.; Fahs, A.; Guentas-Dombrowsky, L.; Culioli, G.; Blache, Y.; Cérantola, S.; Ortalo-Magné, A. Characterization and anti-biofilm activity of extracellular polymeric substances produced by the marine biofilm-forming bacterium pseudoalteromonas ulvae strain TC14. *Biofouling* **2016**, *32*, 547–560. [CrossRef] [PubMed]
127. Augustine, N.; Kumar, P.; Thomas, S. Inhibition of Vibrio cholerae biofilm by AiiA enzyme produced from Bacillus spp. *Arch. Microbiol.* **2010**, *192*, 1019–1022. [CrossRef] [PubMed]
128. Pande, V.; McWhorter, A.R.; Chousalkar, K.K. Anti-bacterial and anti-biofilm activity of commercial organic acid products against *Salmonella enterica* isolates recovered from an egg farm environment. *Avian Pathol.* **2018**, *47*, 189–196. [CrossRef] [PubMed]
129. Francolini, I.; Donelli, G. Prevention and control of biofilm-based medical-device-related infections. *FEMS Immunol. Med. Microbiol.* **2010**, *59*, 227–238. [CrossRef] [PubMed]
130. Junter, G.A.; Thébault, P.; Lebrun, L. Polysaccharide-based antibiofilm surfaces. *Acta Biomater.* **2016**, *30*, 13–25. [CrossRef] [PubMed]
131. Cooper, R. Honey as an effective antimicrobial treatment for chronic wounds: Is there a place for it in modern medicine? *Chronic Wound Care Manag. Res.* **2014**, *1*, 15–22. [CrossRef]
132. Simon, A.; Traynor, K.; Santos, K.; Blaser, G.; Bode, U.; Molan, P. Medical honey for wound care still the latest resort. *Evid.-Based Complement. Altern. Med.* **2009**, *6*, 165–173. [CrossRef] [PubMed]
133. Biglari, B.; Swing, T.; Büchler, A.; Ferbert, T.; Simon, A.; Schmidmaier, G.; Moghaddam, A. Medical honey in professional wound care. *Expert Rev. Dermatol.* **2013**, *8*, 51–56. [CrossRef]
134. Watts, R.; Frehner, E. Evidence Summary: Wound management: Medical-grade honey. *Wound Pract. Res.* **2017**, *25*, 117–120. [CrossRef]
135. Müller, P.; Alber, D.G.; Turnbull, L.; Schlothauer, R.C.; Carter, D.A.; Whitchurch, C.B.; Harry, E.J. Synergism between Medihoney and Rifampicin against Methicillin-Resistant *Staphylococcus aureus* (MRSA). *PLoS ONE* **2013**, *8*, 1–9. [CrossRef] [PubMed]
136. Liu, M.Y.; Cokcetin, N.N.; Lu, J.; Turnbull, L.; Carter, D.A.; Whitchurch, C.B.; Harry, E.J. Rifampicin-manuka honey combinations are superior to other antibiotic-manuka honey combinations in eradicating *Staphylococcus aureus* biofilms. *Front. Microbiol.* **2018**, *8*, 1–12. [CrossRef] [PubMed]
137. Liu, M.; Lu, J.; Müller, P.; Turnbull, L.; Burke, C.M.; Schlothauer, R.C.; Carter, D.A.; Whitchurch, C.B.; Harry, E.J. Antibiotic-specific differences in the response of *Staphylococcus aureus* to treatment with antimicrobials combined with manuka honey. *Front. Microbiol.* **2014**, *5*, 1–9. [CrossRef] [PubMed]
138. Paramasivan, S.; Drilling, A.J.; Jardeleza, C.; Jervis-Bardy, J.; Vreugde, S.; Wormald, P.J. Methylglyoxal-augmented manuka honey as a topical anti-*Staphylococcus aureus* biofilm agent: Safety and efficacy in an in vivo model. *Int. Forum Allergy Rhinol.* **2014**, *4*, 187–195. [CrossRef] [PubMed]
139. El-Kased, R.F.; Amer, R.I.; Attia, D.; Elmazar, M.M. Honey-based hydrogel: In vitro and comparative in vivo evaluation for burn wound healing. *Sci. Rep.* **2017**, *7*, 1–11. [CrossRef]
140. Lu, J.; Carter, D.A.; Turnbull, L.; Rosendale, D.; Hedderley, D.; Stephens, J.; Gannabathula, S.; Steinhorn, G.; Schlothauer, R.C.; Whitchurch, C.B.; et al. The Effect of New Zealand Kanuka, Manuka and Clover The effect of New Zealand kanuka, manuka and clover honeys on bacterial growth dynamics and cellular morphology varies according to the species. *PLoS ONE* **2013**, *8*, e55898. [CrossRef] [PubMed]
141. Abbas, H.A. Comparative Antibacterial and Antibiofilm Activities of Manuka Honey and Egyptian Clover Honey. *Asian J. Appl. Sci.* **2014**, *2*, 110–115.
142. Majtan, J.; Bohova, J.; Horniackova, M.; Klaudiny, J.; Majtan, V. Anti-biofilm effects of honey against wound pathogens proteus mirabilis and enterobacter cloacae. *Phyther. Res.* **2014**, *28*, 69–75. [CrossRef] [PubMed]
143. Campeau, M.E.M.; Patel, R.; Campeau, M.E.M.; Patel, R. Antibiofilm Activity of Manuka Honey in Combination with Antibiotics. *Int. J. Bacteriol.* **2014**, *2014*, 1–7. [CrossRef] [PubMed]
144. Wang, Y.-L.; Yu, Q.-H.; Chen, S.-K.; Wang, Y.-H. In-vitro Activity of Honey and Topical Silver in Wound Care Management. *Drug Res.* **2015**, *65*, 592–596. [CrossRef] [PubMed]
145. Sojka, M.; Valachova, I.; Bucekova, M.; Majtan, J. Antibiofilm efficacy of honey and bee-derived defensin-1 on multispecies wound biofilm. *J. Med. Microbiol.* **2016**, *65*, 337–344. [CrossRef] [PubMed]

146. Halstead, F.D.; Webber, M.A.; Oppenheim, B.A. Use of an engineered honey to eradicate preformed biofilms of important wound pathogens: An in vitro study. *J. Wound Care* **2017**, *26*, 442–450. [CrossRef] [PubMed]
147. Piotrowski, M.; Karpiński, P.; Pituch, H.; van Belkum, A.; Obuch-Woszczatyński, P. Antimicrobial effects of Manuka honey on in vitro biofilm formation by Clostridium difficile. *Eur. J. Clin. Microbiol. Infect. Dis.* **2017**, *36*, 1661–1664. [CrossRef] [PubMed]
148. Emineke, S.; Cooper, A.J.; Fouch, S.; Birch, B.R.; Lwaleed, B.A. Diluted honey inhibits biofilm formation: Potential application in urinary catheter management? *J. Clin. Pathol.* **2017**, *70*, 140–144. [CrossRef] [PubMed]
149. Lu, J.; Turnbull, L.; Burke, C.M.; Liu, M.; Carter, D.A.; Schlothauer, R.C.; Whitchurch, C.B.; Harry, E.J. Manuka-type honeys can eradicate biofilms produced by *Staphylococcus aureus* strains with different biofilm-forming abilities. *PeerJ* **2014**, *2*, e326. [CrossRef] [PubMed]
150. Ceylan, O.; Ugur, A.; Isiloglu, M.; Ozcan, F. Evaluation of the Antibacterial, Antibiofilm, Antioxidant, and Cytotoxic Effects of Some Turkish Honeys. In Proceedings of the XXXXIII International Apicultural Congres, Kyiv, Ukraine, 29 September–4 October 2013.
151. Aissat, S.; Ahmed, M.; Djebli, N. Propolis-Sahara honeys preparation exhibits antibacterial and anti-biofilm activity against bacterial biofilms formed on urinary catheters. *Asian Pac. J. Trop. Dis.* **2016**, *6*, 873–877. [CrossRef]
152. da Silva, C.I.; Aazza, S.; Faleiro, M.L.; Miguel, M.D.G.; Neto, L. Propiedades antibacterianas, anti-biofilm, anti-inflamatorias y de inhibición de la virulencia de mieles portuguesas. *J. Apic. Res.* **2016**, *55*, 292–304. [CrossRef]
153. Hancock, R.E.W.; Sahl, H.G. Antimicrobial and host-defense peptides as new anti-infective therapeutic strategies. *Nat. Biotechnol.* **2006**, *24*, 1551–1557. [CrossRef] [PubMed]
154. Ganz, T.; Lehrer, R.I. Antibiotic peptides from higher eukaryotes: Biology and applications. *Mol. Med. Today* **1999**, *5*, 292–297. [CrossRef]
155. Batoni, G.; Maisetta, G.; Esin, S. Antimicrobial peptides and their interaction with biofilms of medically relevant bacteria. *Biochim. Biophys. Acta -Biomembr.* **2016**, *1858*, 1044–1060. [CrossRef] [PubMed]
156. Pletzer, D.; Hancock, R.E.W.W. Anti-biofilm peptides: Potential as broad-spectrum agents. *J. Bacteriol.* **2016**, *198*, 2572–2578. [CrossRef] [PubMed]
157. Chung, P.Y.; Khanum, R. Antimicrobial peptides as potential anti-biofilm agents against multidrug-resistant bacteria. *J. Microbiol. Immunol. Infect.* **2017**, *50*, 405–410. [CrossRef] [PubMed]
158. Zasloff, M. Antimicrobial peptides of multicellular organisms. *Nature* **2002**, *415*, 389–395. [CrossRef] [PubMed]
159. Wang, J.; Chou, S.; Xu, L.; Zhu, X.; Dong, N.; Shan, A.; Chen, Z. High specific selectivity and Membrane-Active Mechanism of the synthetic centrosymmetric α-helical peptides with Gly-Gly pairs. *Sci. Rep.* **2015**, *5*, 1–19. [CrossRef] [PubMed]
160. De La Fuente-Núñez, C.; Cardoso, M.H.; De Souza Cândido, E.; Franco, O.L.; Hancock, R.E.W. Synthetic antibiofilm peptides. *Biochim. Biophys. Acta -Biomembr.* **2016**, *1858*, 1061–1069. [CrossRef] [PubMed]
161. Di Luca, M.; Maccari, G.; Maisetta, G.; Batoni, G. BaAMPs: The database of biofilm-active antimicrobial peptides. *Biofouling* **2015**, *31*, 193–199. [CrossRef] [PubMed]
162. Takahashi, H.; Nadres, E.T.; Kuroda, K. Cationic amphiphilic polymers with antimicrobial activity for oral care applications: Eradication of *S. mutans* biofilm. *Biomacromolecules* **2017**, *181*, 257–265. [CrossRef] [PubMed]
163. Muñoz-Bonilla, A.; Fernández-García, M. Polymeric materials with antimicrobial activity. *Prog. Polym. Sci.* **2012**, *37*, 281–339. [CrossRef]
164. Li, F.; Chai, Z.G.; Sun, M.N.; Wang, F.; Ma, S.; Zhang, L.; Fang, M.; Chen, J.H. Anti-biofilm effect of dental adhesive with cationic monomer. *J. Dent. Res.* **2009**, *88*, 372–376. [CrossRef] [PubMed]
165. Peng, C.; Vishwakarma, A.; Li, Z.; Miyoshi, T.; Barton, H.; Joy, A. Modification of a conventional polyurethane composition provides significant anti-biofilm activity against Escherichia coli. *Polym. Chem.* **2018**, 776. [CrossRef]
166. Kaehn, K. Polihexanide: A safe and highly effective biocide. *Skin Pharmacol. Physiol.* **2010**, *23*, 7–16. [CrossRef] [PubMed]
167. Kamaruzzaman, N.F.; Pina, M.D.F.; Chivu, A.; Good, L. Polyhexamethylene biguanide and nadifloxacin self-assembled nanoparticles: Antimicrobial effects against intracellular methicillin-resistant *Staphylococcus aureus*. *Polymers (Basel)* **2018**, *10*, 521. [CrossRef]

168. Lefebvre, E.; Lembre, P.; Picard, J.; El-Guermah, L.; Seyer, D.; Larreta Garde, V. Ephemeral biogels to control anti-biofilm agent delivery: From conception to the construction of an active dressing. *Mater. Sci. Eng. C* **2018**, *82*, 210–216. [CrossRef] [PubMed]
169. Cutting, K.F. Addressing the challenge of wound cleansing in the modern era. *Br. J. Nurs.* **2010**, *19*, S24–S29. [CrossRef] [PubMed]

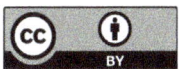

© 2018 by the authors. Licensee MDPI, Basel, Switzerland. This article is an open access article distributed under the terms and conditions of the Creative Commons Attribution (CC BY) license (http://creativecommons.org/licenses/by/4.0/).

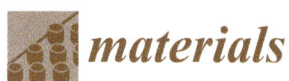

Article

In Vitro Efficacy of Antibiotics Released from Calcium Sulfate Bone Void Filler Beads

Phillip A. Laycock [1], John J. Cooper [1], Robert P. Howlin [2], Craig Delury [1], Sean Aiken [1] and Paul Stoodley [3,4,*]

[1] Biocomposites Ltd., Keele Science Park, Keele, Staffordshire ST5 5NL, UK; pl@biocomposites.com (P.A.L.); jjc@biocomposites.com (J.J.C.); cpd@biocomposites.com (C.D.); sa@biocomposites.com (S.A.)
[2] National Institute for Health Research Southampton Respiratory Biomedical Research Unit, Southampton Centre for Biomedical Research, University of Southampton NHS Foundation Trust, Southampton SO17 1BJ, UK; rhowlin159@gmail.com
[3] National Centre for Advanced Tribology at Southampton (nCATS), Dept, Mechanical Engineering, University of Southampton, Southampton SO17 IBJ, UK
[4] Department of Microbial Infection and Immunity and Orthopedics, The Ohio State University, Columbus, OH 43210, USA
* Correspondence: Paul.Stoodley@osumc.edu.com; Tel.: +1-614-292-7826

Received: 15 October 2018; Accepted: 10 November 2018; Published: 13 November 2018

Abstract: 15 different antibiotics were individually mixed with commercially available calcium sulfate bone void filler beads. The antibiotics were: amikacin, ceftriaxone, cefuroxime, ciprofloxacin, clindamycin, colistamethate sodium, daptomycin, gentamicin, imipenem/cilastatin, meropenem, nafcillin, rifampicin, teicoplanin, tobramycin and vancomycin. The efficacy of specific released antibiotics was validated by zone of inhibition (ZOI) testing using a modified Kirby–Bauer disk diffusion method against common periprosthetic joint infection pathogens. With a subset of experiments (daptomycin, rifampin, vancomycin alone and rifampin and vancomycin in combination), we investigated how release varied over 15 days using a repeated ZOI assay. We also tested the ability of these beads to kill biofilms formed by *Staphylococcus epidermidis* 35984, a prolific biofilm former. The results suggested that certain antibiotics could be combined and released from calcium sulfate with retained antibacterial efficacy. The daptomycin and rifampin plus vancomycin beads showed antimicrobial efficacy for the full 15 days of testing and vancomycin in combination with rifampin prevented resistant mutants. In the biofilm killing assay, all of the antibiotic combinations showed a significant reduction in biofilm bacteria after 24 h. The exposure time was an important factor in the amount of killing, and varied among the antibiotics.

Keywords: calcium sulfate; antibiotics; release; zone of inhibition; biofilm

1. Introduction

Musculoskeletal infection represents a serious problem for patients, operating surgeons and the economic wellbeing of the healthcare system. Infection is a serious and debilitating complication of many clinical conditions and surgical procedures. Increasing resistance to current antibiotics is, according to the World Health Organization (WHO), "a problem so serious that it threatens the achievements of modern medicine" [1]. Reported in the Review of Antimicrobial Resistance, by 2050, "today's already large 700,000 deaths every year would become an extremely disturbing 10 million every year, more people than currently die from cancer" [2]. The levels of antibiotics required to successfully manage infection are rising as bacterial resistance increases, to such a point where systemic levels required to be effective against the infection are increasingly toxic to the patient. An area gaining increasing interest is the combination and local release of antibiotics from suitable implantable materials. The benefits of local release at the site of infection are significant and include the ability to provide very high local levels of antibiotic, many times the minimal inhibitory concentration (MIC), with serum levels and associated toxicity remaining low. Reduced systemic administration may then be possible as, in addition to toxicity, exposure to antibiotics can lead to disruption of the normal human colonic flora and increased susceptibility to colonization and toxin production by *Clostridium difficile* (*C. difficile*). *C. difficile* causes an inflammation of the colon and deadly diarrhea, and is one of the most common microbial causes of healthcare associated infections in USA hospitals [3]. One of the most adopted materials used in combination with antibiotics is poly-methyl methacrylate bone cement (PMMA) [3]. A number of commercially available antibiotic-loaded PMMA bone cements are shown in Table 1, where gentamicin is the most common combined antibiotic.

Table 1. Antibiotic-loaded PMMA cements.

Name	Antibiotic	Manufacturer	CE Mark	FDA 510 (k)
CEMEX® Genta	CEMEX® Genta	CEMEX® Genta	Yes	K043403
Copal® G + C	Gentamicin, Clindamycin	Heraeus GmbH, Hanau, Germany	Yes	No
Copal® G + V	Gentamicin, Vancomycin	Heraeus GmbH, Hanau, Germany	Yes	No
Palacos® R + G	Gentamicin	Heraeus GmbH, Hanau, Germany	Yes	K031673
Palamed® G	Gentamicin	Heraeus GmbH, Hanau, Germany	Yes	K050855
Smartset GHV	Gentamicin	Depuy Orthopaedics, Rosemont, IL, USA	Yes	K033563
Simplex® P	Tobramycin	Stryker, Kalamazoo, MI, USA	Yes	K014199
VancogeneX®	Vancomycin, Gentamicin	Tecres S.P.A, Verona, Italy	Yes	No

There is valid evidence to support the use of antibiotic-loaded PMMA in the form of spacers, bone cement for anchoring a prosthesis or as beads on a wire, however, there are still a number of significant disadvantages. PMMA is not absorbed in the body and needs a further operation for removal. In addition, the dead space following removal of the PMMA beads must be managed. Due to the way the antibiotic is contained within the material, following an initial burst release, it can continue to release sub-inhibitory levels over an extended time period increasing the risk of bacterial resistance [4–6]. PMMA is not suitable for thermosensitive antibiotics because of the high temperatures generated during curing. The combination of antibiotics with alternative biomaterials is now the subject of extensive investigation. A number of antibiotic-loaded biomaterials have received the European CE mark approval (Table 2) but have yet to be approved by the USA FDA (Food and Drug Administration). All these materials have advantages including good biocompatibility and drug/material compatibility but can have inherent disadvantages such as too rapid or inconsistent elution or, in the cases of calcium phosphates and composites, slow to incomplete absorption, which may present a potential nidus for infection. There is also a risk of damage to articulating surfaces from hard, non-absorbable biomaterials such as Hydroxyapatite (HA) with the migration of particles into the joint space, producing third-body wear and subsequent osteolysis [7].

Table 2. Antibiotic-loaded biomaterials (CE marked).

Name	Composition	Antibiotic	Manufacturer
Cerament™ G	Calcium sulfate/HA	Gentamicin	Bonesupport AB, Lund, Sweden
Cerament™ V	Calcium sulfate/HA	Vancomycin	Bonesupport AB, Lund, Sweden
Collatamp® G	Collagen	Gentamicin	EUSAPharma Ltd., Hemel Hempstead, UK
Herafill® beads G	Calcium sulfate/Calcium carbonate	Gentamicin	Heraeus GmbH, Hanau, Germany
Osteoset® T	Calcium sulfate	Tobramycin	Wright Medical Technology, Inc., Memphis, TN, USA

One material with high potential is pure calcium sulfate. It is completely absorbed in the body and is biocompatible. Calcium sulfate has a long history of clinical use. Its first reported use in combination with a medicament was as early as 1892 when Dreesman and colleagues added 5% phenol (carbolic acid) solution to treat bone cavities as a result of tuberculosis osteomyelitis in long bones [8]. A typical residence time for calcium sulfate beads implanted in a contained bone defect is reported as 4 to 13 weeks [9–12]. In a soft tissue site and a site with high fluid exchange this time period may be considerably less (around three weeks) [13–15]. The antibiotic will elute predominantly over the first few days (burst release) followed by a gradual reduction in concentration as the calcium sulfate resorbs [16–18]. As there is a very small temperature rise on curing, mixing of heat labile antibiotics is possible [19,20]. With a well-established biocompatibility and resorption profile, calcium sulfate is increasingly being used in clinical practice for local antibiotic release [21–24].

Recent research has been carried out on the elution of specific antibiotics from calcium sulfate [16] but little work has been reported on the antimicrobial efficacy of the eluted antibiotic. In this study, investigations into the in vitro efficacy of the antibiotic(s) released from the calcium sulfate was carried out through zone of inhibition (ZOI) testing using the disk diffusion method against a range of susceptible pathogens, and compared to the published data according to the European Committee on Antimicrobial Susceptibility Testing (EUCAST) breakpoints [25] and Clinical and Laboratory Standards Institute (CLSI) M100 Standards [26]. In addition, in a subset of experiments, we used a repeated zone of inhibition assay and in vitro grown biofilms to expand on previous experiments with vancomycin and tobramycin [27], and to assess how the local elution of daptomycin and rifampicin alone and in combination with vancomycin may release over time and its efficacy of killing staphylococcal biofilms. Daptomycin has shown promise in treating patients with osteomyelitis or orthopaedic device infections when delivered systemically [28] and rifampicin has been shown to have good activity against staphylococcal biofilms but should be used in combination with other antibiotics due to concerns over resistance [29].

2. Materials and Methods

2.1. Preparation of Calcium Sulfate Beads

All bead/antibiotic combinations were prepared using a commercially available synthetic recrystallized calcium sulfate hemi-hydrate—$CaSO_4 \cdot \frac{1}{2}H_2O$ (SRCS) (Stimulan® Rapid Cure, Biocomposites, Staffordshire, UK). This material is produced from pharmaceutical grade reagents without the addition of other excipients such as steric acid, to give a high purity, hydrophilic material having a physiological pH 10 cc packs of SRCS containing 20 g of calcium sulfate hemihydrate powder were used.

15 different antibiotics were selected based on published or 'data on file' clinical reports of their use with calcium sulfate [11,12,14,15,21–24] (Table 3). A number of bacteria were tested including

S. epidermidis ATCC12228, *P. aeruginosa* NCTC 13437, *S. aureus* ATCC 6538, *Acinetobacter Baumanii* NCTC 134242, *S. aureus* 12493 MRSA, *E. faecalis* NCTC 12202, *P. acnes* NCTC 737 and *E. faecalis* NCTC 12201. For daptomycin, the maximum dose was referenced from the USP (United States Pharmacopeia) [30]. Sterile saline was used in the mixing of amikacin and daptomycin, replacing some or all of the mixing solution provided in the SRCS pack. The use of a 0.9% sodium chloride solution was found to speed up the setting reaction for these retarding antibiotics. The resultant paste, together with added antibiotic was pressed into hemispherical cavities, 6 mm diameter, in a flexible rubber mold where it was allowed to hydrate and set accordingly.

Table 3. Antibiotics tested in this study.

Antibiotic	Manufacturer
Amikacin Sulfate	Hospira Ltd., Maidenhead, UK
Ceftriaxone Sodium	Apotex Corporation, Toronto, ON, Canada
Cefuroxime	Stravencon, London, UK
Ciprofloxacin Hydrochloride	Medisca Inc., Las Vegas, NV, USA
Colistamethane Sodium	Sigma-Aldrich, Dorset, UK
Clindamycin (Dalacin C® Phosphate)	Pfizer, Tadworth, UK
Daptomycin (Cubicin®)	Novartis, Basel, Switzerland
Gentamicin Sulfate	Hospira Ltd., Maidenhead, UK
Imipenem/Cilastatin (Zienam®)	Merck & Co., Inc, Kenilworth, NJ, USA
Meropenem Trihydrate	Fresenius Kabi Ltd., Cestrian, UK
Nafcillin Sodium	Sandoz, Princeton, NJ, USA
Rifampicin	Sigma-Aldrich, Dorset, UK
Teicoplanin (Targocid®)	Sanofi-Aventis, Guildford, UK
Tobramycin Sulfate	Hospira Ltd., Maidenhead, UK
Vancomycin Hydrochloride	Hospira Ltd., Maidenhead, UK

2.2. Zone of Inhibition Testing

Tryptone soya agar (TSA) plates were seeded with a 0.2 mL suspension of the relevant organism containing approximately 10^8 CFU (Colony Forming Units)/mL. The plates were transferred to an incubator operating at $33 \pm 2\ ^\circ\text{C}$ for 30 min. The plates were then removed from the incubator and a single 6 mm antibiotic-loaded bead was placed on the surface of the agar. The plates were then incubated at $33 \pm 2\ ^\circ\text{C}$ for 24 h, after which time they were removed from the incubator and examined for any clear zones around the test sample. Zones were measured to the nearest mm where no obvious growth could be detected by the unaided eye. Samples were tested in triplicate and an average diameter was recorded. Zone diameters were compared to published data according to the European Committee on Antimicrobial Susceptibility Testing (EUCAST) breakpoints and Clinical and Laboratory Standards Institute (CLSI) M100 Standards [26] where applicable. It is important to note that this assay was not designed to determine breakpoint zones of the challenge strains against the various antibiotics. Breakpoint testing is performed using well-defined amounts of antibiotics loaded onto filter papers, which have well-characterized and reproducible release kinetics. Rather this assay was used to determine that the antibiotic was (1) released from the bead and (2) had retained antibiotic potency. Presence of a zone of inhibition was demonstrative that both these conditions were true. The known breakpoints from the standard method guidelines were provided as a reference guide.

2.3. Repeat Zone of Inhibition Testing

To assess how long the beads may release antibiotic, we used a modified Kirby–Bauer disk diffusion assay as previously reported [27]. *Staphylococcus aureus* NCTC 13143 EMRSA-16 (an MRSA strain) and *S. epidermidis* ATCC 35984, a prolific biofilm former was used as the challenge organisms. First, a lawn of bacteria was spread onto TSA plates using 50 µL of an overnight culture grown for 15 h at 37 °C. A single bead containing (in mg/5 cc pack SRCS) either (a) daptomycin (500 mg), (b) vancomycin (500 mg), (c) rifampicin (300 mg) or (d) a combination of vancomycin and rifampicin

(500 mg + 300 mg) were placed on the agar plate using sterile forceps and incubated at 37 °C for 24 h. Zones of inhibition (ZOI) were measured and photographed, and then the beads were aseptically transferred onto a freshly prepared lawn of bacteria in a laminar flow hood as previously described [27]. This process was repeated each day until the ZOI was lost or the beads broke up. The area (cm^2) of the ZOI was calculated using Image J (version 1.48) image analysis package. Area, rather than the diameter of the ZOI for these tests was reported to account for irregularities in the shape of the ZOI as the beads dissolved over time. We assessed the release and antimicrobial activity into agar rather than into an aqueous solution (which is another common method for measuring release kinetics) since we were interested in assessing the area of antimicrobial activity that a single bead might have in a diffusion-dominated environment such as what might be found adjacent to tissue.

2.4. Biofilm Killing Assay

S. epidermidis ATCC 35984 was used as the challenge organism. Overnight broth cultures were diluted in fresh Tryptone soya broth (TSB) to an optical density (OD) corresponding to 10^6 cells/mL. 4 mL of the culture was added to each well of a 6 well plate (for viable cell counts) or tissue culture plates (MatTek, Corp.) (for confocal microscopy). Biofilms were grown for 72 h at 37 °C with a daily TSB nutrient exchange. Ten, 4.8 mm diameter beads were placed into each well plate and incubated at 37 °C for a further 24 h, 72 h or 1 week, with daily media changes. For cell counts, the wells were rinsed with 4 mL Hanks Buffered Salt Solution (HBSS) and a cell scraper was used to transfer the biofilm into 1 mL of HBSS. After scraping into 1 mL HBSS, the cells were vortexed using a lab bench vortexer for 20 s to homogenize the biofilm bacteria. A 10-fold serial dilution was plated onto tryptic soy agar (TSA; Sigma-Aldrich, St. Louis, MI, USA). Following incubation for 24 h at 37 °C, viable cell counts were performed, and the data expressed as CFU/cm^2. Concurrently, confocal scanning laser microscopy (CSLM) of the biofilm was performed after 24h, 72 h and 1-week exposure to the beads. The biofilm was stained with Live/Dead Baclight (Invitrogen), which stains live cells green and dead cells red. After a 30 min incubation the plates were gently rinsed and observed using an inverted confocal laser scanning microscope (Leica DMI600 SP5, Wetzlar, Germany). The images were rendered using the freely downloadable NIH ImageJ. Each channel (green and red) was optimized for contrast using the "auto" setting. The channels were then merged using the "make composite" function. The individual z-sections in the stack were then compressed to show the full biomass in a 2-dimensional representation using "Z-project" with "sum slices", and finally saved as a JPEG image.

2.5. Statistics

Viability CFU data were tested for normality using the Shapiro–Wilk test. Since the data were not normal ($p > 0.05$) they were compared using a Mann–Whitney rank sum test (Sigma-Plot, San Jose, CA, USA) for not normally distributed data, and a difference was considered significant when the p value was <0.05.

3. Results

3.1. Preparation of Calcium Sulfate Beads

Of the 15 antibiotics selected, 12 were in a lyophilized powder form. Where the powdered antibiotics were mixed with the SRCS by combining the powders together and then adding the aqueous mixing solution, all except ceftriaxone, daptomycin and imipenem/cilastatin allowed the SRCS to set hard but extended the setting time out from 4 min to a maximum of 20 min. For the powdered antibiotics that significantly delayed the setting time, the effect was reduced by hydrating the SRCS prior to the addition of the antibiotic thus initiating the calcium sulfate setting reaction whilst unloaded. This technique allowed the SRCS to set when ceftriaxone, daptomycin and imipenem/cilastatin were added. In addition, replacing the mixing solution with sterile saline reduced the set time even further with daptomycin. For the tobramycin and gentamicin liquid formulations, these were supplied in

2 mL vials, each containing 80 mg of antibiotic. For both these antibiotics, 3 vials were used to provide the required 6 mL for hydration of the SRCS, giving a dose of 240 mg. This was a limiting factor in the maximum dose, which may be combined. Two of the liquid antibiotic formulations; amikacin and clindamycin, were commercially provided in volumes of 2 mL and 4 mL. Additional fluid was required to make the volume up to 6 mL, required to fully hydrate the SRCS. For these antibiotics, a quantity of the aqueous mixing solution was accurately added via a syringe to make the volume up to the required 6 mL. Neither of these antibiotic combinations would set hard when the aqueous mixing solution was used, therefore, sterile saline was investigated as an alternative. This method allowed for the production of fully hardened amikacin-loaded beads. The clindamycin, which is in the form of a phosphate, may chemically react with the calcium sulfate, precipitating out as an insoluble calcium phosphate. In addition, this formulation of clindamycin contained benzyl alcohol and EDTA (ethylenediaminetetraacetic acid) as excipients. The ability of SRCS to set hard with Clindamycin in the form tested here was not achieved, therefore was unable to be combined in this way and no microbiology data was obtained.

3.2. Zone of Inhibition Testing

Zone diameters for each antibiotic/SRCS bead combination are shown in Table 4. Where EUCAST clinical breakpoint data [31] or CLSI M100 data [26] were available, they were included for reference. SRCS beads mixed with rifampicin achieved zones which fell below the CLSI M100 breakpoint data for both *S. epidermidis* and a methicillin-resistant strain of *S. aureus*. Interestingly, SRCS beads mixed with ciprofloxacin had varying success, depending on the species of bacteria under investigation. Ciprofloxacin-loaded SRCS beads were tested against a range of Gram-negative species including *P. aeruginosa* and *Acinetobacter Baumanii*. The zones of inhibition recorded for these species, fell below the EUCAST and CLSI breakpoints for the respective bacteria (12 and 15 mm respectively) (Table 4). Conversely, when SRCS were mixed with ciprofloxacin and tested against a range of Gram-positive species, the SRCS-loaded beads were able to generate zones measuring 36 and 25 mm (for *S. epidermidis* and *S. aureus* respectively). The observed zones were greater than the EUCAST and CLSI breakpoint for these bacterial species tested against this antibiotic. All other antibiotic combinations produced a clear zone against susceptible species and where breakpoint data was available, exceeded the breakpoint diameter, demonstrating an above MIC elution concentration and maintained efficacy (Table 4). For the vancomycin SRCS beads with *Enterococcus faecalis*, two vancomycin resistant control strains were used. NCTC 12201 (VanA-type glycopeptide resistance, Erythromycin resistant) and NCTC 12202 (VanA-type glycopeptide resistance). The results demonstrated that the high burst release concentration could exceed the vancomycin MIC of these two strains which are reported to exceed 256 µg/mL [32]. EUCAST and CLSI breakpoints have not been published for these strains but the zones observed were larger than the published breakpoints for susceptible strains of *E. faecalis* (Table 4).

Table 4. Zones of Inhibition (ZOI) data with EUCAST clinical breakpoint tables v 6.0 and CLSI M100 breakpoints.

Antibiotic Conc. per 10cc Pack SRCS	Species	Zone Diameter (mm)	EUCAST/ CLSI M100	Zone Diameter Breakpoint (mm)		Note
				Susceptible $\geq$	Resistant $\leq$	
Amikacin 500 mg/2 mL	*S. epidermidis* (ATCC 12228)	30	EUCAST	22 [a]	19 [a]	[a] Coagulase negative staphylococci
			CLSI	-	-	n/a
	P. aeruginosa (NCTC 13437)	20	EUCAST	18 [c]	15 [c]	[c] *Pseudomonas* spp.
			CLSI	15	12	
Ceftriaxone 1 g	*S. aureus* (ATCC 6538)	47	EUCAST	-	-	n/a
			CLSI	-	-	n/a
	S. epidermidis (ATCC 12228)	31	EUCAST	-	-	n/a
			CLSI	-	-	n/a

Table 4. Cont.

Antibiotic Conc. per 10cc Pack SRCS	Species	Zone Diameter (mm)	EUCAST/ CLSI M100	Zone Diameter Breakpoint (mm)		Note
				Susceptible ≥	Resistant ≤	
Cefuroxime 1.5 g	S. aureus (ATCC 6538)	47	EUCAST CLSI	- -	- -	n/a n/a
	S. epidermidis (ATCC 12228)	22	EUCAST CLSI	- -	- -	n/a n/a
	P. aeruginosa (NCTC 13437)	28	EUCAST CLSI	- -	- -	n/a n/a
	Acinetobacter Baumannii (NCTC 134242)	22	EUCAST CLSI	- -	- -	n/a n/a
Colistamethane Sodium 400 mg	S. aureus (ATCC 6538)	9	EUCAST CLSI	- -	- -	n/a n/a
	S. epidermidis (ATCC 12228)	11	EUCAST CLSI	- -	- -	n/a n/a
	P. aeruginosa (NCTC 13437)	13	EUCAST CLSI	- -	- -	n/a n/a
Ciprofloxacin 1 g	P. aeruginosa (NCTC 13437)	17	EUCAST CLSI	25 [c] 21	22 [c] 15	[c] *Pseudomonas* spp. -
	Acinetobacter Baumannii (NCTC 134242)	15	EUCAST CLSI	21 [d] 21 [d]	21 [d] 15 [d]	[d] *Acinetobacter* spp. [d] *Acinetobacter* spp.
Ciprofloxacin 1 g	S. epidermidis (ATCC 12228) S.aureus (NCTC 12493) MRSA (NCTC 134242)	36 25	EUCAST CLSI EUCAST CLSI	20 [b] 21 [b] 20 [b] 21 [b]	20 [b] 15 [b] 20 [b] 15 [b]	[b] *Staphylococcus* spp. [b] *Staphylococcus* spp. [b] *Staphylococcus* spp. [b] *Staphylococcus* spp.
Daptomycin 1 g	S. epidermidis (ATCC 12228) E. faecalis * (NCTC 12202) P. acnes (NCTC 737) P. aeruginosa (NCTC 13437)	25 13.5 31 11	EUCAST CLSI EUCAST CLSI EUCAST CLSI EUCAST CLSI	- - - - - - - -	- - - - - - - -	n/a n/a n/a n/a n/a n/a n/a n/a
Gentamicin 240 mg	S. aureus (ATCC 6538) S. epidermidis (ATCC 12228)	20 30	EUCAST CLSI EUCAST CLSI	18 15 [b] 22 [a] 15 [b]	18 12 [b] 22 [a] 12 [b]	- [b] *Staphylococcus* spp. [a] Coagulase negative staphylococci [b] *Staphylococcus* spp.
Imipenem & Cilastatin 500 mg	S. aureus (ATCC 6538) S. aureus (NCTC 12493) MRSA	58 49	EUCAST CLSI EUCAST CLSI	- - - -	- - - -	n/a n/a n/a n/a
	S. epidermidis (ATCC 12228)	60	EUCAST CLSI	- -	- -	n/a n/a
Meropenem 1 g	S. epidermidis (ATCC 12228) S. aureus (NCTC 12493) MRSA	56 37	EUCAST CLSI EUCAST CLSI	- - - -	- - - -	n/a n/a n/a n/a
	P. aeruginosa (NCTC 13437) Acinetobacter Baumannii (NCTC 134242)	28 22	EUCAST CLSI EUCAST CLSI	24 [c] 19 21 [d] 18 [d]	18 [c] 15 15 [d] 14 [d]	[c] *Pseudomonas* spp. - [d] *Acinetobacter* spp. [d] *Acinetobacter* spp.

109

Table 4. Cont.

Antibiotic Conc. per 10cc Pack SRCS	Species	Zone Diameter (mm)	EUCAST/ CLSI M100	Zone Diameter Breakpoint (mm) Susceptible ≥	Resistant ≤	Note
Nafcillin 1 g	S. aureus (ATCC 6538)	51	EUCAST CLSI	- 22 [b]	- 21 [b]	n/a [b] Staphylococcus spp. Cefoxitin (Oxicillin surrogate)
	S. epidermidis (ATCC 12228)	57 13	EUCAST CLSI	- 22 [b]	- 21 [b]	n/a [b] Staphylococcus spp. Cefoxitin (Oxicillin surrogate)
	P. aeruginosa (NCTC 13437)		EUCAST CLSI	- -	- -	n/a n/a
Rifampicin 600 mg	S. epidermidis (ATCC 12228)	15	EUCAST CLSI	- 20 [b]	- 16 [b]	n/a [b] Staphylococcus spp.
	S. aureus (NCTC 12493) MRSA	11	EUCAST CLSI	- 20 [b]	- 16 [b]	n/a [b] Staphylococcus spp.
Teicoplanin 400 mg	S. aureus (ATCC 6538)	18	EUCAST CLSI	- -	- -	n/a n/a
	S. aureus (NCTC 12493) MRSA	26 23	EUCAST CLSI	- -	- -	n/a n/a
	S. epidermidis (ATCC 12228)		EUCAST CLSI	- -	- -	n/a n/a
Tobramycin 1.2 g	S. aureus (ATCC 6538)	19	EUCAST CLSI	18 -	18 -	- n/a
	S. epidermidis (ATCC 12228)	28	EUCAST CLSI	22 [a] -	22 [a] -	[a] Coagulase negative staphylococci n/a
Vancomycin 1 g	S. aureus (ATCC 6538)	21	EUCAST CLSI	- -	- -	n/a n/a
	S. epidermidis (ATCC 12228)	23	EUCAST CLSI	- -	- -	n/a n/a
	E. faecalis * (NCTC 12201)	17–18	EUCAST CLSI	12 [e] 17 [e]	12 [e] 14 [e]	[e] Enterococcus spp. [e] Enterococcus spp.
	E. faecalis * (NCTC 12202)	12–13	EUCAST CLSI	12 [e] 17 [e]	12 [e] 14 [e]	[e] Enterococcus spp. [e] Enterococcus spp.

* Denotes Vancomycin Resistant Control Strains. ([a–e]) Represent the breakpoints for that particular species.

3.3. Repeat Zone of Inhibition Testing

In the case of beads tested against *S. aureus* NCTC 13143 EMRSA-16 strains, large ZOIs were maintained for 20 days in the case of rifampicin and rifampicin and vancomycin in the combination beads (Figure 1). In the case of daptomycin-loaded beads, the size of the ZOI was smaller (~4 cm^2) but were also maintained for the 20 days duration. A similar trend was seen for beads tested against a *S. epidermidis* ATCC 35984 strain.

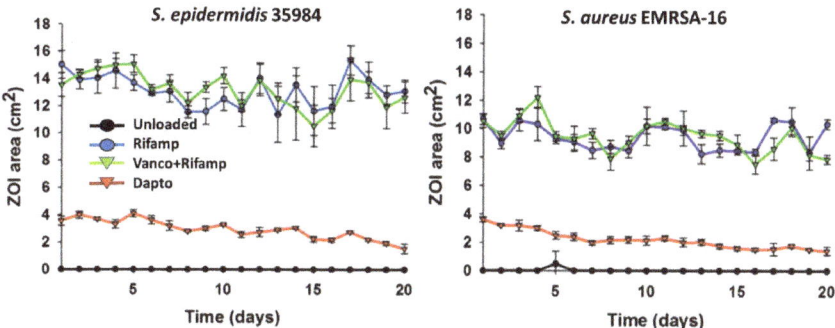

Figure 1. Repeated zone of inhibition (ZOI) of *S. aureus* NCTC 13143 EMRSA-16 and *S. epidermidis* ATCC 35984 Stimulan® beads loaded with rifampicin, rifampicin and vancomycin or daptomycin. Assays were performed in triplicate and data expressed as the mean and 1SD.

At the end of the 20 day assay, suspected resistance was noted developing in the rifampicin-only loaded beads, as shown by an internal ring of viable bacteria within the ZOI (Figure 2A,C). This was not observed on plates that had been exposed to beads containing rifampicin and vancomycin in combination (Figure 2B,D).

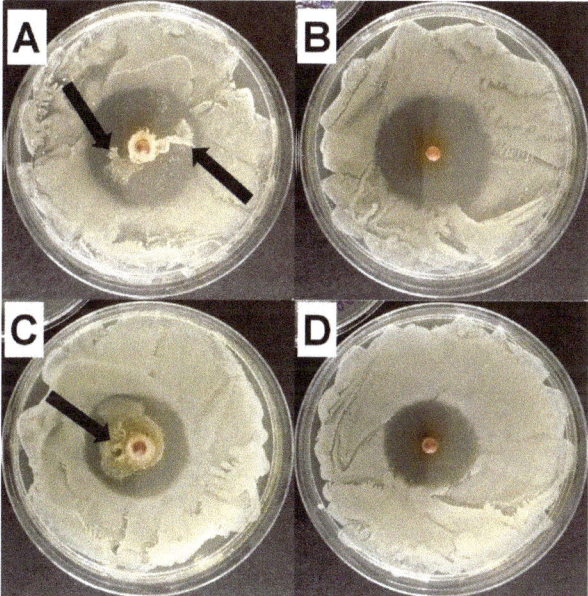

Figure 2. Representative image of the Zones of Inhibition (ZOI) observed with (**A,B**) *S. epidermidis* ATCC 35984 and (**C,D**) *S. aureus* NCTC 13143 EMRSA-16 at day 20 of rifampicin and vancomycin in combination, showing no evidence of resistant colonies (**B,D**) and rifampicin alone (**A,C**) showing potential resistant mutant colonies growing within the ZOI (black arrows).

3.4. Biofilm Killing Assay

Beads loaded with rifampicin, and vancomycin and rifampicin in combination were able to achieve a 2-log reduction in CFU/cm^2 at 24 h (Figure 3) with CSLM imaging showing a concurrent marked reduction in biofilm mass (Figure 4). After 72 h contact time, rifampicin alone achieved a

5-log reduction in CFU/cm^2 (Figure 3) with the combination of vancomycin and rifampicin showing no growth on the plate. CSLM imaging showed almost complete removal of the biofilm with only a few single cells remaining (Figure 4). However, at one week, regrowth was noted in rifampicin and rifampicin and vancomycin treatment groups and reformation of microcolonies noted with CSLM imaging (Figure 4). Additionally, the combination of rifampicin and vancomycin demonstrated a 3-log regrowth relative to CFU/cm^2 data at 72 h suggesting that the regrowth may have been due to some cells that were rendered viable but nonculturable at 72 h. Daptomycin-loaded beads resulted in an approximate 7-log reduction in CFU/cm^2 relative to unloaded beads after 24 h contact time with mature *S. epidermidis* biofilms (Figure 3). There was little further change over the next seven days. CSLM imaging corroborated the CFU data showing a significant reduction in biofilm and total surface coverage observed at day 7 relative to unloaded beads (Figure 4). Interestingly, in the biofilm exposed to the rifampicin only beads, after 7 days there was the appearance of larger aggregates, which had both live (green) and dead (red) cells suggesting the proliferation of resistant mutants. In the control most of the cells were still live (green) however, there were patches of red (dead or compromised) cells suggesting that the cells may have been undergoing starvation due to nutrient limitation. In the biofilms exposed to the combination of vancomycin and rifampicin there was a sparse covering of cells, which were mainly live, while in the daptomycin-exposed biofilm there were very few cells and these were only very faintly stained green (Figure 4).

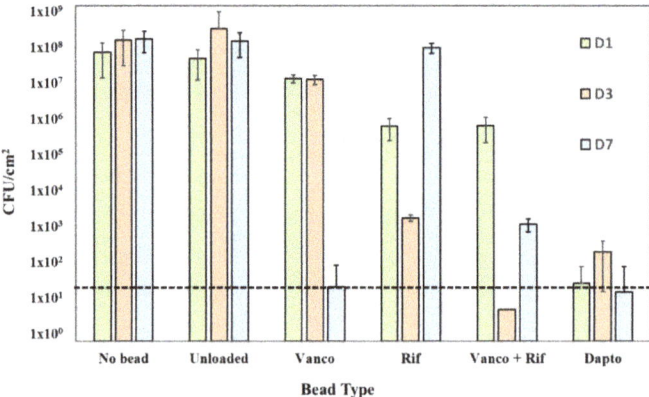

Figure 3. Effect of unloaded beads as well as vancomycin (Vanco), rifampicin (Rif), rifampicin and vancomycin in combination (Vanco + Rif) and daptomycin (Dapto) loaded beads on established *S. epidermidis* ATCC 35984 biofilms at contact times at days (D) 1,3 and 7. Dashed line is the detection limit. No beads were added as a positive control for biofilm growth. Mean and 95% CI (n = 3), *indicates statistically significant differences from the unloaded beads ($p < 0.05$).

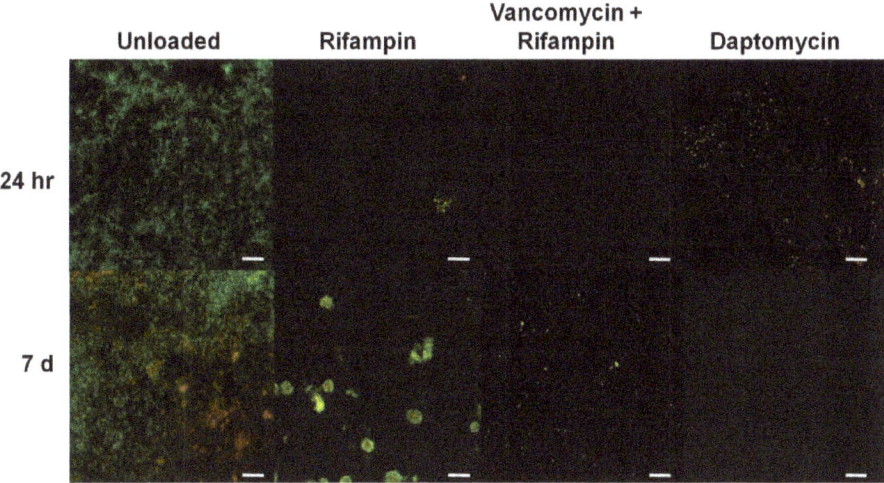

Figure 4. Representative CSLM images showing *S. epidermidis* ATCC 35984 biofilm (live cells stained green and dead and membrane compromised cells stained red or yellow) following treatment for 24 h and 1 week with unloaded beads (negative control) and beads loaded with rifampicin (Rifampin), rifampicin and vancomycin, and daptomycin. Scale bars: 25 µm.

4. Discussion

With the exception of clindamycin, the calcium sulfate in combination with the antibiotics tested, set hard, maintaining its function as a void filler. All antibiotics used in this study were IV formulations. Antibiotic capsules and tablets contain different excipients to IV formulations and these may create additional risks if administered locally. Ceftriaxone, although included here, is contraindicated when mixing with a calcium-containing product such as Ringer's solution, Hartmann's solution or parenteral nutrition containing calcium. The reason for this contraindication is the risk of crystalline precipitates forming in the lungs and kidneys. Although this risk is for IV administration, the risks should be considered if used in combination with calcium sulfate in this application and warrants further investigation. The ability of SRCS or any biomaterial to mix and set with antibiotics, and demonstrate release and potency alone or in combination in in vitro laboratory studies, does not imply safety or efficacy in clinical use, and in vitro results may not be indicative of clinical performance.

A number of independent studies have shown that calcium sulfate beads may be used in revision arthroplasty for PJI (Periprosthetic Joint Infection), with favorable outcomes [21,33,34]. However, their use is not without risk. One potential risk is transitory hypercalcemia in vivo and this has been reported in literature, [15,21] although only when the material has been implanted in soft tissue sites and in larger volumes. More recent studies however, have shown that there is no significant difference in incidences of hypercalcemia when compared with other antibiotic-loaded materials [35].

This study demonstrates that a wide range of antibiotics can be incorporated into the SRCS and retain potency against a wide range of common bacterial pathogens associated with PJI using an *in vitro* zone of inhibition assay. Where EUCAST or CLSI breakpoints were available for specific antibiotics against susceptible pathogens, the same antibiotics when eluted from the SRCS all maintained their antimicrobial activity with the exception of ciprofloxacin and rifampicin. This assay is a relatively simple test which can be used to assess whether antibiotics as monotherapy or in combination, which (a) are currently used to treat orthopedic infections systemically or (b) show promise in in vitro studies also have potential to be eluted locally by SRCS made up as beads or in other forms. Although the standardized Kirby–Bauer disc diffusion method is used as a quick and convenient method of assessing the susceptibility of a given organism to a given antibiotic [36], modifications of the assay allow it to be used to assess the release and maintenance of potency from materials other than filter paper, such as how we have done with materials such as SRCS, and PMMA as detailed in previous studies [27]. The results for ciprofloxacin against *Pseudomonas aerugonisa* (NCTC 13437) and *Acinetobacter baumannii* (NCTC 134242) showed a smaller zone than the breakpoint data for Pseudomonas spp. (Table 4). This may be due to the susceptibility of the specific species or other factors such as compatibility with the SRCS or reduced elution.

The quantity of each antibiotic held in the disks used in the EUCAST or CLSI M100 may differ to the quantity of antibiotic in the SRCS beads, therefore, correlation to the clinical breakpoints should not be inferred and these values are included for reference and demonstration of susceptibility only. Future work should focus on testing the release of antibiotics from SRCS as per the guidance of EUCAST or CLSI in order to make a more direct comparison of the efficacy of released antibiotic from SRCS beads.

We further modified the method to assess the longevity of release in vitro by placing SRCS on new spread plates daily. The ZOI for daptomycin started at approximately 4 cm^2 and slowly reduced to 2 cm^2 after 20 days of the experiment for both the EMRSA and *S. epidermidis* challenge strains. This behavior was very similar to that seen with vancomycin and tobramycin assessed previously [27]. Interestingly the SRCS beads containing vancomycin and rifampicin or rifampicin alone had much greater ZOIs of between 14 cm^2 and 10 cm^2 against EMRSA and *S. epidermidis*, respectively. These remained relatively constant over the full 20 days of testing.

Rifampicin has been noted to have "excellent activity on adherent staphylococci" [37] and biofilms [29]. However, since it is known that there is rapid emergence of resistance when used in monotherapy [38] it is used in combination with other antibiotics. Indeed, in our assay we noted growth within the ZOI of the beads loaded with rifampicin alone (Figure 2). Since the plates were spread freshly every day it was possible that the growth came from bacteria carried over with the bead that had been exposed to rifampicin for an extended period. Interestingly, the beads with both vancomycin and rifampicin showed no evidence of the emergence of resistance. However, to more fully assess the potential for the development of resistance with vancomycin and rifampicin, more stringent studies are required. The *S. epidermidis* biofilm killing assay showed different patterns of killing with the various antibiotics. Vancomycin-alone only caused an approximate 1-log reduction after 1 and 3 days exposure but by 7 days there was a 6-log reduction illustrating the importance of prolonged exposure to high concentrations of antibiotics when treating biofilms. Rifampicin alone was more effective, showing an approximate 2-log reduction after 1 day and 5-log reduction after 3 days, however, there was significant regrowth at day 7. The confocal image showed large cell clusters had formed suggesting the emergence of resistant mutants within this time period (Figure 4). Rifampicin and vancomycin in combination reduced the biofilm to below detectable levels after 3 days (>7-log reduction) but there was a "bounce" back at day 7 to an approximate 5-log reduction compared to the control unloaded beads. Although there was no evidence of new colony formation from the confocal data, more work needs to be done to assess the potential for the emergence of resistance with this combination. However, a combination of vancomycin and rifampicin has been shown to be more effective than vancomycin alone in treating PJI in a mouse model [39], and the local release of rifampicin from SRCS in combination with other antibiotics to treat orthopedic biofilm infections shows promise. Although daptomycin resulted in the lowest ZOI in the diffusion assay, it caused the greatest reduction in biofilm (approximately 6 logs) after only 1-day exposure, however, little further reduction was seen after the longer exposure periods.

5. Conclusions

The use of locally released antibiotics from synthetic recrystallized calcium sulfate may offer significant benefits in the management of surgical site infections. The ability to combine different antibiotics could enable a therapy tailored to the offending pathogens. The exposure time, type of antibiotic(s) released from SRCS and the challenge bacterial strain can all influence the kinetics of biofilm killing and thus, in vitro results with one set of conditions should not be over generalized.

Author Contributions: Conceptualization, P.A.L., J.J.C., S.A., and P.S.; methodology, P.A.L., J.J.C. and R.P.H.; formal analysis, P.A.L., R.H., P.S.; resources, S.A. and P.S.; writing—original draft preparation, P.A.L., P.S. and C.D.; writing—review and editing, P.A.L., C.D., S.A. and P.S.; visualization, P.A.L., R.H., C.D., and P.S.; supervision, P.A.L. and P.S.; project administration, S.A. and P.S.; funding acquisition, S.A. and P.S.

Funding: This research was funded by Biocomposites Ltd.

Acknowledgments: In this section you can acknowledge any support given which is not covered by the author contribution or funding sections. This may include administrative and technical support, or donations in kind (e.g., materials used for experiments).

Conflicts of Interest: P.A.L., J.J.C., C.D. and S.A. are employees of Biocomposites Ltd. R.H. and P.S. consult for Biocomposites Ltd. The funders contributed to the design, collection, analyses or interpretation of data and in the writing of the manuscript for the zone of inhibition study. The funders had no role in the original design, execution, data analysis or writing up of the repeated zone of inhibition and biofilm killing parts of the study. The funders did prepare the beads used in these parts of the study and reviewed the experiments but offered no amendments.

References

1. *Antimicrobial Resistance: Global Report on Surveillance*; World Health Organization: Geneva, Switzerland, 2014.
2. *Tackling Drug-Resistant Infections Globally: Final Report and Recommendations*; Review on Antimicrobial Resistance: London, UK, 2016.
3. Saleh, K.E.O.; El Othmani, M.M.; Tzeng, T.H.; Mihalko, W.M.; Chmabers, M.C.; Grupp, T.M. Acrylic bone cement in total joint arthroplasty: A review. *J. Orthop. Res.* **2016**, *34*, 737–744. [CrossRef] [PubMed]
4. Ma, D.; Shanks, R.M.Q.; Davis, C.M.; Craft, D.W.; Wood, T.K.; Hamlin, B.R.; Urish, K.L. Viable bacteria persist on antibiotic spacers following two-stage revision for periprosthetic joint infection. *J. Orthop. Res.* **2017**. [CrossRef] [PubMed]
5. Van de Belt, H.; Neut, D.; Schenk, W.; van Horn, J.R.; van der Mei, H.C.; Busscher, H.J. Gentamicin release from polymethylmethacrylate bone cements and Staphylococcus aureus biofilm formation. *Acta Orthop. Scand.* **2000**, *71*, 625–629. [CrossRef] [PubMed]
6. Van de Belt, H.; Neut, D.; Schenk, W.; van Horn, J.R.; van der Mei, H.C.; Busscher, H.J. Staphylococcus aureus biofilm formation on different gentamicin-loaded polymethlmethacrylate bone cements. *Biomaterials* **2001**, *22*, 1607–1611. [CrossRef]
7. Morscher, E.W.; Hefti, A.; Aebi, U. Severe osteolysis after third-body wear due to hydroxyapatite particles from acetabular cup coating. *J. Bone Jt. Surg.* **1998**, *80*, 267–272. [CrossRef]
8. Dreesman, H. Über Knochenplombierung. *Beitr Klin Chir.* **1892**, *9*, 804–810.
9. McKee, M.D.; Wild, L.M.; Schemitsch, E.H.; Waddell, J.P. The use of an antibiotic-impregnated, osteoconductive, bioabsorbable bone substitute in the treatment of infected long bone defects: Early results of a prospective trial. *J. Orthop. Trauma* **2002**, *16*, 622–627. [CrossRef] [PubMed]
10. Beuerlein, M.J.; McKee, M.D. Calcium sulfates: What is the evidence? *J. Orthop. Trauma* **2010**, *24* (Suppl. 1), S46–S51. [CrossRef] [PubMed]
11. Ferguson, J.Y.; Dudareva, M.; Riley, N.D.; Stubbs, D.; Atkins, B.L.; McNally, M.A. The use of a biodegradable antibiotic-loaded calcium sulphate carrier containing tobramycin for the treatment of chronic osteomyelitis: A series of 195 cases. *Bone Jt. J.* **2014**, *96*, 829–836. [CrossRef] [PubMed]
12. Cierny, G., III; DiPasquale, D. Comparing OsteoSet and Stimulan as Antibiotic-loaded, Calcium Sulfate Beads in the Management of Musculoskeletal Infection. In Proceedings of the 19th Annual Open Scientific Meeting of the Musculoskeletal Infection Society, San Diego, CA, USA, 7–8 August 2009.
13. Oliver, R.A.; Lovric, V.; Yu, Y.; Christou, C.; Aiken, S.S.; Cooper, J.J.; Walsh, W.R. Development of a Novel Model for the Assessment of Dead-Space Management in Soft Tissue. *PLoS ONE* **2015**, *10*, e0136514. [CrossRef] [PubMed]
14. Maale, G.E.; Casa-Ganem, J.E. The Use of Antibiotic Loaded Synthesized Calcium Sulfate Pellets in the One Stage Treatment for Osteomyelitis. In Proceedings of the 19th Annual Open Scientific Meeting of the Musculoskeletal Infection Society, San Diego, CA, USA, 7–8 August 2009.
15. Kallala, R.; Nizam, I.; Haddad, F. Outcomes Following Use of Antibiotic-Eluting, Absorbable, Calcium Sulphate Beads in Revision Hip and Knee Surgery for Periprosthetic Infection. *Bone Jt. J. Orthop. Proc. Suppl.* **2013**, *95*, 364.

16. Aiken, S.S.; Cooper, J.J.; Florance, H.; Robinson, M.T.; Michell, S. Local release of antibiotics for surgical site infection management using high-purity calcium sulfate: An in vitro elution study. *Surg. Infect.* **2015**, *16*, 54–61. [CrossRef] [PubMed]
17. McConoughey, S.J.; Howlin, R.P.; Wiseman, J.; Stoodley, P.; Calhoun, J.H. Comparing PMMA and calcium sulfate as carriers for the local delivery of antibiotics to infected surgical sites. *J. Biomed. Mater. Res. Part B Appl. Biomater.* **2015**, *103*, 870–877. [CrossRef] [PubMed]
18. Roberts, R.; McConoughey, S.J.; Calhoun, J.H. Size and composition of synthetic calcium sulfate beads influence dissolution and elution rates in vitro. *J. Biomed. Mater. Res. Part B Appl. Biomater.* **2014**, *102*, 667–673. [CrossRef] [PubMed]
19. Traub, W.H.; Leonhard, B. Heat stability of the antimicrobial activity of sixty-two antibacterial agents. *J. Antimicrob. Chemother.* **1995**, *35*, 149–154. [CrossRef] [PubMed]
20. Albright, S.B.; Xue, A.S.; McKnight, A.; Wolfswinkel, E.M.; Hollier, L.H.J.; Brown, R.H.; Bullocks, J.M.; Izaddoost, S.A. Pilot Study: One-Step Salvage of Infected Prosthetic Breast Reconstructions Using Antibiotic-Impregnated Polymethylmethacrylate Plates and Concurrent Tissue Expander Exchange. *Ann. Plast. Surg.* **2016**, *77*, 280–285. [CrossRef] [PubMed]
21. McPherson, E.J.; Dipane, M.V.; Sherif, S.M. Dissolvable Antibiotic Beads in Treatment of Periprosthetic Joint Infection and Revision Arthroplasty. The Use of Synthetic Pure Calcium Sulfate (Stimulan®) Impregnated with Vancomycin & Tobramycin. *Reconstr. Rev.* **2013**, *3*, 32–43.
22. Gauland, C. Managing lower-extremity osteomyelitis locally with surgical debridement and synthetic calcium sulfate antibiotic tablets. *Adv. Skin Wound Care* **2011**, *24*, 515–523. [CrossRef] [PubMed]
23. Agarwal, S.; Healey, B. The use of antibiotic impregnated absorbable calcium sulphate beads in management of infected joint replacement prostheses. *J. Arthrosc. Jt. Surg.* **2014**, *1*, 72–75. [CrossRef]
24. Jogia, R.M.; Modha, D.E.; Nisal, K.; Berrington, R.; Kong, M.-F. Use of Highly Purified Synthetic Calcium Sulfate Impregnated with Antibiotics for the Management of Diabetic Foot Ulcers Complicated by Osteomyelitis. *Diabetes Care* **2015**, *38*, e79–e80. [CrossRef] [PubMed]
25. The European Committee on Antimicrobial Susceptibility Testing. Available online: http://www.eucast.org (accessed on 20 October 2017).
26. Weinstein, M.P. *M100 Performance Standards for Antimicrobial Susceptibility Testing*, 28th ed.; Clinical and Laboratory Standards Institute: Wayne, PA, USA, 2018.
27. Howlin, R.P.; Brayford, M.J.; Webb, J.S.; Cooper, J.J.; Aiken, S.S.; Stoodley, P. Antibiotic-loaded synthetic calcium sulfate beads for the prevention of bacterial colonisation and biofilm formation in periprosthetic infections. *Antimicrob. Agents Chemother.* **2015**, *59*, 111–120. [CrossRef] [PubMed]
28. Malizos, K.; Sarma, J.; Seaton, R.A.; Militz, M.; Menichetti, F.; Riccio, G.; Gaudias, J.; Trostmann, U.; Pathan, R.; Hamed, K. Daptomycin for the treatment of osteomyelitis and orthopaedic device infections: Real-world clinical experience from a European registry. *Eur. J. Clin. Microbiol. Infect. Dis.* **2016**, *35*, 111–118. [CrossRef] [PubMed]
29. Zimmerli, W. Clinical presentation and treatment of orthopaedic impant-associated infection. *J. Intern. Med.* **2014**, *276*, 111–119. [CrossRef] [PubMed]
30. MERCK. Prescribing Information. CUBICIN (Daptmycin for Infection). Available online: https://www.cubicin.com/prescribing-information (accessed on 6 July 2016).
31. Breakpoint Tables for Interpretation of MICs and Zone Diameters. Available online: http://www.eucast.org (accessed on 16 May 2018).
32. Raja, N.S.; Karunakaran, R.; Ngeow, Y.F.; Awang, R. Community-acquired vancomycin-resistant Enterococcus faecium: A case report from Malaysia. *J. Med. Microbiol.* **2005**, *54*, 901–903. [CrossRef] [PubMed]
33. McPherson, E.J. Dissolvable antibiotic beads in treatment of periprosthetic joint infection—The use of commercially pure calcium sulfate (Stimulan™) impregnated with vancomycin & tobramycin. *Reconstr. Rev.* **2012**, *2*, 55–56.
34. Stancil, R.D.; Summers, N.W.; Fernando, N.D.; Chansky, H.A.; Sassoon, A. Prophylactic Use of Antibiotic Impregnated Calcium Sulfate Beads in Revision Hip and Knee Arthroplasty Procedures at High Risk for Prosthetic Joint Infection. In *Discoveries*; Department of Orthopaedics and Sports Medicine, University of Washington: Seattle, WA, USA, 2016; pp. 56–58.

35. Sandiford, N.A.; Veerapen Pierce, R.N.; Fahmy, M.; Dabis, J.; Trompeter, A.; Hutt, J.; Mitchell, P.A. Hypercalcaemia in the management of bone and joint infection—A comparison of 2 calcium sulphate antibiotic delivery systems. In Proceedings of the 7th National Orthopaedic Infection Forum, London, UK, 27 June 2017.
36. Bauer, A.W.; Kirby, W.M.; Sherris, J.C.; Turck, M. Antibiotic susceptibility testing by a standardized single disk method. *Am. J. Clin. Pathol.* **1966**, *45*, 493–496. [CrossRef] [PubMed]
37. Trampuz, A.; Zimmerli, W. Antimicrobial agents in orthopaedic surgery: Prophylaxis and treatment. *Drugs* **2006**, *66*, 1089–1105. [CrossRef] [PubMed]
38. Forrest, G.N.; Tamura, K. Rifampin combination therapy for nonmycobacterial infections. *Clin. Microbiol. Rev.* **2010**, *23*, 14–34. [CrossRef] [PubMed]
39. Niska, J.A.; Shahbazian, J.H.; Ramos, R.I.; Francis, K.P.; Bernthal, N.M.; Miller, L.S. Vancomycin plus Rifampicin Combination Therapy has Enhanced Efficacy Against an Experimental Staphylococcus aureus Prosthetic Joint Infection. *Antimicrob. Agents Chemother.* **2013**, *57*, 5080–5086. [CrossRef] [PubMed]

© 2018 by the authors. Licensee MDPI, Basel, Switzerland. This article is an open access article distributed under the terms and conditions of the Creative Commons Attribution (CC BY) license (http://creativecommons.org/licenses/by/4.0/).

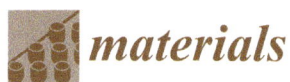

Review

Action of Antimicrobial Peptides against Bacterial Biofilms

Muhammad Yasir, Mark Duncan Perry Willcox * and Debarun Dutta

School of Optometry and Vision Science, University of New South Wales, Sydney, NSW 2052, Australia; m.yasir@unsw.edu.au (M.Y.); debarun.dutta@unsw.edu.au (D.D.)
* Correspondence: m.willcox@unsw.edu.au or mdpwillcox@gmail.com; Tel.: +61-2-93854164

Received: 3 November 2018; Accepted: 1 December 2018; Published: 5 December 2018

Abstract: Microbes are known to colonize surfaces and form biofilms. These biofilms are communities of microbes encased in a self-produced matrix that often contains polysaccharides, DNA and proteins. Antimicrobial peptides (AMPs) have been used to control the formation and to eradicate mature biofilms. Naturally occurring or synthetic antimicrobial peptides have been shown to prevent microbial colonization of surfaces, to kill bacteria in biofilms and to disrupt the biofilm structure. This review systemically analyzed published data since 1970 to summarize the possible anti-biofilm mechanisms of AMPs. One hundred and sixty-two published reports were initially selected for this review following searches using the criteria 'antimicrobial peptide' OR 'peptide' AND 'mechanism of action' AND 'biofilm' OR 'antibiofilm' in the databases PubMed; Scopus; Web of Science; MEDLINE; and Cochrane Library. Studies that investigated anti-biofilm activities without describing the possible mechanisms were removed from the analysis. A total of 17 original reports were included which have articulated the mechanism of antimicrobial action of AMPs against biofilms. The major anti-biofilm mechanisms of antimicrobial peptides are: (1) disruption or degradation of the membrane potential of biofilm embedded cells; (2) interruption of bacterial cell signaling systems; (3) degradation of the polysaccharide and biofilm matrix; (4) inhibition of the alarmone system to avoid the bacterial stringent response; (5) downregulation of genes responsible for biofilm formation and transportation of binding proteins.

Keywords: biofilm; antimicrobial peptides; mechanism of action; medical devices; biomaterials

1. Biofilms

A biofilm is a group of organisms such as fungi, bacteria, and viruses, existing in a sessile form and surrounded by a self-produced extracellular matrix. Costerton et al. [1] proposed a basic definition of biofilm as "a structured community of bacterial cells enclosed in a self-produced polymeric matrix and adherent to an inert or living surface" and Hall-Stoodley et al. [2] defined biofilms as "surface-associated microbial communities, surrounded by an extracellular polymeric substance (EPS) matrix". A biofilm can also be called "an aggregate of microbial cells adherent to a living or nonliving surface, embedded within a matrix of EPS of microbial origin" [3]. Recently, biofilms have been described as complex sessile communities of microbes found either attached to a surface or buried firmly in an extracellular matrix as aggregates [4]. The matrix can be composed of exopolysaccharides, proteins, nucleic acids, and other cellular debris collectively called extra polymeric substances (EPS) [5–7].

1.1. Biofilm Formation

The process of biofilm formation on biomaterials begins by the initial adhesion of planktonic bacteria to surfaces and then aggregation into smaller groups of bacteria known as microcolonies. Following attachment, EPS such as proteins, glycoproteins, glycolipids, and extracellular DNA are synthesized [8]. Glycopeptides, glycolipids and lipopolysaccharides help to keep the biofilms intact [9]. In mature biofilms, the microcolonies differentiate into distinct phenotypes which are significantly different in gene expression than their planktonic counterparts [10]. The differentiation can be triggered by the accumulation of quorum sensing molecules such as N-acyl homoserine lactones that facilitate cell to cell communication [1].

Starvation conditions are known to promote the formation of biofilms, and bacteria grown or living under starvation are known to have higher antibiotic tolerance. Biofilm formation can be an adaptation of microorganisms to hostile environments [11,12]. Under hostile conditions bacteria can activate the stringent response (which can be characterized by the production of "alarmones") by synthesizing the signaling nucleoside guanosine pentaphosphate or tetraphosphate ((p)ppGpp) which can cause the inhibition of RNA synthesis when amino acids are in low concentrations [13]. RelA and SpoT are homologous proteins that are responsible for modulating intracellular concentrations of (p)ppGpp, often conserved among Gram-negative and Gram-positive bacteria, with a few exceptions such as *S. aureus* [14]. This stringent response plays an important role in the development of biofilms as mutants lacking RelA and SpoT produce comparatively fragile and antibiotic sensitive biofilms [15]. The exact role of (p)ppGpp in biofilm formation is not known, but it is likely that hostile conditions trigger transcription of hundreds of genes responsible for altered intracellular metabolism and energy conservation through suspension of cell division [15].

Biofilm formation can occur on a variety of surfaces, including living tissues, medical devices, industrial or potable water system piping, or on surfaces in the natural aquatic environment [16]. Approximately 99% of the microbial world exists as biofilms [17,18] and these biofilms are diverse containing a wide range of microbes [19]. For example, more than 500 types of bacteria are present in biofilms in the oral cavity [20].

1.2. Characteristics of Biofilms

Biofilm embedded cells are not as sensitive to antimicrobials compared with their planktonic counterparts. [21] They are highly resistant to conventional antibiotics, up to 1000 times more than planktonic bacteria. This is related in part to the slow growth rate and low metabolic activity of cells in biofilms [15,22,23]. In addition, the EPS matrix surrounding biofilms, which can make up to 50% to 90% of the total biomass of biofilms, resists the penetration of antimicrobials [16,24–30]. Moreover, microbes in biofilms can have a high rate of mutation and exchange of resistance genes on mobile genetic elements [31,32] which can also lead to increase in the overall resistance of cells in biofilms.

1.3. Biofilm-Associated Infections

Biofilms pose a serious threat to public health because of their potential to cause biomaterial-associated infections due in-part to the high resistance of biofilms to antimicrobials agents [33]. About 80% of bacterial infections in humans are caused by biofilms [1,12,23]. Biofilm mediated infection can be divided into two categories, non-device and device associated infections [34,35].

The first category involves biofilm formation on host tissues such as epithelial, mucosal surfaces, and teeth. These can cause infections associated with cystic fibrosis (CF) patients, foot ulcers in diabetic patients, chronic otitis media or rhinosinusitis, chronic prostatitis, recurrent urinary tract infections, and dental caries and periodontitis [36,37].

The second category of infections arises due to the microbial colonization of abiotic objects, for example indwelling medical devices such as central venous or urinary catheters, joint or dental prostheses, heart valves, endotracheal tubes, intrauterine devices, and dental implants [34,35,38]. Microbes can detach from these biofilms and disseminate to the surrounding tissues or to the bloodstream, further exacerbating the infection [39]. Worldwide production of biomedical devices and tissue engineering-related objects is approximately $180 billion per annum [37]. According to current estimates, over 5 million medical devices or implants are used annually in the U.S.A. alone [37]. About 60–70% of nosocomial infections are associated with biomaterials or implants [37]. Regardless of the sophistication of the biomedical implant and tissue engineering constructs, all medical devices are susceptible to microbial colonization and can cause infections [40–42]. Biofilm growth on medical devices can be extremely difficult to eradicate, with only a few treatment options such as removal of the infected device or use of large doses of antibiotics [43]. However, this increases treatment costs and may increase the potential for the development of antibiotic resistance and cytotoxicity [44]. Moreover, removal may not be an easy option for patients with medical devices for critical care such as pacemakers. The clinical significance of biofilm-associated infections and their inherent resistance to antimicrobials urgently demand development of novel anti-biofilm compounds.

2. Antimicrobial Peptides

Antimicrobial peptides (AMPs) have a varying number (from five to over a hundred) of amino acids, most commonly L forms, with molecular weights between 1–5 KDa. AMPs have a broad spectrum of activity ranging from viruses to parasites [45]. AMPs are generally cationic in nature, and often referred as cationic host defense peptides because of their role in the immune response [46]. They are also known as cationic amphipathic peptides [47], cationic AMPs [48], and α-helical AMPs [49]. Recently, a few anionic antimicrobial peptides have been reported which have a net charge ranging from −1 to −7, and a length from 5 to circa 7 amino acid residues [50]. AMPs have been recognized as promising alternatives to conventional antibiotics due to their multiple target sites and non-specific mechanism of action which reduces the chances of resistance development. AMPs exhibit strong anti-biofilm activity against multidrug resistant as well as clinically isolated bacterial biofilms [51]. AMPs can interfere in the early stages of biofilm formation to prevent the initial adhesion of bacteria to surfaces [51]. They can destroy mature biofilms by encouraging microbial detachment or killing [52]. Here we focus on the anti-biofilm action of AMPs against different Gram-positive and Gram-negative bacteria, with emphasis on their mechanism of action.

Based on their secondary structure, AMPs are generally categorized into four groups (1) α-helical AMPs; (2) β-sheet AMPs; (3) extended AMPs; and (4) cationic loop AMPs [53]. Alpha-helical peptides are the largest group of AMPs representing 30–50% of all AMPs of known secondary structure [54–56]. These peptides commonly consist of 12–40 amino acids and contain an abundance of helix stabilizing amino acids such as alanine, leucine, and lysine [56]. Beta-sheet AMPs usually consist of two to ten cysteine residues that from one to five inter-chain disulfide bonds that help the peptides to form the beta-sheet [57]. Beta-sheet antimicrobial peptides include the defensin family of peptides [58,59]. Defensins consist of two to three antiparallel beta-sheets however, in some cases alpha-helical or unstructured segments can be found at their N- or C-termini [60]. Compared with α-helical antimicrobial peptides, the defensins adopt a globular structure in aqueous solutions [60,61]. Despite extensive variations in length, amino acid composition and net positive charge, β-strands are observed in all α- and β-defensins [62,63]. Extended AMPs are not folded into α-helix or β-sheet structures. These AMPs often contain high numbers of arginine, tryptophan, proline or cystine residues [64]. Some of these AMPs can fold into defined amphipathic molecules in bacterial membranes, but often these are not membrane active [65]. The proline-rich insect-derived pyrrhocoricin, drosocin and apidaecin peptides penetrate membranes and exert their antimicrobial activities by interacting with intracellular proteins such as the heat-shock protein DnaK and GroEL to inhibit the DnaK ATPase and chaperone-assisted protein folding related activities, respectively [66,67]. Cationic loop AMPs are proline-arginine rich peptides, and because of their high numbers of proline residues, they rarely form amphipathic characteristics and tend to adopt polyproline helical type-II structures [68].

2.1. Mechanism of Action of AMPs against Planktonic Bacteria

The mechanism of action of AMPs usually starts by interacting with negatively charged moieties such as lipopolysaccharides (LPS) in the outer membranes of Gram-negative bacteria and lipoteichoic acid (LTA) in the cell wall of Gram-positive bacteria [69–71]. Once AMPs cross or produce pores in the outer membrane or the cell wall of bacteria, disruption of cytoplasmic membranes occurs followed by cell lysis [72]. The mechanisms of action of AMPs have been divided into pore-forming and non-pore models [73]. Pore-forming models include the barrel stave and the toroidal pore models. Non-pore models include the carpet model. AMPs can also inhibit the synthesis of cell walls, DNA, RNA and protein, and activate enzymes such as autolysins that induce autolytic death [66,74,75].

2.2. Mechanism of Action against Biofilms

In this review, we systemically analyzed all published data since 1970 to summarize all the possible anti-biofilm mechanisms of antimicrobial peptides. A total of 162 published reports were initially selected for this review following search criteria using 'antimicrobial peptide' OR 'peptide' AND 'mechanism of action' AND 'biofilm' OR 'antibiofilm' in the databases PubMed, Scopus, Web of Science, MEDLINE, and Cochrane Library. The studies investigated the antimicrobial activity of AMPs against a variety of microorganisms. A total of 17 original reports qualified for our review which have articulated the mechanism of anti-biofilm action of AMPs. These reports are included in this review.

Several overlapping anti-biofilm mechanisms of AMPs are reported in the literature. Following careful consideration, we found five major anti-biofilm mechanisms: (1) disruption or degradation of the membrane potential of biofilm embedded cells; (2) interruption of bacterial cell signaling systems; (3) degradation of the polysaccharide and biofilm matrix; (4) inhibition of the alarmone system to avoid the bacterial stringent response; (5) downregulation of genes responsible for biofilm formation and transportation of binding proteins.

Certain synthetic AMPs can rapidly degrade pre-established biofilms of *P. aeruginosa* [52]. Although the mechanism of biofilm degradation is poorly understood, the rapid destruction of biofilm embedded cells [52] may indicate that they act by disrupting the membranes of the bacteria. Table 1 and Figure 1 summarize the mechanisms of biofilm inhibition and degradation of various AMPs. Mechanistic studies have tended to focus on the membrane-disrupting properties of AMPs [76,77].

(i) disruption or degradation of the membrane potential of biofilm embedded cells

Three bacteriocins (nisin A, lacticin Q, and nukacin ISK-1) can destroy the membrane potential of biofilm embedded cells of *S. aureus* (an MRSA strain) and can cause the release of ATP from the cells [78]. An engineered peptide RN3(5-17P22-36) [79] derived from the cationic proteins of eosinophil granules [80,81] can kill bacteria via membrane disruption. However, this membrane depolarization of cells in biofilms was 2–3-fold less compared with planktonic bacteria at the same concentration [79]. A frog skin-derived AMP esculentin (Esc (1-21)) can permeabilize the cytoplasmic membrane of *P. aeruginosa* PAO1 in biofilms and cause release of β-galactosidase [82]. However, this effect was slower and did not result in comparable β-galactosidase release compared to its action on planktonic cells [82]. The AMP (CSA)-13 can quickly penetrate into biofilms and permeabilize the cell membranes of biofilm cells of *P. aeruginosa* [83].

(ii) interruption of the bacterial cell signaling system

Human cathelicidic LL-37 and indolicidin can prevent biofilm formation of *P. aeruginosa* possibly by down-regulating the transcription of two major quorum-sensing systems, Las and Rhl [84]. Another mechanism by which AMPs have been shown to inhibit the formation of biofilms is by increasing twitching motility in *P. aeruginosa* by stimulating the expression of genes needed for type IV pilli biosynthesis and function [84,85]. The main function of type IV pilli is to increase the movement of bacteria on surfaces, which may facilitate removal of cells [86].

(iii) degradation of the polysaccharide and biofilm matrix

AMPs can also act on the extracellular polymeric matrix of bacterial biofilms. For example, peptide PI can degrade the EPS produced by *Streptococcus mutans* leading to reductions in biofilms formed on polystyrene or and saliva-coated hydroxyapatite [87]. An anti-biofilm peptide derived from maggots of the blowfly *Calliphora vicina* can degrade the biofilm matrix produced by drug resistant

Escherichia coli, *Staphylococcus aureus* and *Acinetobacter baumannii* but the mechanism of degradation was not investigated [88]. Human liver-derived antimicrobial peptide hepcidin 20 can reduce the mass of extracellular matrix and alter the architecture of biofilms of *S. epidermidis* by targeting polysaccharide intercellular adhesin (PIA) [89]. Another peptide S4(1–16) M4Ka, a derivative of S4, has been shown to act against immature *P. aeruginosa* biofilms by disintegration and release of membrane lipids, detachment of bacteria and inhibition of biofilm formation [90]. The fish derived AMP piscidin-3 has nucleosidase activity and can destroy extracellular DNA of *P. aeruginosa* by coordinating with Cu^{2+} through its N-terminus [91].

(iv) inhibition of the alarmone system to avoid the bacterial stringent response

Anti-biofilm peptides may act by targeting an almost universal stringent stress response in both Gram-positive and Gram-negative bacteria [92]. Many bacteria produce the signaling nucleotides guanosine 5′-diphosphate 3′-diphosphate (ppGpp) and (p)ppGpp, that can regulate the expression of a plethora of genes [93,94] and are important in biofilm formation [95]. The AMPs 1018, DJK-5, and DJK-6 can block the synthesis and trigger degradation of (p)ppGpp in both Gram-positive and Gram-negative bacteria, and this can lead to reduction in biofilm formation which in turn increases susceptibility to AMPs [15]. Some other AMPs such as DJK-5 and 1018 can act on the stringent response in *P. aeruginosa* by suppressing spoT promoter activity [96]. DJK-5 and DJK-6 can degrade (p)ppGpp on *P. aeruginosa* biofilms to higher extent than 1018 [14].

(v) downregulation of genes responsible for biofilm formation and transportation of binding proteins

Biofilm formation by staphylococci is an accumulative process which crucially depends upon the synthesis of polysaccharide intercellular adhesin molecule PIA encoded by icaADBC locus in staphylococci [97]. Human β-defensin 3 (hBD-3) can reduce the expression of icaA, icaD and icaR genes of *Staphylococus epidermidis* ATCC 35,984 thereby reducing biofilm formation [98]. AMPs can inhibit genes controlling the mobility of extrachromosomal elements and transport and binding proteins [99]. A peptide Nal-P-113, can inhibit *Porphyromonas* gingivalis biofilm formation by down-regulating genes such as PG0282 and PG1663 which encode ABC transporter and ATP-binding protein [99]. ABC transporters have been involved in cell-to-surface and cell-to-cell interactions in biofilms formation [100,101]. Figure 2 summarizes the targets sites of representative anti-biofilm AMPs.

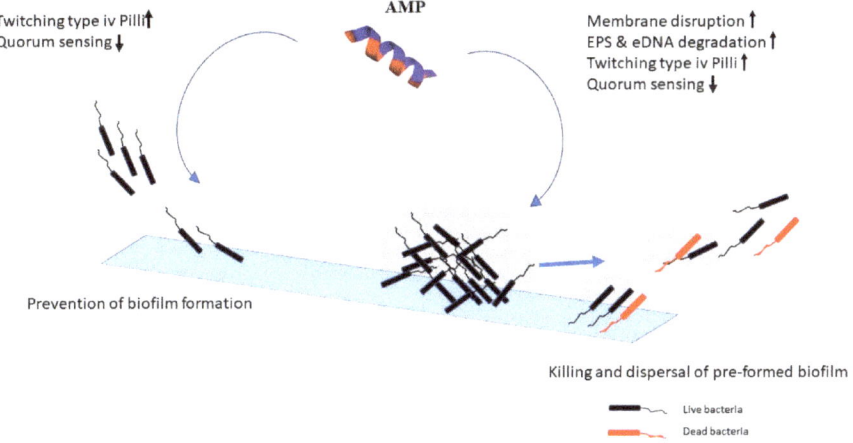

Figure 1. Anti-biofilm activity and mechanism of action of antimicrobial peptides (AMPs). AMPs effect mainly involve prevention of bacterial attachment and inhibition of biofilm formation or disruption of pre-formed biofilms. ↑ activation ▼ inhibition.

Table 1. Representative AMPs and their anti-biofilm mechanism of action

AMPs	Sources	Amino Acids Sequence	Microorganisms	Proposed Mechanism of Action	Ref
LL-37	Human	LLGDFFRKSKEKIGKEFKRIVQRIKDFLRNLVPRTES	Pseudomonas aeruginosa	Reduces swimming and swarming motilities, promotes twitching motility, downregulates the genes required for biofilm formation and influences QS system	[84,85]
1037	Denovo	KRFRIRVRV	Pseudomonas aeruginosa		[14]
1018	Denovo	VRLIVAVRIWRR	Pseudomonas aeruginosa	Decrease intracellular (p) PpGpp	[82]
Esculentin-1a (1-21)	Denovo	GIFSKLAGKKIKNLLISGLKG	Pseudomonas aeruginosa	Disrupts cell membrane	[78]
Nisin A	Denovo	MSTKDFNLDLVSVSKKDSGASPR	Staphylococcus aureus	Depolarizes cell membrane	[78]
lacticin Q	Denovo	MAGFLKVVQLLAKYGSKAVQMAWANKGKILDWLNAGQAIDK VVSKIKQILGIK	Staphylococcus aureus	Depolarizes cell membrane	[78]
Nukacin ISK-1	Denovo	KK-KSGVIPTVSHGCHMNSFQFVFTCC	Staphylococcus aureus	Depolarizes cell membrane	[78]
RN3(5-17P22-36)	Denovo	RPFTRAQWFAIQHISPRTIAMRAINNYRWR	Pseudomonas aeruginosa	Depolarizes and permeabilize cell membrane	[79]
S4 (1-16)	Denovo	ALWKTLLKKVLKAAAK	Pseudomonas aeruginosa	Disintegrates and release membrane lipids	[90]
P1	Calliphora vicina	FVDRNRIPRSNNGPKIPIISNP	Escherichia coli, Staphylococcus aureus, Acinetobacter baumannii	Degrades biofilm matrix	[88]
L-K6L9	Denovo	LKLLKKLLKKLLKLL	Pseudomonas aeruginosa	Degrades biofilms matrix	[52]
Piscidin-3	Fish	FIHHIFRGIVHAGRSIGRFLTG	Pseudomonas aeruginosa	Degrades eDNA	[91]
PI	Tick	PARKARAATAATAATAATAAT	Streptococcus mutans	Interferes and degrade EPS matrix	[87]
Hepcidin 20	Human	ICIFCCGCCHRSHCGMCCKT	Staphylococcus epidermidis	Acts on polysaccharide intercellular adhesin (PIA)	[88]
Nal-P-113	Denovo	AKR-Nal-Nal-GYKRKF-Nal-	Porphyromonas gingivalis	Down regulates genes related to transport and binding proteins	[99]
Human β-defensin 3 (hBD-3)	Human	GIINTLQKYYCRVRGGRCAVLSCLPKEEQIGKCSTRGRKCCRRKK	Staphylococcus epidermidis	Targets icaA, icaD and icaR genes	[98]
DJK-5	Denovo	VQWRAIRVRVIR	Pseudomonas aeruginosa	Suppress spoT promoter activity	[96]

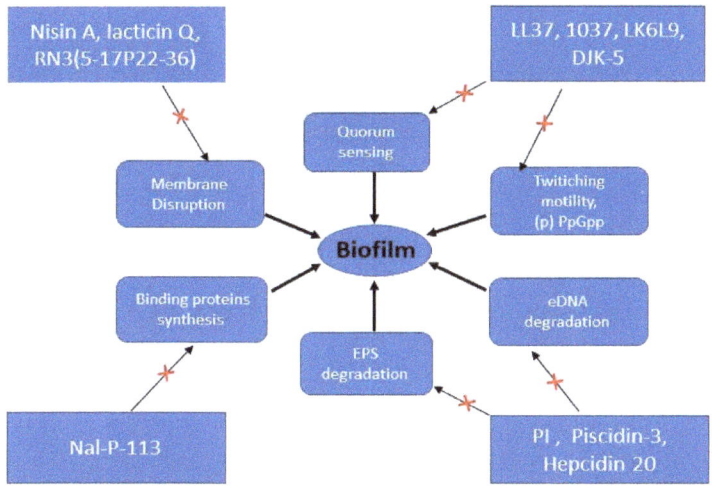

Figure 2. Representation of the different targets of anti-biofilm AMPs. × signs indicate inhibition and/or action on targets sites.

3. Biofilm Resistance to AMPs

3.1. Interaction with EPS

It is thought that biofilm mediated resistance to AMPs is mainly due to their interaction with EPS, however the exact mechanism of interaction remained unknown in large number of cases [102]. Although most of the substances in EPS are negatively charged, the positively charged exopolymer PIA (which is composed of poly-N-acetyl glucosamine) can cause electrostatic repulsion of the cationic AMPs [103]. PIA protects *S. epidermidis* and *S. aureus* from the bactericidal actions of cationic AMPs such as LL-37 and human β-defensin [103]. PIA can also protect bacteria in biofilm from anionic AMP such as dermcidin (a human epithelial secreted) [102]. So, the role of PIA in protection of bacterial biofilms may be due to sequestration of AMPs along with electrostatic repulsion [102].

Gram negative bacteria such as *P. aeruginosa* secrete an anionic extracellular polysaccharide known as alginate which is made up of the uronic acid D-mannuronate and C-5 epimer-L guluronate [104,105]. Alginate can interact with positively charge AMPs and protect *P. aeruginosa* biofilm embedded cells from attack of AMPs [106]. Wild-type strains such as PAO1, PA14 (a mucoid cystic fibrosis strain), and FRD1 (a mutant which lacks alginate producing ability) can be easily killed by human leukocytes and their peptides within 4 h of exposure, [107] but became resistant in the presence of alginate [107]. Alginate can bind and induce an α-helical conformation for AMPs such as magainin II and cecropin P1 which is similar to their interaction with cytoplasmic membranes, suggesting that alginate can mediate hydrophobic interactions with AMPs despite its hydrophilic nature [106]. Alginate can trap AMPs in hydrophobic microdomains which consist of pyranosyl C–H groups that are inducible upon formation of AMPs-alginate complexes due to charge neutralization between the two species [108]. However, with the exception of cystic fibrosis, mucoid strains of *P. aeruginosa* account for only 1% of isolates from infections [109] so the role of mucoid strains in medical device related infections is limited. In contrast to mucoid strains, non-mucoid strains contain low levels of alginate [110] but can use either Pel or Psl (a structural cationic exopolysaccharide) to develop biofilms [111].

3.2. Adaptive Resistance Mechanism

Staphylococci have a peptide sensing system known as *aps*, which was first recognized in *S. epidermidis* [112]. The *aps* consist of two-component system that has a sensor histidine kinase (ApsS) and a DNA-binding response regulator (ApsR). A third component (ApsX) is also found only in some staphylococci species [112]. This *aps* system can protect Gram positive bacteria including methicillin resistant *S. aureus* (MRSA) strains from action of AMPs [113]. The aps system upregulates D-alanylation of teichoic acid and increases the expression of putative AMP efflux pumps [114]. A D-alanine deficient mutant of *E. faecalis* produced less biofilm but was more resistant to AMPs than the wild type [115]. The PhoP/PhoQ genetic system found in *P. aeruginosa* and *Salmonella enterica* [116] is used to sense AMPs [117]. This system tends to change the structure of LPS by addition of aminoarabinose to lipid A, which has the effect of decreasing the net negative charge of lipopolysaccharides [118]. Therefore, this system may also confer resistance of biofilm bacteria to AMPs. A two-component regulatory system pmrA-pmrB identified in *P. aeruginosa* that regulates resistance to polymyxin B, polymyxins E, cattle indolicidin and LL-37 [119] modifies lipopolysaccharides in the outer membrane of bacteria and this reduces the AMPs interaction with the outer membrane [120,121] this confering resistance.

3.3. Heterogeneity

Biofilms consist of structurally and functionally diverse bacterial populations and maintain a micro-environment which controls microbial activity, intracellular signaling and metabolic and genetic material exchange [122]. These properties can establish cellular and communal behaviors which result in tolerance and persistence of cells in the presence of antimicrobials [122]. For example, colistin can kill low metabolically active *P. aeruginosa* in biofilms but cannot destroy metabolically active cells [123]. This resistance to colistin in biofilms may be due to physiological tolerance [124]. *E. coli* possessing IncF plasmids can differentiate into structured and unstructured biofilms and can produce genetically regulated tolerant subpopulations [124]. Colistin can kill a small number of genetically tolerant bacteria in structured biofilms but can kill a high number of bacteria in unstructured biofilms. [124].

3.4. Synergy of Anti-Biofilm AMPs with Antibiotics

The anti-biofilm activity of AMPs can be enhanced against biofilms by combining them with antibiotics [125–128]. Combination strategies are useful since they can target a variety of microbial communities present with different metabolisms cells in low pH, hypoxic or low nutritious environments [129]. AMP-1018 can prevent initial bacterial attachment to surfaces by inhibiting the synthesis of (p)ppGpp [23]. When 1018 was used in combination with ceftazidime, ciprofloxacin, imipenem, or tobramycin, at sub-MIC this combination could inhibit 50% biofilms produced by *P. aeruginosa*, *E. coli*, *A. baumannii*, *K. pneumoniae*, *S. enterica*, and methicillin-resistant *S. aureus* (MRSA) [23]. Similarly, colistin in combination with temporin A (TEMP-A), citropin 1.1 (CIT-1.1) and tachyplesin I (TP-I-L) can eradiate mature biofilms of drug resistant *P. aeruginosa* and *S. aureus* [130]. AMPs can act synergistically with antibiotics against biofilm following two types of mechanism. Firstly, AMPs-antibiotic combinations can degrade biofilms matrix then AMPs act alone and disperse biofilms embedded cells [131]. AMP-antibiotic combinations can also be used against fungal biofilms [132]. An antifungal plant defensin derived peptide HsLin06_18 acts synergistically with caspofungin against *Candida glabrata* and *Candida albicans*. HsLin06_18 was shown to act by permeabilization cell membrane which facilitated caspofungin penetration into the fungal cells, inducing death at a sub-inhibitory concentration [132].

4. Future Considerations

Treating bacterial infections caused by biofilm-producing microorganisms is a troublesome task and a major challenge for health care systems. Antibiotic therapy or antibiotic releasing products are not adequate to control biofilm related infections, particularly due to the emergence of antibiotic resistant infections. Currently, there is no clear answer for the management and prevention of these infections. Use of very high concentrations of antibiotics in attempts to disrupt or prevent biofilm formation can be associated with cytotoxicity and poor prognosis. Hence, finding an alternative class of drugs to address biofilm-related infections represents a promising strategy. AMPs have broad-spectrum antimicrobial activity and are generally immune to development of bacterial resistance [45,133] and can work synergistically with first line antibiotics. AMPs have several promising characteristics that can be used to inhibit biofilms. However, there is limited information on the interaction of AMPs with biofilm components. More research is needed to understand their precise mechanisms of action such as inhibiting QS signals that restrict biofilm formation and interfere with signaling pathways involved in the synthesis of EPS. Molecular modelling approaches may provide insights on action of AMPs on biofilms. AMP-AMP and AMP-drug combinations that can induce biofilm matrix degradation could be the potential areas of future anti-biofilm research.

In conclusion, this review found that AMPs have a variety of active anti-biofilm mechanisms that could be exploited for clinical applications to eradicate biofilms. It is clear that AMPs have high potential for further development as an active anti-biofilm agent, particularly in the high-risk environments such as hospital settings. AMPs could be used as a stand-alone therapy or in combination with other antimicrobials to eradicate biofilms. Further in vivo investigations are warranted to better understand the complex host environment that may affect their efficacy by reducing their activity and stability. Moreover, the role of immunomodulatory activities must be evaluated in complex biofilm environment in vivo.

Funding: This research was funded by Australian Research Council (ARC) discovery project funding scheme (project number DP160101664).

Acknowledgments: The first author received PhD scholarship from Higher Education Commission (HEC) of Pakistan and the University of New South Wales, Australia.

Conflicts of Interest: The authors declare no conflict of interest.

References

1. Costerton, J.W.; Stewart, P.S.; Greenberg, E.P. Bacterial biofilms: A common cause of persistent infections. *Science* **1999**, *284*, 1318–1322. [CrossRef] [PubMed]
2. Hall-Stoodley, L.; Stoodley, P. Evolving concepts in biofilm infections. *Cell. Microbiol.* **2009**, *11*, 1034–1043. [CrossRef] [PubMed]
3. Hall-Stoodley, L.; Stoodley, P.; Kathju, S.; Høiby, N.; Moser, C.; William Costerton, J.; Moter, A.; Bjarnsholt, T. Towards diagnostic guidelines for biofilm-associated infections. *FEMS Immun. Med. Microbiol.* **2012**, *65*, 127–145. [CrossRef] [PubMed]
4. Roy, R.; Tiwari, M.; Donelli, G.; Tiwari, V. Strategies for combating bacterial biofilms: A focus on anti-biofilm agents and their mechanisms of action. *Virulence* **2018**, *9*, 522–554. [CrossRef] [PubMed]
5. Costerton, J.W.; Cheng, K.J.; Geesey, G.G.; Ladd, T.I.; Nickel, J.C.; Dasgupta, M.; Marrie, T.J. Bacterial biofilms in nature and disease. *Annu. Rev. Microbiol.* **1987**, *41*, 435–464. [CrossRef] [PubMed]
6. Anwar, H.; Dasgupta, M.K.; Costerton, J.W. Testing the susceptibility of bacteria in biofilms to antibacterial agents. *Antimicrob. Agents Chemother.* **1990**, *34*, 2043–2046. [CrossRef] [PubMed]
7. Matz, C.; Bergfeld, T.; Rice, S.A.; Kjelleberg, S. Microcolonies, quorum sensing and cytotoxicity determine the survival of Pseudomonas aeruginosa biofilms exposed to protozoan grazing. *Environ. Microbiol.* **2004**, *6*, 218–226. [CrossRef] [PubMed]
8. Shirtliff, M.E.; Peters, B.M.; Jabra-Rizk, M.A. Cross-kingdom interactions: Candida albicans and bacteria. *FEMS Microbiol. Lett* **2009**, *299*, 1–8. [CrossRef] [PubMed]
9. Flemming, H.C.; Wingender, J. The biofilm matrix. *Nat. Rev. Microbiol.* **2010**, *8*, 623–633. [CrossRef] [PubMed]
10. Stoodley, P.; Sauer, K.; Davies, D.G.; Costerton, J.W. Biofilms as complex differentiated communities. *Ann. Rev. Microbiol.* **2002**, *56*, 187–209. [CrossRef]
11. De la Fuente-Núñez, C.; Reffuveille, F.; Fernández, L.; Hancock, R.E. Bacterial biofilm development as a multicellular adaptation: Antibiotic resistance and new therapeutic strategies. *Curr. Opin. Microbiol.* **2013**, *16*, 580–589. [CrossRef] [PubMed]
12. Hall-Stoodley, L.; Costerton, J.W.; Stoodley, P. Bacterial biofilms: From the natural environment to infectious diseases. *Nat. Rev. Microbiol.* **2004**, *2*, 95. [CrossRef] [PubMed]

13. Porat, Y.; Marynka, K.; Tam, A.; Steinberg, D.; Mor, A. Acyl-substituted dermaseptin S4 derivatives with improved bactericidal properties, including on oral microflora. *Antimicrob. Agents Chemother.* **2006**, *50*, 4153–4160. [CrossRef] [PubMed]
14. De la Fuente-Nunez, C.; Reffuveille, F.; Mansour, S.C.; Reckseidler-Zenteno, S.L.; Hernandez, D.; Brackman, G.; Coenye, T.; Hancock, R.E. D-enantiomeric peptides that eradicate wild-type and multidrug-resistant biofilms and protect against lethal *Pseudomonas aeruginosa* infections. *Chem. Biol.* **2015**, *22*, 196–205. [CrossRef] [PubMed]
15. De la Fuente-Núñez, C.; Reffuveille, F.; Haney, E.F.; Straus, S.K.; Hancock, R.E. Broad-spectrum anti-biofilm peptide that targets a cellular stress response. *PloS. Pathog.* **2014**, *10*, e1004152. [CrossRef] [PubMed]
16. Donlan, R.M. Biofilms: Microbial Life on Surfaces. *Emerg. Inf. Dis.* **2002**, *8*, 881–890. [CrossRef] [PubMed]
17. Stoica, P.; Chifiriuc, M.C.; Rapa, M.; Lazăr, V. Overview of biofilm-related problems in medical devices. In *Biofilms and Implantable Medical Devices*; Deng, Y., Lv, W., Eds.; Woodhead Publishing: Cambridge, UK, 2017; pp. 3–23.
18. Dalton, H.M.; March, P.E. Molecular genetics of bacterial attachment and biofouling. *Curr. Opin. Biotechnol.* **1998**, *9*, 252–255. [CrossRef]
19. Garrett, T.R.; Bhakoo, M.; Zhang, Z. Bacterial adhesion and biofilms on surfaces. *Prog. Nat. Sci.* **2008**, *18*, 1049–1056. [CrossRef]
20. Whittaker, C.J.; Klier, C.M.; Kolenbrander, P.E. Mechanisms of adhesion by oral bacteria. *Ann. Rev. Microbiol.* **1996**, *50*, 513–552. [CrossRef] [PubMed]
21. Costerton, J.W. Introduction to biofilm. *Int. J. Antimicrob. Agents.* **1999**, *11*, 217–221. [CrossRef]
22. de la Fuente-Núñez, C.; Cardoso, M.H.; de Souza Cândido, E.; Franco, O.L.; Hancock, R.E. Synthetic antibiofilm peptides. *Biochimic. Biophys. Acta. Biomem.* **2016**, *1858*, 1061–1069. [CrossRef] [PubMed]
23. Reffuveille, F.; de la Fuente-Núñez, C.; Mansour, S.; Hancock, R.E.W. A Broad-Spectrum Antibiofilm Peptide Enhances Antibiotic Action against Bacterial Biofilms. *Antmicrob. Agents Chemother.* **2014**, *58*, 5363–5371. [CrossRef] [PubMed]
24. Stewart, P.S. Theoretical aspects of antibiotic diffusion into microbial biofilms. *Antmicrob. Agents Chemother.* **1996**, *40*, 2517–2522. [CrossRef]
25. Mah, T.-F.C.; O'toole, G.A. Mechanisms of biofilm resistance to antimicrobial agents. *Trends. Microbiol.* **2001**, *9*, 34–39. [CrossRef]
26. Arciola, C.R.; Campoccia, D.; Speziale, P.; Montanaro, L.; Costerton, J.W. Biofilm formation in Staphylococcus implant infections. A review of molecular mechanisms and implications for biofilm-resistant materials. *Biomaterials* **2012**, *33*, 5967–5982. [CrossRef] [PubMed]
27. Lewis, K. Riddle of biofilm resistance. *Antmicrob. Agents Chemother.* **2001**, *45*, 999–1007. [CrossRef] [PubMed]
28. Hoiby, N.; Ciofu, O.; Johansen, H.K.; Song, Z.J.; Moser, C.; Jensen, P.O.; Molin, S.; Givskov, M.; Tolker-Nielsen, T.; Bjarnsholt, T. The clinical impact of bacterial biofilms. *Int. J. Oral Sci.* **2011**, *3*, 55–65. [CrossRef] [PubMed]
29. Stewart, P.S.; Roe, F.; Rayner, J.; Elkins, J.G.; Lewandowski, Z.; Ochsner, U.A.; Hassett, D.J. Effect of catalase on hydrogen peroxide penetration into Pseudomonas aeruginosa biofilms. *Appl. Environ. Microbiol.* **2000**, *66*, 836–838. [CrossRef] [PubMed]
30. Fux, C.; Costerton, J.W.; Stewart, P.S.; Stoodley, P. Survival strategies of infectious biofilms. *Trends Microbiol.* **2005**, *13*, 34–40. [CrossRef] [PubMed]
31. Hoiby, N.; Bjarnsholt, T.; Givskov, M.; Molin, S.; Ciofu, O. Antibiotic resistance of bacterial biofilms. *Int. J. Antimicrob. Agents* **2010**, *35*, 322–332. [CrossRef]
32. Mah, T.F. Biofilm-specific antibiotic resistance. *Future Microbiol.* **2012**, *7*, 1061–1072. [CrossRef] [PubMed]
33. Donlan, R.M. Biofilm formation: A clinically relevant microbiological process. *Clin. Infec. Dis.* **2001**, *33*, 1387–1392. [CrossRef] [PubMed]
34. Høiby, N.; Bjarnsholt, T.; Moser, C.; Bassi, G.; Coenye, T.; Donelli, G.; Hall-Stoodley, L.; Hola, V.; Imbert, C.; Kirketerp-Møller, K. ESCMID∗ guideline for the diagnosis and treatment of biofilm infections. *Clin. Microbiol. Infect.* **2015**, *21*, S1–S25. [CrossRef] [PubMed]
35. Romling, U.; Kjelleberg, S.; Normark, S.; Nyman, L.; Uhlin, B.E.; Akerlund, B. Microbial biofilm formation: A need to act. *J. Intern. Med.* **2014**, *276*, 98–110. [CrossRef] [PubMed]
36. Romling, U.; Balsalobre, C. Biofilm infections, their resilience to therapy and innovative treatment strategies. *J. Intern. Med.* **2012**, *272*, 541–561. [CrossRef] [PubMed]

37. Bryers, J.D. Medical Biofilms. *Biotechnol. Bioeng.* **2008**, *100*, 1–18. [CrossRef] [PubMed]
38. Costerton, J.W.; Montanaro, L.; Arciola, C.R. Biofilm in implant infections: Its production and regulation. *Int. J. Art. Organs* **2005**, *28*, 1062–1068. [CrossRef]
39. Costerton, W.; Veeh, R.; Shirtliff, M.; Pasmore, M.; Post, C.; Ehrlich, G. The application of biofilm science to the study and control of chronic bacterial infections. *J. Clin. Investig.* **2003**, *112*, 1466–1477. [CrossRef] [PubMed]
40. Veerachamy, S.; Yarlagadda, T.; Manivasagam, G.; Yarlagadda, P.K. Bacterial adherence and biofilm formation on medical implants: A review. *Proc. Inst. Mech. Eng. Part. H J. Eng. Med.* **2014**, *228*, 1083–1099. [CrossRef] [PubMed]
41. Bryers, J.D.; Ratner, B.D. Bioinspired implant materials befuddle bacteria. *ASM News-Am. Soc. Microbiol.* **2004**, *70*, 232.
42. Castelli, P.; Caronno, R.; Ferrarese, S.; Mantovani, V.; Piffaretti, G.; Tozzi, M.; Lomazzi, C.; Rivolta, N.; Sala, A. New trends in prosthesis infection in cardiovascular surgery. *Surg. Infect.* **2006**, *7* (Suppl. 2), S45–S47. [CrossRef]
43. Carmen, J.C.; Roeder, B.L.; Nelson, J.L.; Ogilvie, R.L.R.; Robison, R.A.; Schaalje, G.B.; Pitt, W.G. Treatment of biofilm infections on implants with low-frequency ultrasound and antibiotics. *Am. J. Infect. Cont.* **2005**, *33*, 78–82. [CrossRef] [PubMed]
44. Paterson, I.K.; Hoyle, A.; Ochoa, G.; Baker-Austin, C.; Taylor, N.G. Optimising antibiotic usage to treat bacterial infections. *Sci Rep* **2016**, *6*, 37853. [CrossRef] [PubMed]
45. Bahar, A.A.; Ren, D. Antimicrobial peptides. *Pharmaceuticals* **2013**, *6*, 1543–1575. [CrossRef] [PubMed]
46. Brown, K.L.; Hancock, R.E. Cationic host defense (antimicrobial) peptides. *Curr. Opin. Immunol.* **2006**, *18*, 24–30. [CrossRef] [PubMed]
47. Groenink, J.; Walgreen-Weterings, E.; van't Hof, W.; Veerman, E.I.; Nieuw Amerongen, A.V. Cationic amphipathic peptides, derived from bovine and human lactoferrins, with antimicrobial activity against oral pathogens. *FEMS Microbiol. Lett.* **1999**, *179*, 217–222. [CrossRef] [PubMed]
48. Bradshaw, J.P. Cationic antimicrobial peptides. *BioDrugs* **2003**, *17*, 233–240. [CrossRef] [PubMed]
49. Huang, Y.; Huang, J.; Chen, Y. Alpha-helical cationic antimicrobial peptides: Relationships of structure and function. *Protein Cell* **2010**, *1*, 143–152. [CrossRef]
50. Harris, F.; Dennison, S.R.; Phoenix, D.A. Anionic antimicrobial peptides from eukaryotic organisms. *Curr. Prot. Pep. Sci.* **2009**, *10*, 585–606. [CrossRef]
51. Batoni, G.; Maisetta, G.; Esin, S. Antimicrobial peptides and their interaction with biofilms of medically relevant bacteria. *Biochim. Biophys. Acta* **2016**, *1858*, 1044–1060. [CrossRef]
52. Segev-Zarko, L.; Saar-Dover, R.; Brumfeld, V.; Mangoni, M.L.; Shai, Y. Mechanisms of biofilm inhibition and degradation by antimicrobial peptides. *Biochem. J.* **2015**, *468*, 259–270. [CrossRef] [PubMed]
53. Bowdish, D.M.; Davidson, D.J.; Hancock, R.E. A re-evaluation of the role of host defence peptides in mammalian immunity. *Curr. Protein Pept. Sci.* **2005**, *6*, 35–51. [CrossRef] [PubMed]
54. Boman, H.G. Peptide antibiotics and their role in innate immunity. *Ann. Rev. Immunol.* **1995**, *13*, 61–92. [CrossRef] [PubMed]
55. Tossi, A.; Sandri, L.; Giangaspero, A. Amphipathic, alpha-helical antimicrobial peptides. *Biopolymers* **2000**, *55*, 4–30. [CrossRef]
56. Ebenhan, T.; Gheysens, O.; Kruger, H.G.; Zeevaart, J.R.; Sathekge, M.M. Antimicrobial peptides: Their role as infection-selective tracers for molecular imaging. *BioMed. Res. Int.* **2014**, *2014*, 867381. [CrossRef] [PubMed]
57. Tossi, A.; Sandri, L. Molecular diversity in gene-encoded, cationic antimicrobial polypeptides. *Curr. Pharm. Des.* **2002**, *8*, 743–761. [CrossRef] [PubMed]
58. Ganz, T. Defensins: Antimicrobial peptides of innate immunity. *Nat. Rev. Immunol.* **2003**, *3*, 710–720. [CrossRef]
59. Lehrer, R.I. Primate defensins. *Nat. Rev. Microbiol.* **2004**, *2*, 727–738. [CrossRef]
60. Takahashi, D.; Shukla, S.K.; Prakash, O.; Zhang, G. Structural determinants of host defense peptides for antimicrobial activity and target cell selectivity. *Biochimie* **2010**, *92*, 1236–1241. [CrossRef]
61. Zasloff, M. Antimicrobial peptides of multicellular organisms. *Nature* **2002**, *415*, 389. [CrossRef]
62. Selsted, M.E.; Harwig, S.S. Determination of the disulfide array in the human defensin HNP-2. A covalently cyclized peptide. *J. Biol. Chem.* **1989**, *264*, 4003–4007. [PubMed]
63. Tang, Y.Q.; Selsted, M.E. Characterization of the disulfide motif in BNBD-12, an antimicrobial beta-defensin peptide from bovine neutrophils. *J. Biol. Chem.* **1993**, *268*, 6649–6653. [PubMed]

64. Cruz, J.; Ortiz, C.; Guzman, F.; Fernandez-Lafuente, R.; Torres, R. Antimicrobial peptides: Promising compounds against pathogenic microorganisms. *Curr. Med. Chem.* **2014**, *21*, 2299–2321. [CrossRef] [PubMed]
65. Su, L.Y.; Willner, D.L.; Segall, A.M. An antimicrobial peptide that targets DNA repair intermediates in vitro inhibits Salmonella growth within murine macrophages. *Antimicrob. Agents Chemother.* **2010**, *54*, 1888–1899. [CrossRef] [PubMed]
66. Brogden, K.A. Antimicrobial peptides: Pore formers or metabolic inhibitors in bacteria? *Nat. Rev. Microbiol.* **2005**, *3*, 238–250. [CrossRef] [PubMed]
67. Kragol, G.; Lovas, S.; Varadi, G.; Condie, B.A.; Hoffmann, R.; Otvos, L. The antibacterial peptide pyrrhocoricin inhibits the ATPase actions of DnaK and prevents chaperone-assisted protein folding. *Biochemistry* **2001**, *40*, 3016–3026. [CrossRef] [PubMed]
68. Conti, S.; Radicioni, G.; Ciociola, T.; Longhi, R.; Polonelli, L.; Gatti, R.; Cabras, T.; Messana, I.; Castagnola, M.; Vitali, A. Structural and functional studies on a proline-rich peptide isolated from swine saliva endowed with antifungal activity towards Cryptococcus neoformans. *Biochim. Biophys. Acta Biomem.* **2013**, *1828*, 1066–1074. [CrossRef]
69. Shai, Y. Mechanism of the binding, insertion and destabilization of phospholipid bilayer membranes by alpha-helical antimicrobial and cell non-selective membrane-lytic peptides. *Biochimic. Biophys. Acta* **1999**, *1462*, 55–70. [CrossRef]
70. Peschel, A.; Sahl, H.-G. The co-evolution of host cationic antimicrobial peptides and microbial resistance. *Nat. Rev. Microbiol.* **2006**, *4*, 529. [CrossRef]
71. Schuller, F.; Benz, R.; Sahl, H.G. The peptide antibiotic subtilin acts by formation of voltage-dependent multi-state pores in bacterial and artificial membranes. *Eur. J. Biochem.* **1989**, *182*, 181–186. [CrossRef]
72. Tennessen, J.A. Molecular evolution of animal antimicrobial peptides: Widespread moderate positive selection. *J. Evol. Biol.* **2005**, *18*, 1387–1394. [CrossRef] [PubMed]
73. Wimley, W.C.; Hristova, K. Antimicrobial Peptides: Successes, challenges and unanswered questions. *J. Memb. Biol.* **2011**, *239*, 27–34. [CrossRef] [PubMed]
74. Straus, S.K.; Hancock, R.E. Mode of action of the new antibiotic for Gram-positive pathogens daptomycin: Comparison with cationic antimicrobial peptides and lipopeptides. *Biochim. Biophys. Acta* **2006**, *1758*, 1215–1223. [CrossRef]
75. Sang, Y.; Blecha, F. Antimicrobial peptides and bacteriocins: Alternatives to traditional antibiotics. *Anim. Health Res. Rev.* **2008**, *9*, 227–235. [CrossRef] [PubMed]
76. Haney, E.F.; Mansour, S.C.; Hancock, R.E. Antimicrobial Peptides: An Introduction. *Meth. Mol. Biol.* **2017**, *1548*, 3–22. [CrossRef]
77. Sun, E.; Belanger, C.R.; Haney, E.F.; Hancock, R.E. Host defense (antimicrobial) peptides. In *Peptide Applications in Biomedicine, Biotechnology and Bioengineering*; Elsevier: Amsterdam, the Netherlands, 2018; pp. 253–285.
78. Okuda, K.; Zendo, T.; Sugimoto, S.; Iwase, T.; Tajima, A.; Yamada, S.; Sonomoto, K.; Mizunoe, Y. Effects of bacteriocins on methicillin-resistant Staphylococcus aureus biofilm. *Antimicrob. Agents Chemother.* **2013**, *57*, 5572–5579. [CrossRef]
79. Pulido, D.; Prats-Ejarque, G.; Villalba, C.; Albacar, M.; González-López, J.J.; Torrent, M.; Moussaoui, M.; Boix, E. A novel RNase 3/ECP peptide for Pseudomonas aeruginosa biofilm eradication. Combining antimicrobial, lipopolysaccharide binding and cell agglutinating activities. *Antimicrob. Agents Chemother.* **2016**, *60*, 6313–6325. [CrossRef]
80. Venge, P. Eosinophil cationic protein (ECP): Molecular and biological properties and the use of ECP as a marker of eosinophil activation in disease. *Clin. Exp. Allergy* **1999**, *29*, 1172–1186. [CrossRef]
81. Acharya, K.R.; Ackerman, S.J. Eosinophil granule proteins: Form and function. *J. Biol. Chem.* **2014**. [CrossRef]
82. Luca, V.; Stringaro, A.; Colone, M.; Pini, A.; Mangoni, M.L. Esculentin(1-21), an amphibian skin membrane-active peptide with potent activity on both planktonic and biofilm cells of the bacterial pathogen Pseudomonas aeruginosa. *Cell. Mol. Life. Sci.* **2013**, *70*, 2773–2786. [CrossRef]
83. Nagant, C.; Pitts, B.; Stewart, P.S.; Feng, Y.; Savage, P.B.; Dehaye, J.P. Study of the effect of antimicrobial peptide mimic, CSA-13, on an established biofilm formed by P seudomonas aeruginosa. *Microbiologyopen* **2013**, *2*, 318–325. [CrossRef] [PubMed]
84. Overhage, J.; Campisano, A.; Bains, M.; Torfs, E.C.; Rehm, B.H.; Hancock, R.E. Human host defense peptide LL-37 prevents bacterial biofilm formation. *Infect. Immun.* **2008**, *76*, 4176–4182. [CrossRef] [PubMed]

85. de la Fuente-Núñez, C.; Korolik, V.; Bains, M.; Nguyen, U.; Breidenstein, E.B.M.; Horsman, S.; Lewenza, S.; Burrows, L.; Hancock, R.E.W. Inhibition of Bacterial Biofilm Formation and Swarming Motility by a Small Synthetic Cationic Peptide. *Antimicrob. Agents Chemother.* **2012**, *56*, 2696–2704. [CrossRef] [PubMed]
86. Jorge, P.; Lourenco, A.; Pereira, M.O. New trends in peptide-based anti-biofilm strategies: A review of recent achievements and bioinformatic approaches. *Biofouling* **2012**, *28*, 1033–1061. [CrossRef] [PubMed]
87. Ansari, J.M.; Abraham, N.M.; Massaro, J.; Murphy, K.; Smith-Carpenter, J.; Fikrig, E. Anti-biofilm activity of a self-aggregating peptide against Streptococcus mutans. *Front. Microbiol.* **2017**, *8*, 488. [CrossRef] [PubMed]
88. Gordya, N.; Yakovlev, A.; Kruglikova, A.; Tulin, D.; Potolitsina, E.; Suborova, T.; Bordo, D.; Rosano, C.; Chernysh, S. Natural antimicrobial peptide complexes in the fighting of antibiotic resistant biofilms: Calliphora vicina medicinal maggots. *PLoS ONE* **2017**, *12*, e0173559. [CrossRef] [PubMed]
89. Brancatisano, F.L.; Maisetta, G.; Di Luca, M.; Esin, S.; Bottai, D.; Bizzarri, R.; Campa, M.; Batoni, G. Inhibitory effect of the human liver-derived antimicrobial peptide hepcidin 20 on biofilms of polysaccharide intercellular adhesin (PIA)-positive and PIA-negative strains of Staphylococcus epidermidis. *Biofouling* **2014**, *30*, 435–446. [CrossRef]
90. Quiles, F.; Saadi, S.; Francius, G.; Bacharouche, J.; Humbert, F. In situ and real time investigation of the evolution of a Pseudomonas fluorescens nascent biofilm in the presence of an antimicrobial peptide. *Biochimic. Biophys. Acta* **2016**, *1858*, 75–84. [CrossRef]
91. Libardo, M.D.J.; Bahar, A.A.; Ma, B.; Fu, R.; McCormick, L.E.; Zhao, J.; McCallum, S.A.; Nussinov, R.; Ren, D.; Angeles-Boza, A.M.; et al. Nuclease activity gives an edge to host-defense peptide piscidin 3 over piscidin 1, rendering it more effective against persisters and biofilms. *FEBS J.* **2017**, *284*, 3662–3683. [CrossRef]
92. Pletzer, D.; Coleman, S.R.; Hancock, R.E. Anti-biofilm peptides as a new weapon in antimicrobial warfare. *Curr. Opin. Microbiol.* **2016**, *33*, 35–40. [CrossRef]
93. Potrykus, K.; Cashel, M. (p)ppGpp: Still magical? *Ann. Rev. Microbiol.* **2008**, *62*, 35–51. [CrossRef] [PubMed]
94. Braeken, K.; Moris, M.; Daniels, R.; Vanderleyden, J.; Michiels, J. New horizons for (p) ppGpp in bacterial and plant physiology. *Trends Microbiol.* **2006**, *14*, 45–54. [CrossRef] [PubMed]
95. Åberg, A.; Shingler, V.; Balsalobre, C. (p) ppGpp regulates type 1 fimbriation of Escherichia coli by modulating the expression of the site-specific recombinase FimB. *Mol. Microbiol.* **2006**, *60*, 1520–1533. [CrossRef] [PubMed]
96. Pletzer, D.; Wolfmeier, H.; Bains, M.; Hancock, R.E.W. Synthetic Peptides to Target Stringent Response-Controlled Virulence in a Pseudomonas aeruginosa Murine Cutaneous Infection Model. *Front. Microbiol.* **2017**, *8*. [CrossRef] [PubMed]
97. Rohde, H.; Frankenberger, S.; Zähringer, U.; Mack, D. Structure, function and contribution of polysaccharide intercellular adhesin (PIA) to Staphylococcus epidermidis biofilm formation and pathogenesis of biomaterial-associated infections. *Eur. J. Cell. Biol.* **2010**, *89*, 103–111. [CrossRef] [PubMed]
98. Zhu, C.; Tan, H.; Cheng, T.; Shen, H.; Shao, J.; Guo, Y.; Shi, S.; Zhang, X. Human beta-defensin 3 inhibits antibiotic-resistant Staphylococcus biofilm formation. *J. Surg. Res.* **2013**, *183*, 204–213. [CrossRef]
99. Wang, H.-Y.; Lin, L.; Tan, L.-S.; Yu, H.-Y.; Cheng, J.-W.; Pan, Y.-P. Molecular pathways underlying inhibitory effect of antimicrobial peptide Nal-P-113 on bacteria biofilms formation of Porphyromonas gingivalis W83 by DNA microarray. *BMC Microbiol.* **2017**, *17*, 37. [CrossRef]
100. Hinsa, S.M.; Espinosa-Urgel, M.; Ramos, J.L.; O'Toole, G.A. Transition from reversible to irreversible attachment during biofilm formation by Pseudomonas fluorescens WCS365 requires an ABC transporter and a large secreted protein. *Mol. Microbiol.* **2003**, *49*, 905–918. [CrossRef]
101. Andersen, R.N.; Ganeshkumar, N.; Kolenbrander, P.E. Cloning of the Streptococcus gordonii PK488 gene, encoding an adhesin which mediates coaggregation with Actinomyces naeslundii PK606. *Infect. Immun.* **1993**, *61*, 981–987.
102. Otto, M. Bacterial evasion of antimicrobial peptides by biofilm formation. *Curr. Top. Microbiol. Immunol.* **2006**, *306*, 251–258.
103. Vuong, C.; Voyich, J.M.; Fischer, E.R.; Braughton, K.R.; Whitney, A.R.; DeLeo, F.R.; Otto, M. Polysaccharide intercellular adhesin (PIA) protects Staphylococcus epidermidis against major components of the human innate immune system. *Cell. Microbiol.* **2004**, *6*, 269–275. [CrossRef] [PubMed]
104. Gacesa, P. Bacterial alginate biosynthesis-recent progress and future prospects. *Microbiology* **1998**, *144*, 1133–1143. [CrossRef] [PubMed]

105. Evans, L.R.; Linker, A. Production and characterization of the slime polysaccharide of Pseudomonas aeruginosa. *J. Bacteriol.* **1973**, *116*, 915–924. [PubMed]
106. Chan, C.; Burrows, L.L.; Deber, C.M. Helix induction in antimicrobial peptides by alginate in biofilms. *J. Biol. Chem.* **2004**, *279*, 38749–38754. [CrossRef] [PubMed]
107. Leid, J.G.; Willson, C.J.; Shirtliff, M.E.; Hassett, D.J.; Parsek, M.R.; Jeffers, A.K. The exopolysaccharide alginate protects Pseudomonas aeruginosa biofilm bacteria from IFN-gamma-mediated macrophage killing. *J. Immunol.* **2005**, *175*, 7512–7518. [CrossRef] [PubMed]
108. Kuo, H.H.; Chan, C.; Burrows, L.L.; Deber, C.M. Hydrophobic interactions in complexes of antimicrobial peptides with bacterial polysaccharides. *Chem. Biol. Drug. Des.* **2007**, *69*, 405–412. [CrossRef]
109. Doggett, R.G.; Harrison, G.M.; Stillwell, R.N.; Wallis, E.S. An atypical Pseudomonas aeruginosa associated with cystic fibrosis of the pancreas. *J. Ped.* **1966**, *68*, 215–221. [CrossRef]
110. Stapper, A.P.; Narasimhan, G.; Ohman, D.E.; Barakat, J.; Hentzer, M.; Molin, S.; Kharazmi, A.; Hoiby, N.; Mathee, K. Alginate production affects Pseudomonas aeruginosa biofilm development and architecture, but is not essential for biofilm formation. *J. Med. Microbiol.* **2004**, *53*, 679–690. [CrossRef] [PubMed]
111. Colvin, K.M.; Irie, Y.; Tart, C.S.; Urbano, R.; Whitney, J.C.; Ryder, C.; Howell, P.L.; Wozniak, D.J.; Parsek, M.R. The Pel and Psl polysaccharides provide Pseudomonas aeruginosa structural redundancy within the biofilm matrix. *Environ. Microbiol.* **2012**, *14*, 1913–1928. [CrossRef] [PubMed]
112. Li, M.; Lai, Y.; Villaruz, A.E.; Cha, D.J.; Sturdevant, D.E.; Otto, M. Gram-positive three-component antimicrobial peptide-sensing system. *Proc. Natl. Acad. Sci. USA* **2007**, *104*, 9469–9474. [CrossRef] [PubMed]
113. Yang, S.-J.; Bayer, A.S.; Mishra, N.N.; Meehl, M.; Ledala, N.; Yeaman, M.R.; Xiong, Y.Q.; Cheung, A.L. The Staphylococcus aureus two-component regulatory system, GraRS, senses and confers resistance to selected cationic antimicrobial peptides. *Infect. Immun.* **2012**, *80*, 74–81. [CrossRef] [PubMed]
114. Otto, M. Bacterial sensing of antimicrobial peptides. *Cont. Microbiol.* **2009**, *16*, 136–149. [CrossRef]
115. Fabretti, F.; Theilacker, C.; Baldassarri, L.; Kaczynski, Z.; Kropec, A.; Holst, O.; Huebner, J. Alanine esters of enterococcal lipoteichoic acid play a role in biofilm formation and resistance to antimicrobial peptides. *Infect. Immun.* **2006**, *74*, 4164–4171. [CrossRef] [PubMed]
116. Skiada, A.; Markogiannakis, A.; Plachouras, D.; Daikos, G.L. Adaptive resistance to cationic compounds in Pseudomonas aeruginosa. *Int. J. Antimicrob. Aents* **2011**, *37*, 187–193. [CrossRef] [PubMed]
117. Bader, M.W.; Sanowar, S.; Daley, M.E.; Schneider, A.R.; Cho, U.; Xu, W.; Klevit, R.E.; Le Moual, H.; Miller, S.I. Recognition of antimicrobial peptides by a bacterial sensor kinase. *Cell* **2005**, *122*, 461–472. [CrossRef] [PubMed]
118. Ramsey, M.M.; Whiteley, M. Pseudomonas aeruginosa attachment and biofilm development in dynamic environments. *Mol. Microbiol.* **2004**, *53*, 1075–1087. [CrossRef]
119. McPhee, J.B.; Lewenza, S.; Hancock, R.E. Cationic antimicrobial peptides activate a two-component regulatory system, PmrA-PmrB, that regulates resistance to polymyxin B and cationic antimicrobial peptides in Pseudomonas aeruginosa. *Mol. Microbiol.* **2003**, *50*, 205–217. [CrossRef] [PubMed]
120. Gunn, J.S.; Lim, K.B.; Krueger, J.; Kim, K.; Guo, L.; Hackett, M.; Miller, S.I. PmrA-PmrB-regulated genes necessary for 4-aminoarabinose lipid A modification and polymyxin resistance. *Mol. Microbiol.* **1998**, *27*, 1171–1182. [CrossRef] [PubMed]
121. Gunn, J.S.; Miller, S.I. PhoP-PhoQ activates transcription of pmrAB, encoding a two-component regulatory system involved in Salmonella typhimurium antimicrobial peptide resistance. *J. Bacteriol.* **1996**, *178*, 6857–6864. [CrossRef]
122. Koo, H.; Allan, R.N.; Howlin, R.P.; Hall-Stoodley, L.; Stoodley, P. Targeting microbial biofilms: Current and prospective therapeutic strategies. *Nat. Rev. Microbiol.* **2017**, *15*, 740–755. [CrossRef]
123. Pamp, S.J.; Gjermansen, M.; Johansen, H.K.; Tolker-Nielsen, T. Tolerance to the antimicrobial peptide colistin in Pseudomonas aeruginosa biofilms is linked to metabolically active cells, and depends on the pmr and mexAB-oprM genes. *Mol. Microbiol.* **2008**, *68*, 223–240. [CrossRef] [PubMed]
124. Folkesson, A.; Haagensen, J.A.; Zampaloni, C.; Sternberg, C.; Molin, S. Biofilm induced tolerance towards antimicrobial peptides. *PLoS ONE* **2008**, *3*, e1891. [CrossRef] [PubMed]
125. Mishra, N.M.; Briers, Y.; Lamberigts, C.; Steenackers, H.; Robijns, S.; Landuyt, B.; Vanderleyden, J.; Schoofs, L.; Lavigne, R.; Luyten, W. Evaluation of the antibacterial and antibiofilm activities of novel CRAMP–vancomycin conjugates with diverse linkers. *Org. Biomol. Chem.* **2015**, *13*, 7477–7486. [CrossRef] [PubMed]

126. Rudilla, H.; Fusté, E.; Cajal, Y.; Rabanal, F.; Vinuesa, T.; Viñas, M. Synergistic antipseudomonal effects of synthetic peptide AMP38 and carbapenems. *Molecules* **2016**, *21*, 1223. [CrossRef] [PubMed]
127. Ribeiro, S.M.; de la Fuente-Núñez, C.; Baquir, B.; Faria-Junior, C.; Franco, O.L.; Hancock, R.E. Antibiofilm peptides increase the susceptibility of carbapenemase-producing Klebsiella pneumoniae clinical isolates to β-lactam antibiotics. *Antimicrob. Agents Chemother.* **2015**, *59*, 3906–3912. [CrossRef]
128. Gopal, R.; Kim, Y.G.; Lee, J.H.; Lee, S.K.; Chae, J.D.; Son, B.K.; Seo, C.H.; Park, Y. Synergistic effects and antibiofilm properties of chimeric peptides against multidrug-resistant Acinetobacter baumannii strains. *Antimicrob. Agents Chemother.* **2014**, *58*, 1622–1629. [CrossRef] [PubMed]
129. Grassi, L.; Maisetta, G.; Esin, S.; Batoni, G. Combination Strategies to Enhance the Efficacy of Antimicrobial Peptides against Bacterial Biofilms. *Front. Microbiol.* **2017**, *8*, 2409. [CrossRef] [PubMed]
130. Jorge, P.; Grzywacz, D.; Kamysz, W.; Lourenço, A.; Pereira, M.O. Searching for new strategies against biofilm infections: Colistin-AMP combinations against Pseudomonas aeruginosa and Staphylococcus aureus single-and double-species biofilms. *PLoS ONE* **2017**, *12*, e0174654. [CrossRef] [PubMed]
131. Chung, P.Y.; Khanum, R. Antimicrobial peptides as potential anti-biofilm agents against multidrug-resistant bacteria. *J. Microbiol. Immunol. Infect.* **2017**, *50*, 405–410. [CrossRef] [PubMed]
132. Cools, T.L.; Struyfs, C.; Drijfhout, J.W.; Kucharikova, S.; Lobo Romero, C.; Van Dijck, P.; Ramada, M.H.S.; Bloch, C., Jr.; Cammue, B.P.A.; Thevissen, K. A Linear 19-Mer Plant Defensin-Derived Peptide Acts Synergistically with Caspofungin against Candida albicans Biofilms. *Front. Microbiol.* **2017**, *8*, 2051. [CrossRef] [PubMed]
133. Mahlapuu, M.; Håkansson, J.; Ringstad, L.; Björn, C. Antimicrobial Peptides: An Emerging Category of Therapeutic Agents. *Front. Cell. Infect. Microbiol.* **2016**, *6*, 194. [CrossRef] [PubMed]

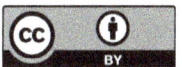

© 2018 by the authors. Licensee MDPI, Basel, Switzerland. This article is an open access article distributed under the terms and conditions of the Creative Commons Attribution (CC BY) license (http://creativecommons.org/licenses/by/4.0/).

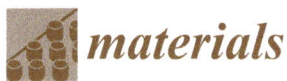

Review

Control of Biofilm Formation in Healthcare: Recent Advances Exploiting Quorum-Sensing Interference Strategies and Multidrug Efflux Pump Inhibitors

Bindu Subhadra, Dong Ho Kim, Kyungho Woo, Surya Surendran and Chul Hee Choi *

Department of Microbiology and Medical Science, Chungnam National University School of Medicine, Daejeon 35015, Korea; bindu.subhadra@gmail.com (B.S.); casiopea1208@naver.com (D.H.K.); khwoo1991@gmail.com (K.W.); tankz93@gmail.com (S.S.)
* Correspondence: choich@cnu.ac.kr; Tel.: +82-42-580-8246

Received: 5 June 2018; Accepted: 7 September 2018; Published: 10 September 2018

Abstract: Biofilm formation in healthcare is an issue of considerable concern, as it results in increased morbidity and mortality, imposing a significant financial burden on the healthcare system. Biofilms are highly resistant to conventional antimicrobial therapies and lead to persistent infections. Hence, there is a high demand for novel strategies other than conventional antibiotic therapies to control biofilm-based infections. There are two approaches which have been employed so far to control biofilm formation in healthcare settings: one is the development of biofilm inhibitors based on the understanding of the molecular mechanism of biofilm formation, and the other is to modify the biomaterials which are used in medical devices to prevent biofilm formation. This review will focus on the recent advances in anti-biofilm approaches by interrupting the quorum-sensing cellular communication system and the multidrug efflux pumps which play an important role in biofilm formation. Research efforts directed towards these promising strategies could eventually lead to the development of better anti-biofilm therapies than the conventional treatments.

Keywords: biofilm formation; healthcare; biofilm inhibition; quorum sensing; multidrug efflux pumps

1. Introduction

Biofilms are surface-attached groups of microbial cells that are embedded in a self-produced extracellular matrix and are highly resistant to antimicrobial agents [1–3]. Biofilms can attach to all kinds of surfaces, including metals, plastics, plant and body tissue, medical devices and implant materials [4]. Biofilm formation on indwelling medical devices and implants such as heart valves, pacemakers, vascular grafts, catheters, prosthetic joints, intrauterine devices, sutures and contact lenses poses a critical problem of infection [5]. The use of intravascular catheters for patient care can give rise to central line-associated blood stream infection (CLABSI), and approximately 250,000 cases of primary blood stream infections are reported each year in the USA [6]. Thus, CLABSI results in significant morbidity and mortality and huge increases in healthcare costs. The bacteria most frequently associated with healthcare-associated infections include *Staphylococcus aureus*, *Staphylococcus epidermidis*, *Enterococcus faecalis*, *Escherichia coli*, *Klebsiella pneumoniae*, *Proteus mirabilis*, *Pseudomonas aeruginosa* and *Acinetobacter* spp. [5,7]. Among the biofilm-forming bacteria, *S. aureus* and *S. epidermidis* are predominantly isolated from cardiovascular devices [8,9]. It has been estimated that *S. aureus* and *S. epidermidis* contribute to 40–50% of prosthetic heart valve infections and 50–70% of the catheter biofilm infections [10]. In recent years, *Acinetobacter* spp. have emerged as the most important nosocomial pathogens involved in a variety of nosocomial infections, including bacteremia, urinary tract infection, soft-tissue infections and secondary meningitis [11–14]. The *Acinetobacter* spp.

have the ability to colonize and form biofilms on medical devices such as implants, cardiac valves, artificial joints, catheters, etc. [11,15].

Biofilm formation is initiated when the cells attach and adhere to surfaces. The attachment of microbial cells to biomaterials can be facilitated by factors such as bacterial motility, increased shear forces, and hydrodynamic and electrostatic interactions between the microorganism and surface [16]. The adherence of bacteria to biomaterials through cell-surface and biomaterial-surface interactions is mediated by multiple factors, which include cell surface proteins, capsular polysaccharide/adhesin, protein autolysin, etc. [17,18]. For example, Staphylococcal species display cell-surface proteins, namely staphylococcal surface protein-1 and -2 (SSP-1 and SSP-2) [17], which are essential for adhesion of *S. epidermidis* to polystyrene [19]. In addition, host factors can also mediate the adherence of bacterial cells to implants, as the implant surfaces are usually covered by host plasma and other extracellular components [20]. Once attached to the surfaces, the bacterial cells will proliferate, aggregate and differentiate into biofilm structures [21]. Bacterial cells can detach from mature biofilms and spread to other organ systems, thereby contributing to persistent chronic infections [21,22].

Biofilms are complex structures with customized living environments with differing pH, nutrient availability and oxygen [23]. A worrying feature of biofilm-based infections is the increased tolerance of biofilm cells to biocides compared to planktonic bacteria [24]. The increased drug resistance could be attributed to plasmids containing genes for multidrug resistance, as biofilms form an ideal niche for plasmid exchange [25]. The mechanisms by which biofilms represent increased drug resistance also include slow or incomplete penetration of antimicrobial agents through the extracellular polymeric matrix, the formation of persister or dormant cells in a spore-like non-dividing state, slow growth rate of cells in the biofilm, thereby reducing the number of targets for antimicrobial molecules, etc. [26–28]. In addition to the difficulty in treating biofilm with conventional antimicrobial therapy, the treatment is further hindered by increased antibiotic resistance, as bacterial cells acquire resistance under antibiotic selective pressure [29]. For example, it has been reported that more than 70% of hospital isolates of *S. epidermidis* are methicillin resistant [30]. Thus, there is a high demand for alternative strategies to control biofilm-based infections other than antibiotic therapy. Considering the number of patients suffering from biofilm-based device-related infections, several strategies have been developed in the past few decades. This review will discuss the most successful antibiofilm approaches so far, as well as some of the more promising prospects for the control of these biofilm-based infections.

2. Strategies for the Control of Biofilms

There have been three major strategies considered so far to control biofilm formation or to target different stages of biofilm development. The first approach is inhibiting the initial attachment of bacteria to biofilm-forming surfaces, thereby reducing the chances of biofilm development. The second approach targets the disruption of biofilm during the maturation process [31]. The third strategy is the signal interference approach, in which the bacterial communication system or the quorum sensing (QS) system is interfered with as QS coordinates biofilm formation/maturation in pathogenic bacteria [32]. The different antibiofilm strategies and agents discussed in this review are summarized in Table 1.

Table 1. Various strategies for the control of biofilms.

Strategy	Methods/Agents	Examples	References
Inhibition of initial biofilm attachment	(i) Altering chemical properties of biomaterials	(i) Antibiotics, biocides, iron coatings	(i) [33–43]
	(ii) Changing physical properties of biomaterials	(ii) Use of hydrophilic polymers, superhydrophobic coatings, hydrogel coatings, heparin coatings	(ii) [44–49]

Table 1. Cont.

Strategy	Methods/Agents	Examples	References
Removal of biofilms	(i) Matrix degrading enzymes	(i) Polysaccharide-degrading enzymes (Dispersin B, Endolysins); Nucleases (Deoxyribonuclease I) and Proteases (Proteinase K, trypsin)	(i) [50–55]
	(ii) Surfactants	(ii) Sodium dodecyl sulfate (SDS), cetyltrimethylammonium bromide (CTAB), Tween 20 and Triton X-100, surfactin, rhamnolipids	(ii) [56–60]
	(iii) Free fatty acids, amino acids and nitric oxide donors	(iii) Cis-2-decenoic acid, D-amino acids, nitric oxide generators such as sodium nitroprusside (SNP), S-nitroso-L-glutathione (GSNO) and S-nitroso-N-acetylpenicillamine (SNAP)	(iii) [61–64]
Biofilm inhibition by quorum quenching	(i) Degradation of QS signals	(i) Lactonases, acylases and oxidoreductases	(i) [65–71]
	(ii) Inhibition of signal synthesis	(ii) Use of analogues of AHL precursor S-adenosyl-methionine (SAM), S-adenosyl-homocysteine (SAH), sinefugin, 5-methylthioadenosine (MTA), butyryl-SAM; SAM biosynthesis inhibitor cycloleucine, AHL synthesis inhibitors such as nickel and cadmium	(ii) [72–79]
	(iii) Antagonizing signal molecules	(iii) AHL analogues (bergamottin, dihydroxybergamottin, cyclic sulfur compounds, phenolic compounds including baicalin hydrate and epigallocatechin); AI-2 analogues (ursolic acid, isobutyl-4,5-dihydroxy-2,3-pentanedione (isobutyl-DPD) and phenyl-DPD); AIP analogues (cyclic peptides such as cyclo (L-Phe-L-Pro) and cyclo(L-Tyr-L-Pro), RNAIII inhibiting peptide (RIP) and its homologues)	(iii) [80–96]
	(iv) Inhibition of signal transduction	(iv) Use of halogenated furanone or fimbrolide, cinnamaldehyde, virstatin	(iv) [97–103]
	(v) Inhibition of signal transport	(v) Use of copper or silver nanoparticles, Phe-Arg-β-naphthylamide (PAβN)	(v) [104–106]

2.1. Inhibition of Initial Attachment

The initial attachment of cells to the biofilm-forming surfaces happens within an average of the first 2 days of biofilm formation. Inhibition of initial attachment of cells to the surfaces is a potential strategy to prevent biofilm formation rather than targeting the dispersal of established biofilms. The attachment of bacteria to surfaces is mediated by several factors, including adhesion surface proteins, pili or fimbriae, and exopolysaccharides [107,108]. The surfaces that are rough, coated with surface conditioning films and more hydrophobic are prone to ease biofilm formation [109–111]. Thus, the initial attachment of cells can be prevented by altering the chemical or physical properties of indwelling medical devices.

2.1.1. By Altering the Chemical Properties of Biomaterials

The commonly used chemical methods to modify the surface of biomedical devices in order to prevent biofilm formation include antibiotics, biocides and ion coatings [33]. Catheters coated with antibiotics such as minocycline and rifampin have been shown to decrease the incidence of biofilm-associated bloodstream infection by *S. aureus* in healthcare [34]. In addition, catheters impregnated with different antibiotics, including nitrofurazone, gentamicin, norfloxacin, etc., are suggested to have a role in preventing biofilm-associated urinary tract infections [35].

High-throughput screening of chemical libraries has led to the identification of several small chemical molecules as potential drug candidates for controlling biofilm formation and infection. These molecules do not elicit antimicrobial activity, and thus decrease the likelihood of the development of resistance due to the absence of selective pressure against biofilm formation. In *Streptococcus pyogenes* and *S. aureus*, a series of small molecules inhibited the expression of many key virulence factors that are involved in biofilm formation and infection [112,113]. The early stages of biofilm formation in *S. aureus*, *S. epidermidis* and *E. faecalis* were inhibited by several aryl rhodamines [114]. In *Vibrio cholerae*, small molecules inhibited the induction of cyclic di-GMP, which is a second messenger controlling the switch between planktonic and sessile lifestyle of bacteria [115,116]. In addition, N-acetylcysteine, a mucolytic agent, was reported to inhibit the production of exopolysaccharides in biofilms in *S. epidermidis* [36].

Several antimicrobial peptides are also known to interfere with biofilm formation in different bacterial pathogens. For example, peptide 1018 is considered to be a biofilm inhibitor in *P. aeruginosa*, *E. coli*, *A. baumannii*, *K. pneumoniae*, *S. aureus*, *Salmonella typhimurium*, *Burkholderia cenocepacia* [37]. In addition, lantibiotics (nisin, subtilin, epidermin and gallidermin), a class of peptide antibiotics, are reported to inhibit biofilm formation in *S. aureus*, *Lactococcus lactis* and *S. epidermidis* [38,39].

Chelators that interfere with the function of metal ions in biofilm formation are also considered to be biofilm inhibitors [117]. Metallic silver, silver salts, and silver nanoparticles have been widely used as antimicrobial agents in medical implants against bacteria such as *E. coli*, *S. aureus*, *Klebsiella* species, *P. aeruginosa*, *S. typhimurium*, and *Candida albicans* [118,119]. The silver treatment inhibits the replication of DNA, expression of ribosomal and cellular proteins, and respiration process, leading to cell death [40–42]. It has been reported that silver ion-coated implants inhibited *S. aureus* biofilm formation without causing silver accumulation in host tissues [120]. In addition, in the presence of nanoparticles, antibiotics such as penicillin G, amoxicillin, erythromycin, clindamycin, and vancomycin displayed increased antibacterial activity against *S. aureus* [121].

The antibacterial agent coatings on medical devices are typically effective for a short time period due to the leaching of the agent over the course of time [33]. Thus, the immobilization of antimicrobial agents on device surfaces using long, flexible polymeric chains has been an effective contribution in controlling biofilm formation in the long run. For example, the attachment of N-alkylpyridinium bromide, an antibacterial agent, to a polymer, poly(4-vinyl-N-hexylpyridine) was capable of inactivating 99% of *S. epidermidis*, *E. coli*, and *P. aeruginosa* on medical devices [43].

2.1.2. By Changing the Physical Properties of Biomaterials

Biofilm formation begins with a weak reversible adhesion of bacterial cells to the surface of medical devices. If bacteria are not immediately detached from the surface of devices, they anchor permanently, using cell adhesion structures such as pili, and form biofilms [44]. Hydrophobicity and surface charge of implant materials play an important role in determining the ability of bacteria to anchor to surfaces [43]. Thus, modification of the surface charge and hydrophobicity of polymeric materials using several backbone compounds and antimicrobial agents has proven to be effective for biofilm prevention [43]. Hydrophilic polymers such as hyaluronic acid [45] and poly N-vinylpyrrolidone [46] on polyurethane catheters and silicone shuts, respectively, have been known to reduce the adhesion of *S. epidermidis*. In addition, various hydrogel coatings which reduce bacterial adhesion due to their hydrophilic properties have also been developed especially for ureteral stents [47]. Superhydrophobic surfaces are reported to reduce bacterial adhesion and biofilm formation due to their extremely low wettability [49,122,123]. Tang et al. observed reduced adherence of *S. aureus* on superhydrophobic titanium surfaces [124]. Also, the adhesion of *S. aureus* and *P. aeruginosa* was significantly reduced on superhydrophobic fluorinated silica coating [125]. Crick et al.demonstrated reduced adhesion of *S. aureus* and *E. coli* on AACVD (aerosol assisted chemical vapor deposition)-coated superhydrophobic surfaces compared to uncoated plain glass [123]. It has been reported that heparin interferes with bacterial adhesion and colonization [48]. The heparin coating makes the vascular catheter negatively charged, thereby preventing thrombosis and microbial colonization, eventually contributing to reduction of catheter-related infections [126,127]. Surface roughness can also influence biofilm formation, as rough, high-energy surfaces are more conducive to biofilm formation compared to smooth surfaces [128]. It is noted that the surface roughness can alter the hydrophobicity, thus in turn affecting bacterial adherence [128].

2.2. Biofilm Removal

Mature biofilms are highly tolerant to antimicrobials due to the altered growth rate of cells in the biofilm and the emergence of resistant subpopulations [129,130]. Also, biofilms favor the horizontal transfer of antibiotic resistance genes among cells [131]. Thus, it is of utmost importance to understand the antibiotic resistance properties of strains in biofilms when designing new drug treatments. Though conventional antibiotics have been proven to be critical in eliminating bacterial pathogens, they extensively damage the host microbiota, making the environment favorable for opportunistic pathogens. Hence, the agents that interfere with the initial biofilm development or biofilm structure have great potential in controlling biofilm-related infections.

2.2.1. Matrix-Degrading Enzymes

The biofilm matrix is usually composed of exopolysaccharides (EPS), extracellular DNAs (eDNAs), and proteins [132–134]. The EPS and eDNAs contribute to antibiotic resistance by preventing the diffusion of antimicrobials or by inducing antibiotic resistance [135,136]. Dissociation of the biofilm matrix is an effective antibiofilm approach, as the matrix accounts for more than 90% of dry mass, and dissociation of the same will expose the sessile cells to antibiotics and host immune defence [137]. Biofilm matrix-degrading enzymes fall into three categories: polysaccharide-degrading enzymes, nucleases and proteases [50]. Dispersin B is a bacterial glycoside hydrolase produced by *Actinobacillus actinomycetemcomitans* which hydrolyzes poly-*N*-acetylglucosamine (PNAG), a major matrix exopolysaccharide of *Staphylococcus* spp. and *E. coli* [138]. In addition, the application of Dispersin B in combination with triclosan effectively reduced biofilm formation in *S. aureus*, *S. epidermidis*, and *E. coli* [51]. Endolysins, a class of peptidoglycan hydolases produced by bacteriophages are reported to digest the cell wall of bacteria thereby disrupting biofilms [52]. Deoxyribonuclease I which is capable of digesting eDNA is known to disperse biofilms in several bacteria including *Staphylococcus* strains, *A. baumannii*, *E. coli*, *Haemophilus influenzae*, *Klebsiella pneumoniae*, *Psuedomonas aeruginosa*, etc. [53,54]. The matrix proteins can be effectively cleaved by Proteinase K contributing to biofilm prevention and biofilm dispersal [55]. It was demonstrated that the treatment with dispersin B followed by Proteinase K or trypsin successfully eradicated *Staphylococcus* biofilms [55]. The *in vivo* application of matrix-degrading enzymes is limited, as the treatment can elicit inflammatory and allergic reactions in the host against these enzymes [139].

2.2.2. Surfactants

Surfactants are reported to have antimicrobial and antibiofilm activities [140]. The surfactants sodium dodecyl sulfate (SDS), cetyltrimethylammonium bromide (CTAB), Tween 20 and Triton X-100 are known to promote either biofilm dispersal or detachment [56–58]. A biosurfactant, surfactin, which is a cyclic lipopeptide produced by *B. subtilis*, is reported to inhibit biofilm formation and induce biofilm dispersal in *S. typhimurium*, *E. coli* and *P. mirabilis* [59]. Rhamnolipids are principal glycolipids produced by many bacteria, including *P. aeruginosa*, and cause biofilm dispersal in a number bacterial strains [57,60].

2.2.3. Free Fatty Acids, Amino Acids and Nitric Oxide Donors

Free fatty acids are shown to have antibiofilm activity against several pathogenic bacteria. It was reported that *P. aeruginosa* produces an organic compound *cis*-2-decenoic acid which is capable of dispersing the already established biofilms by *E. coli*, *K. pneumoniae*, *P. mirabilis*, *S. pyogenes*, *B. subtilis*, *S. aureus*, and *C. albicans* [61]. The diffusible signal factor, *cis*-11-methyl-2-decanoic acid produced by *Xanthomonas campestris* induces biofilm dispersal by controlling the production of exopolysaccharide-degrading enzyme [141]. However, it has also been reported that fatty acids play an important role in the initial stages of biofilm formation in *B. subtilis*, as the lipids form structural component of extracellular matrix of biofilms [142]. In *S. aureus*, *B. subtilis* and *P. aeruginosa*, a mixture of D-amino acids triggered the disassembly of biofilm by releasing amyloid fibers, which are the proteinaceous component of the extracellular matrix [62,63]. While many L-amino acids promote biofilm formation in *P. aeruginosa*, in the case of tryptophan, both D- and L-isoforms inhibited biofilm formation and caused biofilm dispersal [143,144]. Nitric oxide (NO) generators such as sodium nitroprusside (SNP), S-nitroso-L-glutathione (GSNO) and S-nitroso-N-acetylpenicillamine (SNAP) are reported to induce biofilm dispersal in *P. aeruginosa* [64]. A low dose of NO generators dispersed *P. aeruginosa* biofilms both *in vitro* and in cystic fibrosis sputum, and enhanced the effect of antibiotics on biofilm-dispersed cells [145].

2.3. Biofilm Inhibition by Quorum Quenching

Quorum sensing (QS) is an important cellular communication system in many Gram-negative and Gram-positive bacteria. QS mediates the regulation of various genes according to the density of signaling molecules in the surrounding environment [146]. The signaling molecules of the QS system are denoted as autoinducers [147]. Based on signaling molecules, the QS system is categorized into three; N-acyl homoserine lactones (AHLs)-based (Gram-negative bacteria), autoinducing peptide (AIP)-based (Gram-positive bacteria), and autoinducer-2 (AI-2)-based (both Gram-negative and Gram-positive bacteria) [148,149]. During biofilm formation, following the initial attachment, the cells secrete QS molecules, which modulate bacterial gene expression, transforming planktonic lifestyle into a sessile form [150–152]. Since QS plays a crucial role in biofilm formation [153], it has been suggested that QS inhibition (quorum quenching; QQ) would be an interesting strategy to prevent biofilm formation [154]. In addition, QS regulates the production of virulence factors and pathogenesis factors in most pathogens, and thus the QS system can be considered a potential target for the development of new antimicrobial agents [155,156]. The various quorum-quenching strategies that can be beneficial for controlling biofilm formation are depicted in Figure 1. The major advantage of controlling biofilm by QQ is that this strategy reduces the risk of multidrug resistance, making the strategy of great clinical interest for use in the prevention of biofilm-based infections.

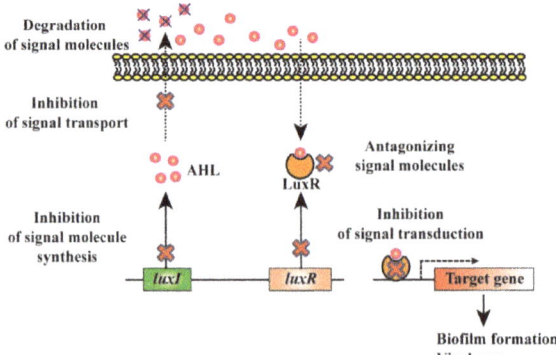

Figure 1. Schematic representation of various quorum-quenching strategies to control biofilm formation. *LuxI* and *luxR* genes encode AHL signal synthase and AHL receptor/activator protein respectively. AHL signal synthase is responsible for the production of AHLs, which are diffused (short chain) or pumped (long chain) out of the bacterial cell to the surrounding medium before being taken up into the nearby bacterial cells. The AHL binds to the receptor protein and the AHL-receptor complex activates the expression of quorum-sensing target genes. The quorum-quenching strategies that have been used for attenuating AHL-mediated phenotypes include the inhibition of AHL synthesis, inhibition of signal transport, degradation of signal molecules, inhibition of AHL receptor synthesis, inhibition of AHL-receptor complex formation, inhibition of the binding of AHL-receptor complex to the promoters of target genes etc.

2.3.1. Degradation of QS Signals

AHLs can be degraded by specific enzymes such as lactonases that hydrolyze the lactone ring in the homoserine moiety and acylases that cleave off the acyl side chain, and the activity can be altered by reductases and oxidases [157]. Most of the AHL-degrading enzymes were discovered in bacterial species [158], though some are found in eukaryotes [159,160]. It has been reported that the application of QQ enzymes inhibits biofilm formation in several bacterial strains [65–70]. Quorum-quenching enzymes disrupt the biofilm architecture, which increases the antibiotic susceptibility of the cells [71]. Significant reduction of biofilm formation and increased sensitivity to antibiotics was noticed in *P. aeruginosa* after treatment with lactonase [71]. The oxidoreductases reduced the signaling molecules AHL and AI-2 to QS-inactive hydroxy-derivatives in *K. oxytoca* and *K. pneumoniae* [70].

2.3.2. Inhibition of Signal Synthesis

Several reports have shown that mutations affecting AHL synthesis have an adverse effect on biofilm formation. For example, *P. aeruginosa* strain that lacked the production of 3-oxo-C12-HSL resulted in impaired biofilm formation [161]. The mutation in the gene encoding for AHL synthesis enzyme in *B. cenocepacia* K56-2, *B. cenocepacia* J2315, *Aeromonas hydrophila* and *Serratia liquefaciens* led to defective biofilm formation [162–165]. In addition, the mutants of several *Vibrio* spp., *Streptococcus* spp. and *Staphylococcus* spp. that are deficient in AI-2 synthesis were not able to produce biofilms properly. Thus, blocking signal production has been considered as a promising strategy to control biofilm formation. Analogues of AHL precursor molecule, S-adenosyl-methionine (SAM), such as S-adenosyl-homocysteine (SAH), sinefugin, 5-methylthioadenosine (MTA), and butyryl-SAM, are known to inhibit biofilm formation in *P. aeruginosa* [72]. Also, the SAM biosynthesis inhibitor cycloleucine is reported to inhibit AHL production [73]. The antibiotic azithromycin interferes with signal synthesis in *P. aeruginosa*, and thus significantly clears biofilm in mouse model of cystic fibrosis [74,75]. In addition, several inhibitors for the key enzymes (5′-methylthioadenosine/S-adenosylhomo-cysteine nucleosidase (MTAN) and S-ribosylhomocysteinase (LuxS) involved in AI-2 synthesis are shown to reduce biofilm formation [76,77]. In *B. multivorans*, nickel (Ni^{2+}) and cadmium (Cd^{2+}) inhibited the expression of genes responsible for AHL production thereby inhibiting cell-cell signaling and subsequently biofilm formation [79]. The inhibitory effect of Cd^{2+} in quorum sensing was also reported in *Chromobacterium violaceum* [78].

2.3.3. Antagonizing the Signal Molecules

Researchers have screened for many signal analogues that antagonize QS signaling, thereby preventing biofilm formation [166–168]. AHL analogues in which the lactone ring was replaced by a cyclopentyl or a cyclohexanone ring adversely affected biofilm formation in *Serratia marcescens* and *P. aeruginosa* [169,170]. Many natural compounds are also reported to antagonize AHL-based QS signaling, and those include bergamottin and dihydroxybergamottin from grapefruit juice, cyclic sulfur compounds from garlic, patulin, and penicillic acid from a variety of fungi, etc. [80–82]. Treatment with patulin, ajoene and garlic extracts resulted in increased antibiotic susceptibility of *P. aeruginosa* biofilms and increased clearance of *P. aeruginosa* in *in vivo* pulmonary infection model [83–85]. In addition, some phenolic compounds including baicalin hydrate and epigallocatechin blocked AHL QS and affected biofilm formation of *B. cenocepacia*, *B. multivorans* and *P. aeruginosa* [86–88]. It was noted that the antibiotic susceptibility of *B. cenocepacia* and *P. aeruginosa* increased after treatment with baicalin hydrate in different *in vitro* biofilm models [86–88]. Thus, the concept of combining QS inhibitor (QSI) and antibiotics would be a better strategy to control biofilm formation by pathogenic bacteria. In addition, it has been noticed that biofilm formation can be effectively controlled by combining QSIs and QQ enzymes. Recently, Fong et al. reported the synergistic effect of a QS inhibitor, G1, which competes with AHL to bind to the response regulator and QQ enzyme, AHL lactonase, to effectively control biofilm formation and virulence by *P. aeruginosa* [171].

Several compounds that antagonize AI-2 signaling have also been reported to exhibit antibiofilm activity. The AI-2 analogues ursolic acid, isobutyl-4,5-dihydroxy-2,3-pentanedione (isobutyl-DPD) and phenyl-DPD inhibited biofilm formation and removed preformed biofilms in *E. coli* and *P. aeruginosa* [89,90]. Although other compounds, including pyrogallol and its derivatives, some nucleoside analogues, boronic acids, and sulfones have been identified to antagonize AI-2 signaling, only a few have been investigated for their antibiofilm activity [172,173].

Several AIP analogues, such as truncated forms of AIP, and probiotic bacteria-producing natural cyclic dipeptides, such as cyclo(l-Phe-l-Pro) and cyclo(l-Tyr-l-Pro), have been developed to antagonize QS signaling in Gram-positive bacteria. However, the experimental evidence on the anti-biofilm activities of these compounds is highly limited [91–93]. The most investigated QS inhibiting peptide is the RNAIII inhibiting peptide (RIP), which is produced by coagulase-negative *Staphylococci*. RIP interferes with the QS response by inhibiting the production of RNAIII, a key component of QS response in *S. aureus* [94]. RIP and several RIP homologues have been reported to have anti-QS and anti-biofilm activity against *Staphylococcus* spp. A RIP analogue, FS3, prevented *S. aureus* biofilm formation in a rat vascular graft model [95]. In addition, a non-peptide RIP analogue, hamamelitannin, blocked QS in *Staphylococcus* spp., and potentially inhibited biofilm formation in *in vitro* and *in vivo* rat model of graft infection [96]. Several natural compounds, including phytol, anthocyanidins, extracts from *Ricinus communis*, freshwater bryozoan *Hyalinella punctata* and selected sponges, and ricinine derivatives, are also known to exhibit anti-biofilm or anti-microbial and anti-quorum sensing activities in *P. aeruginosa* [174–178]. However, the exact mechanisms by which these compounds display anti-quorum sensing activities are not known.

2.3.4. Inhibition of Signal Transduction by Interfering with Response Regulator Activity

The QS system can also be hindered at the level of signal transduction cascade. The natural compounds, halogenated furanone or fimbrolide and cinnamaldehyde which are isolated from red algae *Delisea pulchra* and cinnamon bark, respectively, interfere with signal transduction and affect biofilm formation, thereby increasing antibiotic susceptibility in several pathogenic bacteria [97–100]. Both compounds block AI-2 and AHL-type QS systems, and thereby affect biofilm formation in *V. harveyi* [101,102]. The halogenated furanone and cinnamaldehyde inhibits AI-2 QS and AHL QS by decreasing the DNA-binding ability of the response regulator LuxR, which is important for the signal transduction cascade, or by displacing AHL from its receptor, respectively [101,102,179,180]. In addition, the natural furanone inactivates LuxS and accelerates LuxR turnover, thereby blocking AI-2 and AHL QS signaling system, respectively [181,182]. Cinnamaldehyde is widely used as a flavoring agent in food and beverages, while the application of furanones is limited because of their toxicity [100,183]. We reported previously that virstatin, a small organic molecule, prevents biofilm formation by interfering with the QS system in *A. nosocomialis* [103]. It was noticed that virstatin inhibits the expression of the response regulator, AnoR, which is a positive regulator of the AHL synthase gene, *anoI* in *A. nosocomialis* [103]. The repression of AnoR leads to decreased synthesis of AHL (Figure 2), adversely affecting the signal transduction cascade. Virstatin or its derivatives can be considered potential agents to inhibit the QS system and to control biofilm-based infections, and further studies in this direction could lead to the development of better antibacterial therapeutics.

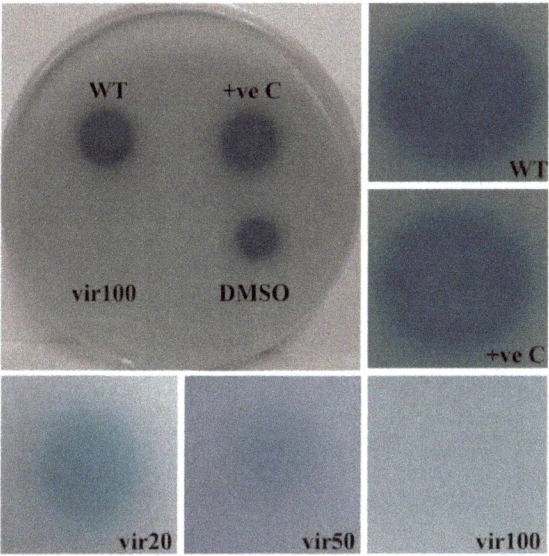

Figure 2. Effect of virstatin on the production of AHL. Bioassay was carried out to check the effect of virstatin on the production of AHLs in *A. nosocomialis*. For this, the strain was cultivated overnight in Luria Bertani (LB) medium at 30 °C, and the cells were washed with LB and diluted to an OD_{600} of 1. The cells were treated with different concentrations of virstatin (20, 50, 100 mM), which was dissolved in dimethyl sulfoxide (DMSO), and 5 µL of the samples were spotted onto chromoplate overlaid with *A. tumefaciens* NT1 (pDCI41E33) [184,185]. Synthetic *N*-(3-hydroxy-dodecanoyl)-L-homoserine lactone (OH-dDHL) was spotted as a positive control. The plates were incubated at 30 °C for 22 h, followed by the detection of the color zone surrounding the bacteria. A representative chromoplate image with 100 mM virstatin and images of color zones from different concentrations of virstatin are shown. WT, *A. nosocomialis* wild type; +ve C, OH-dDHL; vir20, vir50 and vir100; wild-type cells treated with 20, 50 and 100 mM virstatin respectively.

2.3.5. Inhibition of Signal Transport

The signaling molecules need to be exported and released into the extracellular space to be sensed by other bacteria for effective cell-to-cell communication. The role of multidrug-resistant (MDR) efflux pumps in signal traffic was first reported in *P. aeruginosa*, in which AHLs with long side chains are actively transported across the cell membrane through the MexAB-OprM efflux pump [186]. In *P. aeruginosa*, the expression of the autoinducer-producing gene and the genes encoding the virulence factors is limited by the intracellular concentration of the autoinducer [187]. The involvement of the MDR efflux pump in the QS system has also been reported in *E. coli*, in which the overexpression of the QS regulator SdiA led to the increased expression of the AcrAB efflux pump [188]. In *Bacteroides fragilis*, an opportunistic pathogen of the gastrointestinal tract, the BmeB efflux pump controls the intracellular AHL concentration by effluxing AHL outside of cells [189]. In addition, the expression of the MDR efflux pump, BpeAB-OprB, was reported to be essential for the export of six AHL inducers to the extracellular environment in *B. pseudomallei* [190,191]. Thus, the inhibition of the efflux pump would be a promising strategy to alter QS signaling cascade, thereby preventing biofilm formation and virulence.

Several studies have provided evidence to show the link between the physiological function of efflux pump and biofilm formation. In *E. coli* and *Klebsiella* strains, the inhibition of the efflux pump activity using efflux pump inhibitors (EPIs) reduced biofilm formation [192]. The genetic inactivation or the chemical inhibition of efflux pump activity resulted in impaired biofilm formation in *S. enterica* serovar *typhimurium* [193]. The effect of efflux pump inhibitors to prevent biofilm formation was also demonstrated in *P. aeruginosa* and *S. aureus* [105], in which copper nanoparticles work well as EPI and anti-biofilm agents [104]. In addition, in *P. aeruginosa*, the MDR efflux pump, MexAM-OPrM was disrupted by silver nanoparticles [194]. Recently, it was observed that the well-characterized EPI, Phe-Arg-β-naphthylamide (PAβN) alter the expression of QS molecules and QS-dependent virulence phenotypes in *P. aeruginosa* PAO1, as well as in clinical isolates [106]. The application of EPIs not only helps to reduce the biofilm-forming capacity of bacteria, but also to revive the bactericidal effect of conventional antibiotics [195].

It has been reported previously that AHLs with long side chains are exported out through the MexAB-OprM pump in *P. aeruginosa* [186], and the expression of the pump is modulated by the intracellular concentration of autoinducer molecules [196]. In addition, we have identified previously that *A. nosocomialis* produces AHL with long side chain, N-(3-hydroxy-dodecanoyl)-L-homoserine lactone (3OH-C12-AHL) as signaling molecules [103], and these AHLs might be actively transported through the efflux pumps. Thus, it can be postulated that the QS system controls the activity of the efflux system, contributing to the effective transport of AHLs across the cell membrane, in turn contributing to virulence and biofilm formation. Further studies in this direction would unravel in depth the role of the QS system in controlling the activity of these efflux pumps. The MDR efflux pumps and the regulators modulating them would be potential targets for the development of better therapeutics for biofilm-based infections.

3. Conclusions

In this review, we discuss the current strategies and future perspectives for developing improved therapeutics for controlling biofilm-based infections. The various approaches for modulating biofilm formation on medical devices are addressed in detail, with special emphasis on quorum-quenching strategies. Significant advances have been made in understanding the role of quorum sensing in biofilm formation in the past few years. In addition, several studies have shown that multidrug efflux pumps play a potential role in controlling biofilm formation. However, the fundamental mechanisms by which the QS systems exert the regulatory functions on biofilm formation are poorly understood. In this review, we postulate that QS systems regulate the activity of multidrug efflux pumps in transporting QS molecules across the cell membrane, thereby affecting biofilm formation. We propose that the transcriptional factors modulating the QS system and/or efflux pumps would be potential targets for developing QSIs. It is of utmost importance to improve our understanding of the molecular mechanism by which QS systems regulate biofilm formation and multidrug efflux pumps, as it will eventually be of help in developing better therapeutics for the treatment of problematic biofilm-related infections. Furthermore, detailed research is needed to understand the effect of these QSIs on different stages of biofilm formation and to validate their applicability on humans. Since QSIs do not induce any antibiotic resistance, they can be of great potential in the future for the treatment of biofilm-based infections in healthcare settings.

Funding: This research was funded by the research fund of Chungnam National University (2017). Also, this research was supported by the Basic Science Research Program through the National Research Foundation of Korea (NRF) funded by the Ministry of Education (NRF-2014R1A61029617).

Conflicts of Interest: The authors declare no conflict of interest.

References

1. Costerton, J.W.; Irvin, R.T.; Cheng, K.J. The bacterial glycocalyx in nature and disease. *Annu. Rev. Microbiol.* **1981**, *35*, 299–324. [CrossRef] [PubMed]
2. Kunin, C.M.; Steele, C. Culture of the surfaces of urinary catheters to sample urethral flora and study the effect of antimicrobial therapy. *J. Clin. Microbiol.* **1985**, *21*, 902–908. [PubMed]

3. Nickel, J.C.; Ruseska, I.; Wright, J.B.; Costerton, J.W. Tobramycin resistance of Pseudomonas aeruginosa cells growing as a biofilm on urinary catheter material. *Antimicrob. Agents Chemother.* **1985**, *27*, 619–624. [CrossRef] [PubMed]
4. Donlan, R.M. Biofilms: Microbial life on surfaces. *Emerg. Infect. Dis.* **2002**, *8*, 881–890. [CrossRef] [PubMed]
5. Donlan, R.M. Biofilms and device-associated infections. *Emerg. Infect. Dis.* **2001**, *7*, 277–281. [CrossRef] [PubMed]
6. Haddadin, Y.; Regunath, H. *Central Line Associated Blood Stream Infections (CLABSI)*; StatPearls Publishing: Treasure Island, FL, USA, 2017.
7. Tien, H.C.; Battad, A.; Bryce, E.A.; Fuller, J.; Mulvey, M.; Bernard, K.; Brisebois, R.; Doucet, J.J.; Rizoli, S.B.; Fowler, R.; et al. Multi-drug resistant *Acinetobacter* infections in critically injured Canadian forces soldiers. *BMC Infect. Dis.* **2007**, *7*, 95. [CrossRef] [PubMed]
8. Otto, M. Staphylococcal biofilms. In *Bacterial Biofilms*; Romeo, T., Ed.; Current Topics in Microbiology and Immunology book series; Springer: Berlin, Germany, 2008; Volume 322, pp. 207–228.
9. Otto, M. *Staphylococcus epidermidis*—The 'accidental' pathogen. *Nat. Rev. Microbiol.* **2009**, *7*, 555–567. [CrossRef] [PubMed]
10. Agarwal, A.; Singh, K.P.; Jain, A. Medical significance and management of staphylococcal biofilm. *FEMS Immunol. Med. Microbiol.* **2010**, *58*, 147–160. [CrossRef] [PubMed]
11. Pour, N.K.; Dusane, D.H.; Dhakephalkar, P.K.; Zamin, F.R.; Zinjarde, S.S.; Chopade, B.A. Biofilm formation by *Acinetobacter baumannii* strains isolated from urinary tract infection and urinary catheters. *FEMS Immunol. Med. Microbiol.* **2011**, *62*, 328–338. [CrossRef] [PubMed]
12. Dijkshoorn, L.; Nemec, A.; Seifert, H. An increasing threat in hospitals: Multidrug-resistant *Acinetobacter baumannii*. *Nat. Rev. Microbiol.* **2007**, *5*, 939–951. [CrossRef] [PubMed]
13. Patwardhan, R.B.; Dhakephalkar, P.K.; Niphadkar, K.B.; Chopade, B.A. A study on nosocomial pathogens in ICU with special reference to multiresistant *Acinetobacter baumannii* harbouring multiple plasmids. *Indian J. Med. Res.* **2008**, *128*, 178–187. [PubMed]
14. Bergogne-Bérézin, E.; Towner, É.K.J. *Acinetobacter* spp. as nosocomial pathogens: Microbiological, clinical and epidemiological features. *Clin. Microiol. Rev.* **1996**, *9*, 148–165.
15. Litzler, P.Y.; Benard, L.; Barbier-Frebourg, N.; Vilain, S.; Jouenne, T.; Beucher, E.; Bunel, C.; Lemeland, J.F.; Bessou, J.P. Biofilm formation on pyrolytic carbon heart valves: Influence of surface free energy, roughness, and bacterial species. *J. Thorac. Cardiovasc. Surg.* **2007**, *134*, 1025–1032. [CrossRef] [PubMed]
16. Percival, S.L.; Suleman, L.; Vuotto, C.; Donelli, G. Healthcare-associated infections, medical devices and biofilms: Risk, tolerance and control. *J. Med. Microbiol.* **2015**, *64*, 323–334. [CrossRef] [PubMed]
17. Von Eiff, C.; Heilmann, C.; Peters, G. New aspects in the molecular basis of polymer-associated infections due to *Staphylococci*. *Eur. J. Clin. Microbiol. Infect. Dis.* **1999**, *18*, 843–846. [CrossRef] [PubMed]
18. Muller, E.; Hübner, J.; Gutierrez, N.; Takeda, S.; Goldmann, D.A.; Pier, G.B. Isolation and characterization of transposon mutants of *Staphylococcus epidermidis* deficient in capsular polysaccharide/adhesin and slime. *Infect. Immun.* **1993**, *61*, 551–558. [PubMed]
19. Veenstra, G.J.; Cremers, F.F.; van Dijk, H.; Fleer, A. Ultrastructural organization and regulation of a biomaterial adhesin of *Staphylococcus epidermidis*. *J. Bacteriol.* **1996**, *178*, 537–541. [CrossRef] [PubMed]
20. Götz, F. *Staphylococcus* and biofilms. *Mol. Microbiol.* **2002**, *43*, 1367–1378. [CrossRef] [PubMed]
21. Stoodley, P.; Sauer, K.; Davies, D.G.; Costerton, J.W. Biofilms as complex differentiated communities. *Annu. Rev. Microbiol.* **2002**, *56*, 187–209. [CrossRef] [PubMed]
22. Fey, P.D.; Olson, M.E. Current concepts in biofilm formation of *Staphylococcus epidermidis*. *Future Microbiol.* **2010**, *5*, 917–933. [CrossRef] [PubMed]
23. Lawrence, J.R.; Korber, D.R.; Wolfaardt, G.M. Heterogeneity of natural biofilm communities. *Cells Mater.* **1996**, *6*, 175–191.
24. Aslam, S. Effect of antibacterials on biofilms. *Am. J. Infect. Control* **2008**, *36*, S175.e9–S175.e11. [CrossRef] [PubMed]
25. Francolini, I.; Donelli, G. Prevention and control of biofilm-based medical-device-related infections. *FEMS Immunol. Med. Microbiol.* **2010**, *59*, 227–238. [CrossRef] [PubMed]
26. Stewart, P.S.; Davison, W.M.; Steenbergen, J.N. Daptomycin rapidly penetrates a *Staphylococcus epidermidis* biofilm. *Antimicrob. Agents Chemother.* **2009**, *53*, 3505–3507. [CrossRef] [PubMed]

27. Borriello, G.; Werner, E.; Roe, F.; Kim, A.M.; Ehrlich, G.D.; Stewart, P.S. Oxygen limitation contributes to antibiotic tolerance of *Pseudomonas aeruginosa* in biofilms. *Antimicrob. Agents Chemother.* **2004**, *48*, 2659–2664. [CrossRef] [PubMed]
28. Lewis, K. Persister cells, dormancy and infectious disease. *Nat. Rev. Microbiol.* **2007**, *5*, 48–56. [CrossRef] [PubMed]
29. Martínez, J.L.; Baquero, F. Interactions among strategies associated with bacterial infection: Pathogenicity, epidemicity, and antibiotic resistance. *Clin. Microbiol. Rev.* **2002**, *15*, 647–679. [CrossRef] [PubMed]
30. Diekema, D.J.; Pfaller, M.A.; Schmitz, F.J.; Smayevsky, J.; Bell, J.; Jones, R.N.; Beach, M.; Group, S.P. Survey of infections due to *Staphylococcus* species: Frequency of occurrence and antimicrobial susceptibility of isolates collected in the United States, Canada, Latin America, Europe, and the Western Pacific region for the SENTRY antimicrobial surveillance program, 1997–1999. *Clin. Infect. Dis.* **2001**, *32*, S114–S132. [CrossRef] [PubMed]
31. Kalia, V.C.; Purohit, H.J. Quenching the quorum sensing system: Potential antibacterial drug targets. *Crit. Rev. Microbiol.* **2011**, *37*, 121–140. [CrossRef] [PubMed]
32. Wright, J.S., III; Lyon, G.J.; George, E.A.; Muir, T.W.; Novick, R.P. Hydrophobic interactions drive ligand-receptor recognition for activation and inhibition of staphylococcal quorum sensing. *Proc. Natl. Acad. Sci. USA* **2004**, *101*, 16168–16173. [CrossRef] [PubMed]
33. Dror, N.; Mandel, M.; Hazan, Z.; Lavie, G. Advances in microbial biofilm prevention on indwelling medical devices with emphasis on usage of acoustic energy. *Sensors* **2009**, *9*, 2538–2554. [CrossRef] [PubMed]
34. Ramos, E.R.; Reitzel, R.; Jiang, Y.; Hachem, R.Y.; Chaftari, A.M.; Chemaly, R.F.; Hackett, B.; Pravinkumar, S.E.; Nates, J.; Tarrand, J.J.; et al. Clinical effectiveness and risk of emerging resistance associated with prolonged use of antibiotic-impregnated catheters: More than 0.5 million catheter days and 7 years of clinical experience. *Crit. Care Med.* **2011**, *39*, 245–251. [CrossRef] [PubMed]
35. Schumm, K.; Lam, T.B. Types of urethral catheters for management of short-term voiding problems in hospitalised adults. *Cochrane Database Syst. Rev.* **2008**, CD004013. [CrossRef]
36. Pérez-Giraldo, C.; Rodríguez-Benito, A.; Morán, F.J.; Hurtado, C.; Blanco, M.T.; Gómez-García, A.C. Influence of N-acetylcysteine on the formation of biofilm by *Staphylococcus epidermidis*. *J. Antimicrob. Chemother.* **1997**, *39*, 643–646. [CrossRef] [PubMed]
37. De la Fuente-Núñez, C.; Reffuveille, F.; Haney, E.F.; Straus, S.K.; Hancock, R.E. Broad-spectrum anti-biofilm peptide that targets a cellular stress response. *PLoS Pathog.* **2014**, *10*, e1004152. [CrossRef] [PubMed]
38. Parisot, J.; Carey, S.; Breukink, E.; Chan, W.C.; Narbad, A.; Bonev, B. Molecular mechanism of target recognition by subtilin, a class I lanthionine antibiotic. *Antimicrob. Agents Chemother.* **2008**, *52*, 612–618. [CrossRef] [PubMed]
39. Saising, J.; Dube, L.; Ziebandt, A.K.; Voravuthikunchai, S.P.; Nega, M.; Götz, F. Activity of gallidermin on *Staphylococcus aureus* and *Staphylococcus epidermidis* biofilms. *Antimicrob. Agents Chemother.* **2012**, *56*, 5804–5810. [CrossRef] [PubMed]
40. Feng, Q.L.; Wu, J.; Chen, G.Q.; Cui, F.Z.; Kim, T.N.; Kim, J.O. A mechanistic study of the antibacterial effect of silver ions on *Escherichia coli* and *Staphylococcus aureus*. *J. Biomed. Mater. Res.* **2000**, *52*, 662–668. [CrossRef]
41. Yamanaka, M.; Hara, K.; Kudo, J. Bactericidal actions of a silver ion solution on *Escherichia coli*, studied by energy-filtering transmission electron microscopy and proteomic analysis. *Appl. Environ. Microbiol.* **2005**, *71*, 7589–7593. [CrossRef] [PubMed]
42. Klasen, H.J. A historical review of the use of silver in the treatment of burns. II. Renewed interest for silver. *Burns* **2000**, *26*, 131–138. [CrossRef]
43. Jansen, B.; Kohnen, W. Prevention of biofilm formation by polymer modification. *J. Ind. Microbiol.* **1995**, *15*, 391–396. [CrossRef] [PubMed]
44. Marlow, V.L.; Porter, M.; Hobley, L.; Kiley, T.B.; Swedlow, J.R.; Davidson, F.A.; Stanley-Wall, N.R. Phosphorylated DegU manipulates cell fate differentiation in the *Bacillus subtilis* biofilm. *J. Bacteriol.* **2014**, *196*, 16–27. [CrossRef] [PubMed]
45. Cassinelli, C.; Morra, M.; Pavesio, A.; Renier, D. Evaluation of interfacial properties of hyaluronan coated poly(methylmethacrylate) intraocular lenses. *J. Biomater. Sci. Polym. Ed.* **2000**, *11*, 961–977. [CrossRef] [PubMed]
46. Boelens, J.J.; Tan, W.F.; Dankert, J.; Zaat, S.A. Antibacterial activity of antibiotic-soaked polyvinylpyrrolidone-grafted silicon elastomer hydrocephalus shunts. *J. Antimicrob. Chemother.* **2000**, *45*, 221–224. [CrossRef] [PubMed]
47. John, T.; Rajpurkar, A.; Smith, G.; Fairfax, M.; Triest, J. Antibiotic pretreatment of hydrogel ureteral stent. *J. Endourol.* **2007**, *21*, 1211–1216. [CrossRef] [PubMed]

48. Appelgren, P.; Ransjö, U.; Bindslev, L.; Espersen, F.; Larm, O. Surface heparinization of central venous catheters reduces microbial colonization in vitro and in vivo: Results from a prospective, randomized trial. *Crit. Care Med.* **1996**, *24*, 1482–1489. [CrossRef] [PubMed]
49. Falde, E.J.; Yohe, S.T.; Colson, Y.L.; Grinstaff, M.W. Superhydrophobic materials for biomedical applications. *Biomaterials* **2016**, *104*, 87–103. [CrossRef] [PubMed]
50. Li, X.H.; Lee, J.H. Antibiofilm agents: A new perspective for antimicrobial strategy. *J. Microbiol.* **2017**, *55*, 753–766. [CrossRef] [PubMed]
51. Darouiche, R.O.; Mansouri, M.D.; Gawande, P.V.; Madhyastha, S. Antimicrobial and antibiofilm efficacy of triclosan and dispersinb combination. *J. Antimicrob. Chemother.* **2009**, *64*, 88–93. [CrossRef] [PubMed]
52. Shen, Y.; Köller, T.; Kreikemeyer, B.; Nelson, D.C. Rapid degradation of *Streptococcus pyogenes* biofilms by PlyC, a bacteriophage-encoded endolysin. *J. Antimicrob. Chemother.* **2013**, *68*, 1818–1824. [CrossRef] [PubMed]
53. Kaplan, J.B.; LoVetri, K.; Cardona, S.T.; Madhyastha, S.; Sadovskaya, I.; Jabbouri, S.; Izano, E.A. Recombinant human DNase I decreases biofilm and increases antimicrobial susceptibility in *Staphylococci*. *J. Antibiot.* **2012**, *65*, 73–77. [CrossRef] [PubMed]
54. Tetz, G.V.; Artemenko, N.K.; Tetz, V.V. Effect of DNase and antibiotics on biofilm characteristics. *Antimicrob. Agents Chemother.* **2009**, *53*, 1204–1209. [CrossRef] [PubMed]
55. Chaignon, P.; Sadovskaya, I.; Ragunah, C.; Ramasubbu, N.; Kaplan, J.B.; Jabbouri, S. Susceptibility of staphylococcal biofilms to enzymatic treatments depends on their chemical composition. *Appl. Microbiol. Biotechnol.* **2007**, *75*, 125–132. [CrossRef] [PubMed]
56. Simões, M.; Pereira, M.O.; Vieira, M.J. Action of a cationic surfactant on the activity and removal of bacterial biofilms formed under different flow regimes. *Water Res.* **2005**, *39*, 478–486. [CrossRef] [PubMed]
57. Boles, B.R.; Thoendel, M.; Singh, P.K. Rhamnolipids mediate detachment of *Pseudomonas aeruginosa* from biofilms. *Mol. Microbiol.* **2005**, *57*, 1210–1223. [CrossRef] [PubMed]
58. Chen, X.; Stewart, P.S. Biofilm removal caused by chemical treatments. *Water Res.* **2000**, *34*, 4229–4233. [CrossRef]
59. Mireles, J.R., 2nd; Toguchi, A.; Harshey, R.M. *Salmonella enterica* serovar typhimurium swarming mutants with altered biofilm-forming abilities: Surfactin inhibits biofilm formation. *J. Bacteriol.* **2001**, *183*, 5848–5854. [CrossRef] [PubMed]
60. Abdel-Mawgoud, A.M.; Lépine, F.; Déziel, E. Rhamnolipids: Diversity of structures, microbial origins and roles. *Appl. Microbiol. Biotechnol.* **2010**, *86*, 1323–1336. [CrossRef] [PubMed]
61. Davies, D.G.; Marques, C.N. A fatty acid messenger is responsible for inducing dispersion in microbial biofilms. *J. Bacteriol.* **2009**, *191*, 1393–1403. [CrossRef] [PubMed]
62. Kolodkin-Gal, I.; Romero, D.; Cao, S.; Clardy, J.; Kolter, R.; Losick, R. D-amino acids trigger biofilm disassembly. *Science* **2010**, *328*, 627–629. [CrossRef] [PubMed]
63. Jermy, A. Biofilms: Disassembly instructions included. *Nat. Rev. Microbiol.* **2012**, *10*, 376. [CrossRef]
64. Barraud, N.; Schleheck, D.; Klebensberger, J.; Webb, J.S.; Hassett, D.J.; Rice, S.A.; Kjelleberg, S. Nitric oxide signaling in *Pseudomonas aeruginosa* biofilms mediates phosphodiesterase activity, decreased cyclic di-GMP levels, and enhanced dispersal. *J. Bacteriol.* **2009**, *191*, 7333–7342. [CrossRef] [PubMed]
65. dos Reis Ponce, A.; Martins, M.L.; de Araujo, E.F.; Mantovani, H.C.; Vanetti, M.C. AiiA quorum-sensing quenching controls proteolytic activity and biofilm formation by *Enterobacter cloacae*. *Curr. Microbiol.* **2012**, *65*, 758–763. [CrossRef] [PubMed]
66. Ivanova, K.; Fernandes, M.M.; Francesko, A.; Mendoza, E.; Guezguez, J.; Burnet, M.; Tzanov, T. Quorum-quenching and matrix-degrading enzymes in multilayer coatings synergistically prevent bacterial biofilm formation on urinary catheters. *ACS Appl. Mater. Interfaces* **2015**, *7*, 27066–27077. [CrossRef] [PubMed]
67. Jo, S.J.; Kwon, H.; Jeong, S.Y.; Lee, S.H.; Oh, H.S.; Yi, T.; Lee, C.H.; Kim, T.G. Effects of quorum quenching on the microbial community of biofilm in an anoxic/oxic mbr for wastewater treatment. *J. Microbiol. Biotechnol.* **2016**, *26*, 1593–1604. [CrossRef] [PubMed]
68. Lee, J.; Lee, I.; Nam, J.; Hwang, D.S.; Yeon, K.M.; Kim, J. Immobilization and stabilization of acylase on carboxylated polyaniline nanofibers for highly effective antifouling application via quorum quenching. *ACS Appl. Mater. Interfaces* **2017**, *9*, 15424–15432. [CrossRef] [PubMed]
69. Vinoj, G.; Vaseeharan, B.; Thomas, S.; Spiers, A.J.; Shanthi, S. Quorum-quenching activity of the AHL-lactonase from *Bacillus licheniformis* DAHB$_1$ inhibits vibrio biofilm formation in vitro and reduces shrimp intestinal colonisation and mortality. *Mar. Biotechnol.* **2014**, *16*, 707–715. [CrossRef] [PubMed]

70. Weiland-Bräuer, N.; Kisch, M.J.; Pinnow, N.; Liese, A.; Schmitz, R.A. Highly effective inhibition of biofilm formation by the first metagenome-derived AI-2 quenching enzyme. *Front. Microbiol.* **2016**, *7*, 1098. [CrossRef] [PubMed]
71. Kiran, S.; Sharma, P.; Harjai, K.; Capalash, N. Enzymatic quorum quenching increases antibiotic susceptibility of multidrug resistant *Pseudomonas aeruginosa*. *Iran. J. Microbiol.* **2011**, *3*, 1–12. [PubMed]
72. Parsek, M.R.; Val, D.L.; Hanzelka, B.L.; Cronan, J.E., Jr.; Greenberg, E.P. Acyl homoserine-lactone quorum-sensing signal generation. *Proc. Natl. Acad. Sci. USA* **1999**, *96*, 4360–4365. [CrossRef] [PubMed]
73. Hanzelka, B.L.; Greenberg, E.P. Quorum sensing in *Vibrio fischeri*: Evidence that S-adenosylmethionine is the amino acid substrate for autoinducer synthesis. *J. Bacteriol.* **1996**, *178*, 5291–5294. [CrossRef] [PubMed]
74. Favre-Bonté, S.; Köhler, T.; Van Delden, C. Biofilm formation by *Pseudomonas aeruginosa*: Role of the C_4-HSL cell-to-cell signal and inhibition by azithromycin. *J. Antimicrob. Chemother.* **2003**, *52*, 598–604. [CrossRef] [PubMed]
75. Hoffmann, N.; Lee, B.; Hentzer, M.; Rasmussen, T.B.; Song, Z.; Johansen, H.K.; Givskov, M.; Høiby, N. Azithromycin blocks quorum sensing and alginate polymer formation and increases the sensitivity to serum and stationary-growth-phase killing of *Pseudomonas aeruginosa* and attenuates chronic *P. aeruginosa* lung infection in $Cftr^{-/-}$ mice. *Antimicrob. Agents Chemother.* **2007**, *51*, 3677–3687. [CrossRef] [PubMed]
76. Shen, G.; Rajan, R.; Zhu, J.; Bell, C.E.; Pei, D. Design and synthesis of substrate and intermediate analogue inhibitors of S-ribosylhomocysteinase. *J. Med. Chem.* **2006**, *49*, 3003–3011. [CrossRef] [PubMed]
77. Gutierrez, J.A.; Crowder, T.; Rinaldo-Matthis, A.; Ho, M.C.; Almo, S.C.; Schramm, V.L. Transition state analogs of 5′-methylthioadenosine nucleosidase disrupt quorum sensing. *Nat. Chem. Biol.* **2009**, *5*, 251–257. [CrossRef] [PubMed]
78. Thornhill, S.G.; Kumar, M.; Vega, L.M.; McLean, R.J.C. Cadmium ion inhibition of quorum signalling in *Chromobacterium violaceum*. *Microbiology* **2017**, *163*, 1429–1435. [CrossRef] [PubMed]
79. Vega, L.M.; Mathieu, J.; Yang, Y.; Pyle, B.H.; McLean, R.J.C.; Alvarez, P.J.J. Nickel and cadmium ions inhibit quorum sensing and biofilm formation without affecting viability in *Burkholderia multivorans*. *Int. Biodeterior. Biodegrad.* **2014**, *91*, 82–87. [CrossRef]
80. Kim, C.; Kim, J.; Park, H.Y.; Park, H.J.; Lee, J.H.; Kim, C.K.; Yoon, J. Furanone derivatives as quorum-sensing antagonists of *Pseudomonas aeruginosa*. *Appl. Microbiol. Biotechnol.* **2008**, *80*, 37–47. [CrossRef] [PubMed]
81. Rasmussen, T.B.; Skindersoe, M.E.; Bjarnsholt, T.; Phipps, R.K.; Christensen, K.B.; Jensen, P.O.; Andersen, J.B.; Koch, B.; Larsen, T.O.; Hentzer, M.; et al. Identity and effects of quorum-sensing inhibitors produced by *Penicillium* species. *Microbiology* **2005**, *151*, 1325–1340. [CrossRef] [PubMed]
82. Galloway, W.R.; Hodgkinson, J.T.; Bowden, S.D.; Welch, M.; Spring, D.R. Quorum sensing in Gram-negative bacteria: Small-molecule modulation of AHL and AI-2 quorum sensing pathways. *Chem. Rev.* **2011**, *111*, 28–67. [CrossRef] [PubMed]
83. Bjarnsholt, T.; Jensen, P.Ø.; Rasmussen, T.B.; Christophersen, L.; Calum, H.; Hentzer, M.; Hougen, H.P.; Rygaard, J.; Moser, C.; Eberl, L.; et al. Garlic blocks quorum sensing and promotes rapid clearing of pulmonary *Pseudomonas aeruginosa* infections. *Microbiology* **2005**, *151*, 3873–3880. [CrossRef] [PubMed]
84. Rasmussen, T.B.; Bjarnsholt, T.; Skindersoe, M.E.; Hentzer, M.; Kristoffersen, P.; Köte, M.; Nielsen, J.; Eberl, L.; Givskov, M. Screening for quorum-sensing inhibitors (QSI) by use of a novel genetic system, the QSI selector. *J. Bacteriol.* **2005**, *187*, 1799–1814. [CrossRef] [PubMed]
85. Jakobsen, T.H.; van Gennip, M.; Phipps, R.K.; Shanmugham, M.S.; Christensen, L.D.; Alhede, M.; Skindersoe, M.E.; Rasmussen, T.B.; Friedrich, K.; Uthe, F.; et al. Ajoene, a sulfur rich molecule from garlic, inhibits genes controlled by quorum sensing. *Antimicrob. Agents Chemother.* **2012**, *56*, 2314–2325. [CrossRef] [PubMed]
86. Brackman, G.; Cos, P.; Maes, L.; Nelis, H.J.; Coenye, T. Quorum sensing inhibitors increase the susceptibility of bacterial biofilms to antibiotics in vitro and in vivo. *Antimicrob. Agents Chemother.* **2011**, *55*, 2655–2661. [CrossRef] [PubMed]
87. Brackman, G.; Hillaert, U.; Van Calenbergh, S.; Nelis, H.J.; Coenye, T. Use of quorum sensing inhibitors to interfere with biofilm formation and development in *Burkholderia multivorans* and *Burkholderia cenocepacia*. *Res. Microbiol.* **2009**, *160*, 144–151. [CrossRef] [PubMed]
88. Huber, B.; Eberl, L.; Feucht, W.; Polster, J. Influence of polyphenols on bacterial biofilm formation and quorum-sensing. *Z. Naturforsch. C* **2003**, *58*, 879–884. [CrossRef] [PubMed]
89. Ren, D.; Zuo, R.; González Barrios, A.F.; Bedzyk, L.A.; Eldridge, G.R.; Pasmore, M.E.; Wood, T.K. Differential gene expression for investigation of *Escherichia coli* biofilm inhibition by plant extract ursolic acid. *Appl. Environ. Microbiol.* **2005**, *71*, 4022–4034. [CrossRef] [PubMed]

90. Roy, V.; Meyer, M.T.; Smith, J.A.; Gamby, S.; Sintim, H.O.; Ghodssi, R.; Bentley, W.E. AI-2 analogs and antibiotics: A synergistic approach to reduce bacterial biofilms. *Appl. Microbiol. Biotechnol.* **2013**, *97*, 2627–2638. [CrossRef] [PubMed]
91. George, E.A.; Novick, R.P.; Muir, T.W. Cyclic peptide inhibitors of staphylococcal virulence prepared by Fmoc-based thiolactone peptide synthesis. *J. Am. Chem. Soc.* **2008**, *130*, 4914–4924. [CrossRef] [PubMed]
92. Li, J.; Wang, W.; Xu, S.X.; Magarvey, N.A.; McCormick, J.K. *Lactobacillus reuteri*-produced cyclic dipeptides quench *agr*-mediated expression of toxic shock syndrome toxin-1 in *Staphylococci*. *Proc. Natl. Acad. Sci. USA* **2011**, *108*, 3360–3365. [CrossRef] [PubMed]
93. Scott, R.J.; Lian, L.Y.; Muharram, S.H.; Cockayne, A.; Wood, S.J.; Bycroft, B.W.; Williams, P.; Chan, W.C. Side-chain-to-tail thiolactone peptide inhibitors of the staphylococcal quorum-sensing system. *Bioorg. Med. Chem. Lett.* **2003**, *13*, 2449–2453. [CrossRef]
94. Gov, Y.; Bitler, A.; Dell'Acqua, G.; Torres, J.V.; Balaban, N. RNAIII inhibiting peptide (RIP), a global inhibitor of *Staphylococcus aureus* pathogenesis: Structure and function analysis. *Peptides* **2001**, *22*, 1609–1620. [CrossRef]
95. Cirioni, O.; Mocchegiani, F.; Cacciatore, I.; Vecchiet, J.; Silvestri, C.; Baldassarre, L.; Ucciferri, C.; Orsetti, E.; Castelli, P.; Provinciali, M.; et al. Quorum sensing inhibitor FS3-coated vascular graft enhances daptomycin efficacy in a rat model of staphylococcal infection. *Peptides* **2013**, *40*, 77–81. [CrossRef] [PubMed]
96. Kiran, M.D.; Adikesavan, N.V.; Cirioni, O.; Giacometti, A.; Silvestri, C.; Scalise, G.; Ghiselli, R.; Saba, V.; Orlando, F.; Shoham, M.; et al. Discovery of a quorum-sensing inhibitor of drug-resistant staphylococcal infections by structure-based virtual screening. *Mol. Pharmacol.* **2008**, *73*, 1578–1586. [CrossRef] [PubMed]
97. Ren, D.; Sims, J.J.; Wood, T.K. Inhibition of biofilm formation and swarming of *Bacillus subtilis* by (5Z)-4-bromo-5-(bromomethylene)-3-butyl-2(5H)-furanone. *Lett. Appl. Microbiol.* **2002**, *34*, 293–299. [CrossRef] [PubMed]
98. Hume, E.B.H.; Baveja, J.; Muir, B.W.; Schubert, T.L.; Kumar, N.; Kjelleberg, S.; Griesser, H.J.; Thissen, H.; Read, R.; Poole-Warren, L.A.; et al. The control of *Staphylococcus epidermidis* biofilm formation and in vivo infection rates by covalently bound furanones. *Biomaterials* **2004**, *25*, 5023–5030. [CrossRef] [PubMed]
99. He, Z.Y.; Wang, Q.; Hu, Y.J.; Liang, J.P.; Jiang, Y.T.; Ma, R.; Tang, Z.S.; Huang, Z.W. Use of the quorum sensing inhibitor furanone C-30 to interfere with biofilm formation by *Streptococcus mutans* and its *luxS* mutant strain. *Int. J. Antimicrob. Agents* **2012**, *40*, 30–35. [CrossRef] [PubMed]
100. Janssens, J.C.; Steenackers, H.; Robijns, S.; Gellens, E.; Levin, J.; Zhao, H.; Hermans, K.; De Coster, D.; Verhoeven, T.L.; Marchal, K.; et al. Brominated furanones inhibit biofilm formation by *Salmonella enterica* serovar typhimurium. *Appl. Environ. Microbiol.* **2008**, *74*, 6639–6648. [CrossRef] [PubMed]
101. Niu, C.; Afre, S.; Gilbert, E.S. Subinhibitory concentrations of cinnamaldehyde interfere with quorum sensing. *Lett. Appl. Microbiol.* **2006**, *43*, 489–494. [CrossRef] [PubMed]
102. Defoirdt, T.; Miyamoto, C.M.; Wood, T.K.; Meighen, E.A.; Sorgeloos, P.; Verstraete, W.; Bossier, P. The natural furanone (5Z)-4-bromo-5-(bromomethylene)-3-butyl-2(5H)-furanone disrupts quorum sensing-regulated gene expression in *Vibrio harveyi* by decreasing the DNA-binding activity of the transcriptional regulator protein luxR. *Environ. Microbiol.* **2007**, *9*, 2486–2495. [CrossRef] [PubMed]
103. Oh, M.H.; Choi, C.H. Role of LuxIR homologue AnoIR in *Acinetobacter nosocomialis* and the effect of virstatin on the expression of *anoR* gene. *J. Microbiol. Biotechnol.* **2015**, *25*, 1390–1400. [CrossRef] [PubMed]
104. Christena, L.R.; Mangalagowri, V.; Pradheeba, P.; Ahmed, K.B.; Shalini, B.I.; Vidyalakshmi, M.; Anbazhagan, V.; Sai subramanian, N. Copper nanoparticles as an efflux pump inhibitor to tackle drug resistant bacteria. *RSC Adv.* **2015**, *5*, 12899–12909. [CrossRef]
105. Baugh, S.; Phillips, C.R.; Ekanayaka, A.S.; Piddock, L.J.; Webber, M.A. Inhibition of multidrug efflux as a strategy to prevent biofilm formation. *J. Antimicrob. Chemother.* **2014**, *69*, 673–681. [CrossRef] [PubMed]
106. Rampioni, G.; Pillai, C.R.; Longo, F.; Bondì, R.; Baldelli, V.; Messina, M.; Imperi, F.; Visca, P.; Leoni, L. Effect of efflux pump inhibition on *Pseudomonas aeruginosa* transcriptome and virulence. *Sci. Rep.* **2017**, *7*, 11392. [CrossRef] [PubMed]
107. Conrady, D.G.; Brescia, C.C.; Horii, K.; Weiss, A.A.; Hassett, D.J.; Herr, A.B. A zinc-dependent adhesion module is responsible for intercellular adhesion in staphylococcal biofilms. *Proc. Natl. Acad. Sci. USA* **2008**, *105*, 19456–19461. [CrossRef] [PubMed]
108. Maira-Litrán, T.; Kropec, A.; Abeygunawardana, C.; Joyce, J.; Mark, G., 3rd; Goldmann, D.A.; Pier, G.B. Immunochemical properties of the staphylococcal poly-N-acetylglucosamine surface polysaccharide. *Infect. Immun.* **2002**, *70*, 4433–4440. [CrossRef] [PubMed]

109. Mittelman, M.W. Adhesion to biomaterials. In *Bacterial Adhesion: Molecular and Ecological Diversity*; Fletcher, M., Ed.; Wiley-Liss, Inc.: New York, NY, USA, 1996.
110. Characklis, W.G.; McFeters, G.A.; Marshall, K.C. Physiological ecology in biofilm systems. In *Biofilms*; Characklis, W.G., Marshall, K.C., Eds.; John Wiley & Sons: New York, NY, USA, 1990.
111. Fletcher, M.; Loeb, G.I. Influence of substratum characteristics on the attachment of a marine pseudomonad to solid surfaces. *Appl. Environ. Microbiol.* **1979**, *37*, 67–72. [PubMed]
112. Sun, H.; Xu, Y.; Sitkiewicz, I.; Ma, Y.; Wang, X.; Yestrepsky, B.D.; Huang, Y.; Lapadatescu, M.C.; Larsen, M.J.; Larsen, S.D.; et al. Inhibitor of streptokinase gene expression improves survival after group A *Streptococcus* infection in mice. *Proc. Natl. Acad. Sci. USA* **2012**, *109*, 3469–3474. [CrossRef] [PubMed]
113. Ma, Y.; Xu, Y.; Yestrepsky, B.D.; Sorenson, R.J.; Chen, M.; Larsen, S.D.; Sun, H. Novel inhibitors of *Staphylococcus aureus* virulence gene expression and biofilm formation. *PLoS ONE* **2012**, *7*, e47255. [CrossRef] [PubMed]
114. Opperman, T.J.; Kwasny, S.M.; Williams, J.D.; Khan, A.R.; Peet, N.P.; Moir, D.T.; Bowlin, T.L. Aryl rhodanines specifically inhibit staphylococcal and enterococcal biofilm formation. *Antimicrob. Agents Chemother.* **2009**, *53*, 4357–4367. [CrossRef] [PubMed]
115. Jenal, U.; Dorman, C.J. Small molecule signaling. *Curr. Opin. Microbiol.* **2009**, *12*, 125–128. [CrossRef] [PubMed]
116. Römling, U.; Balsalobre, C. Biofilm infections, their resilience to therapy and innovative treatment strategies. *J. Intern. Med.* **2012**, *272*, 541–561. [CrossRef] [PubMed]
117. Abraham, N.M.; Lamlertthon, S.; Fowler, V.G.; Jefferson, K.K. Chelating agents exert distinct effects on biofilm formation in *Staphylococcus aureus* depending on strain background: Role for clumping factor B. *J. Med. Microbiol.* **2012**, *61*, 1062–1070. [CrossRef] [PubMed]
118. Chernousova, S.; Epple, M. Silver as antibacterial agent: Ion, nanoparticle, and metal. *Angew. Chem. Int. Ed.* **2013**, *52*, 1636–1653. [CrossRef] [PubMed]
119. Besinis, A.; Hadi, S.D.; Le, H.R.; Tredwin, C.; Handy, R.D. Antibacterial activity and biofilm inhibition by surface modified titanium alloy medical implants following application of silver, titanium dioxide and hydroxyapatite nanocoatings. *Nanotoxicology* **2017**, *11*, 327–338. [CrossRef] [PubMed]
120. Secinti, K.D.; Özalp, H.; Attar, A.; Sargon, M.F. Nanoparticle silver ion coatings inhibit biofilm formation on titanium implants. *J. Clin. Neurosci.* **2011**, *18*, 391–395. [CrossRef] [PubMed]
121. Shahverdi, A.R.; Fakhimi, A.; Shahverdi, H.R.; Minaian, S. Synthesis and effect of silver nanoparticles on the antibacterial activity of different antibiotics against *Staphylococcus aureus* and *Escherichia coli*. *Nanomedicine* **2007**, *3*, 168–171. [CrossRef] [PubMed]
122. Liu, T.; Yin, B.; He, T.; Guo, N.; Dong, L.; Yin, Y. Complementary effects of nanosilver and superhydrophobic coatings on the prevention of marine bacterial adhesion. *ACS Appl. Mater. Interfaces* **2012**, *4*, 4683–4690. [CrossRef] [PubMed]
123. Crick, C.R.; Ismail, S.; Pratten, J.; Parkin, I.P. An investigation into bacterial attachment to an elastomeric superhydrophobic surface prepared via aerosol assisted deposition. *Thin Solid Films* **2011**, *519*, 3722–3727. [CrossRef]
124. Tang, P.; Zhang, W.; Wang, Y.; Zhang, B.; Wang, H.; Lin, C.; Zhang, L. Effect of superhydrophobic surface of titanium on *Staphylococcus aureus* adhesion. *J. Nanomater.* **2011**, *2011*, 2. [CrossRef]
125. Privett, B.J.; Youn, J.; Hong, S.A.; Lee, J.; Han, J.; Shin, J.H.; Schoenfisch, M.H. Antibacterial fluorinated silica colloid superhydrophobic surfaces. *Langmuir* **2011**, *27*, 9597–9601. [CrossRef] [PubMed]
126. Russell, P.B.; Kline, J.; Yoder, M.C.; Polin, R.A. Staphylococcal adherence to polyvinyl chloride and heparin-bonded polyurethane catheters is species dependent and enhanced by fibronectin. *J. Clin. Microbiol.* **1987**, *25*, 1083–1087. [PubMed]
127. Abdelkefi, A.; Achour, W.; Ben Othman, T.; Ladeb, S.; Torjman, L.; Lakhal, A.; Ben Hassen, A.; Hsairi, M.; Ben Abdeladhim, A. Use of heparin-coated central venous lines to prevent catheter-related bloodstream infection. *J. Support. Oncol.* **2007**, *5*, 273–278. [PubMed]
128. Meiron, T.S.; Saguy, I.S. Adhesion modeling on rough low linear density polyethylene. *J. Food Sci.* **2007**, *72*, E485–E491. [CrossRef] [PubMed]
129. Donlan, R.M.; Costerton, J.W. Biofilms: Survival mechanisms of clinically relevant microorganisms. *Clin. Microbiol. Rev.* **2002**, *15*, 167–193. [CrossRef] [PubMed]
130. Ito, A.; Taniuchi, A.; May, T.; Kawata, K.; Okabe, S. Increased antibiotic resistance of *Escherichia coli* in mature biofilms. *Appl. Environ. Microbiol.* **2009**, *75*, 4093–4100. [CrossRef] [PubMed]

131. Savage, V.J.; Chopra, I.; O'Neill, A.J. *Staphylococcus aureus* biofilms promote horizontal transfer of antibiotic resistance. *Antimicrob. Agents Chemother.* **2013**, *57*, 1968–1970. [CrossRef] [PubMed]
132. Flemming, H.C.; Wingender, J. The biofilm matrix. *Nat. Rev. Microbiol.* **2010**, *8*, 623–633. [CrossRef] [PubMed]
133. Mann, E.E.; Wozniak, D.J. *Pseudomonas* biofilm matrix composition and niche biology. *FEMS Microbiol. Rev.* **2012**, *36*, 893–916. [CrossRef] [PubMed]
134. Whitchurch, C.B.; Tolker-Nielsen, T.; Ragas, P.C.; Mattick, J.S. Extracellular DNA required for bacterial biofilm formation. *Science* **2002**, *295*, 1487. [CrossRef] [PubMed]
135. Mulcahy, H.; Charron-Mazenod, L.; Lewenza, S. Extracellular DNA chelates cations and induces antibiotic resistance in *Pseudomonas aeruginosa* biofilms. *PLoS Pathog.* **2008**, *4*, e1000213. [CrossRef] [PubMed]
136. Mah, T.F.C.; O'Toole, G.A. Mechanisms of biofilm resistance to antimicrobial agents. *Trends Microbiol.* **2001**, *9*, 34–39. [CrossRef]
137. Kaplan, J.B. Therapeutic potential of biofilm-dispersing enzymes. *Int. J. Artif. Organs* **2009**, *32*, 545–554. [CrossRef] [PubMed]
138. Ramasubbu, N.; Thomas, L.M.; Ragunath, C.; Kaplan, J.B. Structural analysis of dispersin B, a biofilm-releasing glycoside hydrolase from the periodontopathogen *Actinobacillus actinomycetemcomitans*. *J. Mol. Biol.* **2005**, *349*, 475–486. [CrossRef] [PubMed]
139. Chen, M.; Yu, Q.; Sun, H. Novel strategies for the prevention and treatment of biofilm related infections. *Int. J. Mol. Sci.* **2013**, *14*, 18488–18501. [CrossRef] [PubMed]
140. Van Hamme, J.D.; Singh, A.; Ward, O.P. Physiological aspects. Part 1 in a series of papers devoted to surfactants in microbiology and biotechnology. *Biotechnol. Adv.* **2006**, *24*, 604–620. [CrossRef] [PubMed]
141. Deng, Y.; Lim, A.; Lee, J.; Chen, S.; An, S.; Dong, Y.H.; Zhang, L.H. Diffusible signal factor (DSF) quorum sensing signal and structurally related molecules enhance the antimicrobial efficacy of antibiotics against some bacterial pathogens. *BMC Microbiol.* **2014**, *14*, 51. [CrossRef] [PubMed]
142. Pedrido, M.E.; de Oña, P.; Ramirez, W.; Leñini, C.; Goñi, A.; Grau, R. Spo0a links de novo fatty acid synthesis to sporulation and biofilm development in *Bacillus subtilis*. *Mol. Microbiol.* **2013**, *87*, 348–367. [CrossRef] [PubMed]
143. Bernier, S.P.; Ha, D.G.; Khan, W.; Merritt, J.H.; O'Toole, G.A. Modulation of *Pseudomonas aeruginosa* surface-associated group behaviors by individual amino acids through c-di-GMP signaling. *Res. Microbiol.* **2011**, *162*, 680–688. [CrossRef] [PubMed]
144. Brandenburg, K.S.; Rodriguez, K.J.; McAnulty, J.F.; Murphy, C.J.; Abbott, N.L.; Schurr, M.J.; Czuprynski, C.J. Tryptophan inhibits biofilm formation by *Pseudomonas aeruginosa*. *Antimicrob. Agents Chemother.* **2013**, *57*, 1921–1925. [CrossRef] [PubMed]
145. Howlin, R.P.; Cathie, K.; Hall-Stoodley, L.; Cornelius, V.; Duignan, C.; Allan, R.N.; Fernandez, B.O.; Barraud, N.; Bruce, K.D.; Jefferies, J.; et al. Low-dose nitric oxide as targeted anti-biofilm adjunctive therapy to treat chronic *Pseudomonas aeruginosa* infection in cystic fibrosis. *Mol. Ther.* **2017**, *25*, 2104–2116. [CrossRef] [PubMed]
146. Socransky, S.S.; Haffajee, A.D. Dental biofilms: Difficult therapeutic targets. *Periodontol* **2000**, *28*, 12–55. [CrossRef]
147. Frias, J.; Olle, E.; Alsina, M. Periodontal pathogens produce quorum sensing signal molecules. *Infect. Immun.* **2001**, *69*, 3431–3434. [CrossRef] [PubMed]
148. Eberhard, A.; Burlingame, A.L.; Eberhard, C.; Kenyon, G.L.; Nealson, K.H.; Oppenheimer, N.J. Structural identification of autoinducer of *Photobacterium fischeri* luciferase. *Biochemistry* **1981**, *20*, 2444–2449. [CrossRef] [PubMed]
149. Waters, C.M.; Bassler, B.L. Quorum sensing: Cell-to-cell communication in bacteria. *Annu. Rev. Cell Dev. Biol.* **2005**, *21*, 319–346. [CrossRef] [PubMed]
150. Brözel, V.S.; Strydom, G.M.; Cloete, T.E. A method for the study of de novo protein synthesis in *Pseudomonas aeruginosa* after attachment. *Biofouling* **1995**, *8*, 195–210. [CrossRef]
151. Davies, D.G.; Chakrabarty, A.M.; Geesey, G.G. Exopolysaccharide production in biofilms: Substratum activation of alginate gene expression by *Pseudomonas aeruginosa*. *Appl. Environ. Microbiol.* **1993**, *59*, 1181–1186. [PubMed]
152. Sauer, K.; Camper, A.K. Characterization of phenotypic changes in *Pseudomonas putida* in response to surface-associated growth. *J. Bacteriol.* **2001**, *183*, 6579–6589. [CrossRef] [PubMed]
153. Parsek, M.R.; Greenberg, E.P. Sociomicrobiology: The connections between quorum sensing and biofilms. *Trends Microbiol.* **2005**, *13*, 27–33. [CrossRef] [PubMed]

154. Brackman, G.; Coenye, T. Quorum sensing inhibitors as anti-biofilm agents. *Curr. Pharm. Des.* **2015**, *21*, 5–11. [CrossRef] [PubMed]
155. Hentzer, M.; Riedel, K.; Rasmussen, T.B.; Heydorn, A.; Andersen, J.B.; Parsek, M.R.; Rice, S.A.; Eberl, L.; Molin, S.; Høiby, N.; et al. Inhibition of quorum sensing in *Pseudomonas aeruginosa* biofilm bacteria by a halogenated furanone compound. *Microbiology* **2002**, *148*, 87–102. [CrossRef] [PubMed]
156. Hentzer, M.; Wu, H.; Andersen, J.B.; Riedel, K.; Rasmussen, T.B.; Bagge, N.; Kumar, N.; Schembri, M.A.; Song, Z.; Kristoffersen, P.; et al. Attenuation of *Pseudomonas aeruginosa* virulence by quorum sensing inhibitors. *EMBO J.* **2003**, *22*, 3803–3815. [CrossRef] [PubMed]
157. Uroz, S.; Chhabra, S.R.; Cámara, M.; Williams, P.; Oger, P.; Dessaux, Y. N-acylhomoserine lactone quorum-sensing molecules are modified and degraded by *Rhodococcus erythropolis* W2 by both amidolytic and novel oxidoreductase activities. *Microbiology* **2005**, *151*, 3313–3322. [CrossRef] [PubMed]
158. Tang, K.; Zhang, X.H. Quorum quenching agents: Resources for antivirulence therapy. *Mar. Drugs* **2014**, *12*, 3245–3282. [CrossRef] [PubMed]
159. Yang, F.; Wang, L.H.; Wang, J.; Dong, Y.H.; Hu, J.Y.; Zhang, L.H. Quorum quenching enzyme activity is widely conserved in the sera of mammalian species. *FEBS Lett.* **2005**, *579*, 3713–3717. [CrossRef] [PubMed]
160. Uroz, S.; Heinonsalo, J. Degradation of N-acyl homoserine lactone quorum sensing signal molecules by forest root-associated fungi. *FEMS Microbiol. Ecol.* **2008**, *65*, 271–278. [CrossRef] [PubMed]
161. Bjarnsholt, T.; Tolker-Nielsen, T.; Høiby, N.; Givskov, M. Interference of *Pseudomonas aeruginosa* signalling and biofilm formation for infection control. *Expert Rev. Mol. Med.* **2010**, *12*, e11. [CrossRef] [PubMed]
162. Tomlin, K.L.; Malott, R.J.; Ramage, G.; Storey, D.G.; Sokol, P.A.; Ceri, H. Quorum-sensing mutations affect attachment and stability of *Burkholderia cenocepacia* biofilms. *Appl. Environ. Microbiol.* **2005**, *71*, 5208–5218. [CrossRef] [PubMed]
163. Huber, B.; Riedel, K.; Hentzer, M.; Heydorn, A.; Gotschlich, A.; Givskov, M.; Molin, S.; Eberl, L. The *cep* quorum-sensing system of *Burkholderia cepacia* H111 controls biofilm formation and swarming motility. *Microbiology* **2001**, *147*, 2517–2528. [CrossRef] [PubMed]
164. Lynch, M.J.; Swift, S.; Kirke, D.F.; Keevil, C.W.; Dodd, C.E.; Williams, P. The regulation of biofilm development by quorum sensing in *Aeromonas hydrophila*. *Environ. Microbiol.* **2002**, *4*, 18–28. [CrossRef] [PubMed]
165. Labbate, M.; Queck, S.Y.; Koh, K.S.; Rice, S.A.; Givskov, M.; Kjelleberg, S. Quorum sensing-controlled biofilm development in *Serratia liquefaciens* MG1. *J. Bacteriol.* **2004**, *186*, 692–698. [CrossRef] [PubMed]
166. Smith, K.M.; Bu, Y.; Suga, H. Induction and inhibition of *Pseudomonas aeruginosa* quorum sensing by synthetic autoinducer analogs. *Chem. Biol.* **2003**, *10*, 81–89. [CrossRef]
167. Smith, K.M.; Bu, Y.; Suga, H. Library screening for synthetic agonists and antagonists of a *Pseudomonas aeruginosa* autoinducer. *Chem. Biol.* **2003**, *10*, 563–571. [CrossRef]
168. Kim, C.; Kim, J.; Park, H.Y.; Park, H.J.; Kim, C.K.; Yoon, J.; Lee, J.H. Development of inhibitors against TraR quorum-sensing system in *Agrobacterium tumefaciens* by molecular modeling of the ligand-receptor interaction. *Mol. Cells* **2009**, *28*, 447–453. [CrossRef] [PubMed]
169. Ishida, T.; Ikeda, T.; Takiguchi, N.; Kuroda, A.; Ohtake, H.; Kato, J. Inhibition of quorum sensing in *Pseudomonas aeruginosa* by N-acyl cyclopentylamides. *Appl. Environ. Microbiol.* **2007**, *73*, 3183–3188. [CrossRef] [PubMed]
170. Morohoshi, T.; Shiono, T.; Takidouchi, K.; Kato, M.; Kato, N.; Kato, J.; Ikeda, T. Inhibition of quorum sensing in *Serratia marcescens* AS-1 by synthetic analogs of N-acylhomoserine lactone. *Appl. Environ. Microbiol.* **2007**, *73*, 6339–6344. [CrossRef] [PubMed]
171. Fong, J.; Zhang, C.; Yang, R.; Boo, Z.Z.; Tan, S.K.; Nielsen, T.E.; Givskov, M.; Wu, B.; Su, H.; Yang, L. Synergy of quorum quenching enzyme and quorum sensing inhibitor in inhibiting *P. aeruginosa* quorum sensing. *bioRxiv* **2017**, 182543. [CrossRef]
172. Ni, N.T.; Choudhary, G.; Li, M.Y.; Wang, B.H. Pyrogallol and its analogs can antagonize bacterial quorum sensing in *Vibrio harveyi*. *Bioorg. Med. Chem. Lett.* **2008**, *18*, 1567–1572. [CrossRef] [PubMed]
173. Brackman, G.; Celen, S.; Baruah, K.; Bossier, P.; Van Calenbergh, S.; Nelis, H.J.; Coenye, T. AI-2 quorum-sensing inhibitors affect the starvation response and reduce virulence in several *Vibrio* species, most likely by interfering with LuxPQ. *Microbiology* **2009**, *155*, 4114–4122. [CrossRef] [PubMed]
174. El-Naggar, M.H.; Elgaml, A.; Abdel Bar, F.M.; Badria, F.A. Antimicrobial and antiquorum-sensing activity of *Ricinus communis* extracts and ricinine derivatives. *Nat. Prod. Res.* **2018**, *32*, 1–7. [CrossRef] [PubMed]

175. Pejin, B.; Ciric, A.; Dimitric Markovic, J.; Glamoclija, J.; Nikolic, M.; Sokovic, M. An insight into anti-biofilm and anti-quorum sensing activities of the selected anthocyanidins: The case study of *Pseudomonas aeruginosa* PAO1. *Nat. Prod. Res.* **2017**, *31*, 1177–1180. [CrossRef] [PubMed]
176. Pejin, B.; Ciric, A.; Glamoclija, J.; Nikolic, M.; Sokovic, M. *In vitro* anti-quorum sensing activity of phytol. *Nat. Prod. Res.* **2015**, *29*, 374–377. [CrossRef] [PubMed]
177. Pejin, B.; Talevska, A.; Ciric, A.; Glamoclija, J.; Nikolic, M.; Talevski, T.; Sokovic, M. Anti-quorum sensing activity of selected sponge extracts: A case study of *Pseudomonas aeruginosa*. *Nat. Prod. Res.* **2014**, *28*, 2330–2333. [CrossRef] [PubMed]
178. Pejin, B.; Ciric, A.; Karaman, I.; Horvatovic, M.; Glamoclija, J.; Nikolic, M.; Sokovic, M. *In vitro* antibiofilm activity of the freshwater bryozoan *Hyalinella punctata*: A case study of *Pseudomonas aeruginosa* PAO1. *Nat. Prod. Res.* **2016**, *30*, 1847–1850. [CrossRef] [PubMed]
179. Brackman, G.; Defoirdt, T.; Miyamoto, C.; Bossier, P.; Van Calenbergh, S.; Nelis, H.; Coenye, T. Cinnamaldehyde and cinnamaldehyde derivatives reduce virulence in *Vibrio* spp. by decreasing the DNA-binding activity of the quorum sensing response regulator LuxR. *BMC Microbiol.* **2008**, *8*, 149. [CrossRef] [PubMed]
180. Manefield, M.; de Nys, R.; Kumar, N.; Read, R.; Givskov, M.; Steinberg, P.; Kjelleberg, S. Evidence that halogenated furanones from *Delisea pulchra* inhibit acylated homoserine lactone (AHL)-mediated gene expression by displacing the AHL signal from its receptor protein. *Microbiology* **1999**, *145*, 283–291. [CrossRef] [PubMed]
181. Kuehl, R.; Al-Bataineh, S.; Gordon, O.; Luginbuehl, R.; Otto, M.; Textor, M.; Landmann, R. Furanone at subinhibitory concentrations enhances staphylococcal biofilm formation by *luxS* repression. *Antimicrob. Agents Chemother.* **2009**, *53*, 4159–4166. [CrossRef] [PubMed]
182. Manefield, M.; Rasmussen, T.B.; Henzter, M.; Andersen, J.B.; Steinberg, P.; Kjelleberg, S.; Givskov, M. Halogenated furanones inhibit quorum sensing through accelerated LuxR turnover. *Microbiology* **2002**, *148*, 1119–1127. [CrossRef] [PubMed]
183. Han, Y.; Hou, S.; Simon, K.A.; Ren, D.; Luk, Y.Y. Identifying the important structural elements of brominated furanones for inhibiting biofilm formation by *Escherichia coli*. *Bioorg. Med. Chem. Lett.* **2008**, *18*, 1006–1010. [CrossRef] [PubMed]
184. Zhang, L.; Murphy, P.J.; Kerr, A.; Tate, M.E. *Agrobacterium* conjugation and gene regulation by N-acyl-L-homoserine lactones. *Nature* **1993**, *362*, 446–448. [CrossRef] [PubMed]
185. Park, S.Y.; Lee, S.J.; Oh, T.K.; Oh, J.W.; Koo, B.T.; Yum, D.Y.; Lee, J.K. AhlD, an N-acylhomoserine lactonase in *Arthrobacter* sp., and predicted homologues in other bacteria. *Microbiology* **2003**, *149*, 1541–1550. [CrossRef] [PubMed]
186. Pearson, J.P.; Van Delden, C.; Iglewski, B.H. Active efflux and diffusion are involved in transport of *Pseudomonas aeruginosa* cell-to-cell signals. *J. Bacteriol.* **1999**, *181*, 1203–1210. [PubMed]
187. Evans, K.; Passador, L.; Srikumar, R.; Tsang, E.; Nezezon, J.; Poole, K. Influence of the MexAB-OprM multidrug efflux system on quorum sensing in *Pseudomonas aeruginosa*. *J. Bacteriol.* **1998**, *180*, 5443–5447. [PubMed]
188. Rahmati, S.; Yang, S.; Davidson, A.L.; Zechiedrich, E.L. Control of the AcrAB multidrug efflux pump by quorum-sensing regulator SdiA. *Mol. Microbiol.* **2002**, *43*, 677–685. [CrossRef] [PubMed]
189. Pumbwe, L.; Skilbeck, C.A.; Wexler, H.M. Presence of quorum-sensing systems associated with multidrug resistance and biofilm formation in *Bacteroides fragilis*. *Microb. Ecol.* **2008**, *56*, 412–419. [CrossRef] [PubMed]
190. Chan, Y.Y.; Chua, K.L. The *Burkholderia pseudomallei* BpeAB-OprB efflux pump: Expression and impact on quorum sensing and virulence. *J. Bacteriol.* **2005**, *187*, 4707–4719. [CrossRef] [PubMed]
191. Chan, Y.Y.; Bian, H.S.; Tan, T.M.; Mattmann, M.E.; Geske, G.D.; Igarashi, J.; Hatano, T.; Suga, H.; Blackwell, H.E.; Chua, K.L. Control of quorum sensing by a *Burkholderia pseudomallei* multidrug efflux pump. *J. Bacteriol.* **2007**, *189*, 4320–4324. [CrossRef] [PubMed]
192. Kvist, M.; Hancock, V.; Klemm, P. Inactivation of efflux pumps abolishes bacterial biofilm formation. *Appl. Environ. Microbiol.* **2008**, *74*, 7376–7382. [CrossRef] [PubMed]
193. Baugh, S.; Ekanayaka, A.S.; Piddock, L.J.; Webber, M.A. Loss of or inhibition of all multidrug resistance efflux pumps of *Salmonella enterica* serovar typhimurium results in impaired ability to form a biofilm. *J. Antimicrob. Chemother.* **2012**, *67*, 2409–2417. [CrossRef] [PubMed]

194. Nallathamby, P.D.; Lee, K.J.; Desai, T.; Xu, X.H. Study of the multidrug membrane transporter of single living *Pseudomonas aeruginosa* cells using size-dependent plasmonic nanoparticle optical probes. *Biochemistry* **2010**, *49*, 5942–5953. [CrossRef] [PubMed]
195. Gupta, D.; Singh, A.; Khan, A.U. Nanoparticles as efflux pump and biofilm inhibitor to rejuvenate bactericidal effect of conventional antibiotics. *Nanoscale Res. Lett.* **2017**, *12*, 454. [CrossRef] [PubMed]
196. Maseda, H.; Sawada, I.; Saito, K.; Uchiyama, H.; Nakae, T.; Nomura, N. Enhancement of the *mexAB-oprM* efflux pump expression by a quorum-sensing autoinducer and its cancellation by a regulator, MexT, of the *mexEF-oprN* efflux pump operon in *Pseudomonas aeruginosa*. *Antimicrob. Agents Chemother.* **2004**, *48*, 1320–1328. [CrossRef] [PubMed]

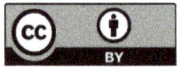

© 2018 by the authors. Licensee MDPI, Basel, Switzerland. This article is an open access article distributed under the terms and conditions of the Creative Commons Attribution (CC BY) license (http://creativecommons.org/licenses/by/4.0/).

MDPI
St. Alban-Anlage 66
4052 Basel
Switzerland
Tel. +41 61 683 77 34
Fax +41 61 302 89 18
www.mdpi.com

Materials Editorial Office
E-mail: materials@mdpi.com
www.mdpi.com/journal/materials

www.ingramcontent.com/pod-product-compliance
Lightning Source LLC
LaVergne TN
LVHW071953080526
838202LV00064B/6735